The International Libra

T0227835

MORBID FEARS AND
COMPULSIONS

Founded by C. K. Ogden

The International Library of Psychology

PSYCHOANALYSIS
In 28 Volumes

MORBID FEARS AND COMPULSIONS

Their Psychology and Psychoanalytic Treatment

HW FRINK

Introduction by James J Putnam

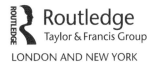

Routledge
Taylor & Francis Group

LONDON AND NEW YORK

First published in 1918 by
Routledge, Trench, Trubner & Co., Ltd.
2 Park Square, Milton Park, Abingdon, Oxfordshire OX14 4RN
711 Third Avenue, New York, NY 10017

First issued in paperback 2014

Routledge is an imprint of the Taylor and Francis Group, an informa business

British Library Cataloguing in Publication Data
A CIP catalogue record for this book
is available from the British Library

Morbid Fears and Compulsions
ISBN 0415-21092-5
Psychoanalysis: 28 Volumes
ISBN 0415-21132-8
The International Library of Psychology: 204 Volumes
ISBN 0415-19132-7

ISBN 13: 978-1-138-88262-1 (pbk)
ISBN 13: 978-0-415-21092-8 (hbk)

INTRODUCTION

The day has fortunately gone by when the far-reaching investigations associated with the name of Sigmund Freud need to be introduced, as if for the first time, to any such circle of readers as that to which this book is likely to appeal. Indeed, so familiar have men grown with the more salient features of the so-called psychoanalytic movement, and so pronounced is the interest which it has evoked, that one feels a sense of lack, if, on looking through a volume or a magazine where human motives are discussed, one does not find some reference to the doctrines here at stake.

That this increased and growing interest is not due to curiosity alone is shown by the fact that many eminent scientific men—psychologists, biologists and educators—have used Freud's generalizations largely, in connection with their own inquiries. Not only have these men published books and papers of which the psychoanalytic movement was the text, but they have made it the basis of discussion in academic courses.

This is an important indication. For these able men stand as representatives of the so-called "normal" members of the community; it is "normal" psychology, both individual and social, and "normal" life processes and the education of "normal" people that they study.

But what is "normal," and to what extent is it possible to distinguish it from what, for one or another reason, we call "abnormal"?

Much has been written on this point, and practically always the answer to the above question has been that there are no means of distinguishing these two states. That which goes by the name of "evil" or "disease" finds its analogue in the instability that is inseparable from life and progress; and the forms that disease takes in the so-called "pervert" or the nervous invalid, or even the criminal, do but represent, in an accentuated form, tendencies of which traces are to be discovered in the history, and as an element in the make-up, of every member of the community. There is then good reason why all those who wish to understand the weaknesses of society and work for the betterment of the race, should take interest in this movement.

What is it (over and above external conditions) that causes the terrible misery in our social life, of which the dramatists and novelists have so much to say and which breaks out in the form of strikes and anarchy, and lies widespread, just beneath the surface, in the form of superstitions, depressions, unreasonable fears, or of "hatred, malice and all uncharitableness"? Why is it that some persons are so much more overwhelmed than others by the recitals of the horrors of the war?

People afflicted with these tendencies present, frequently, the same front to the community that is presented by the happiest and most prosperous of men. But they present this front, in many cases, not from deliberate and reasoned choice, but because, separated in feeling from their assumedly happier or more successful fellows, they feel impelled to seek, as if through a sort of "protective coloration," to preserve every outward sign that is possible, of good health, good fellowship and success. Close observers realize more or less of what is going on with such persons, and the more intelligent of these observers see also that the facts and doctrines that have been brought out through the psychoanalytic movement afford a better explanation of these situations than is provided in any other way.

The present book does not make it one of its main purposes to take up these social problems; but the author has a keen sense for the analogies to which I have referred, and in both parts of his treatise—that is, in the part in which the history and fundamental doctrines are laid down, and in that in which the compulsions and obsessions are more specifically studied—he gives illustrations which every social student may well take to heart, of the varied and significant modes of action of men's unconscious motives.

And yet so difficult is the subject; so hard is it to really grasp these elusive motives that play so large a part in all our lives, to exchange a "knowledge about" them for a real "acquaintance with" them, that there will be room and welcome, during many years to come, for any book that deals consciously and clearly with the problems here involved.

The present volume fulfills these requirements admirably within the limits which the author sets for himself, and inspires confidence by evidences of abundant knowledge and of conscientiousness in forming judgments. Dr. Frink is evidently writing for physicians and those who are ready to take the physician's point of view. This has always been Freud's method, also; and in following it,—that is, through keeping before his mind that he would choose for his imagined audience those only who were ready to gaze at the truth without shrinking,—he was able to cultivate his power of accurate observation to a remarkable degree. If his statements became now and then too blunt, or too one-sided, or extreme, that fact should and will be forgiven, when it is borne in mind that unless he had trained himself to be keenly alive to the presence of certain special motives rather than a judicial evaluer of all motives, the psychoanalytic movement would never have attained the position that it holds.

This is an important consideration in Freud's intellectual history and that of the most stalwart of his followers. If their work has been marked by "defects," they have shown, as a rule, "qualities" enough to justify these defects. It has often been urged against Freud, for example, that his analyses of characters in history and fiction,—such as those of Leonardo, Hamlet and Œdipus, —give a distorted idea of their lives and personalities. In itself this criticism is just, and analogous comments can be made on the psychoanalytic movement as a whole. But they should be made in the light of what I have just now said. The time has perhaps arrived, it is true, when the leaders of this movement should be called upon to cease being monographic, and, instead of this, to take their places, consciously, as students of the mind and its sources of energy from all points of view, even if they continued to emphasize especially one aspect of these matters. And yet, even now, it must be kept in view that knowledge moves forward by a zigzag path, and that the most important thing, where the contributions of men of genius are in question, is that nothing of value shall be lost of what they have to give. The errors of omission of important men and important movements can easily be forgiven.

This consideration should be especially borne in mind when one is dealing with the sex problem,—which Dr. Frink discusses clearly, in a simple and straightforward manner, proposing at the same time a new name, in order to call attention afresh to the very important generalization, that when one uses the word "sexual" one should have in mind all the connotations that go with the word "love," understood as he defines it.

It is true that other emotions are "repressed" besides those classifiable as sexual. But the point mainly at stake is the pragmatic one that the sexual emotions involve a peculiarly large number of dominant, unreasoning passions, of a sort that each individual is least willing to acknowledge (or else, it may be, is over-zealous in asserting) and the subtle signs of which it is especially important that the student of medicine should train himself to detect.

Having said this much about those characteristics of Freud's work which perhaps more than any others have laid its author open to criticism, and having thereby, I trust, made it clear that I am not inclined to deal with Freud's conclusions in anything but a friendly spirit, I shall claim the privilege of indicating some of the points with regard to which I think his critics are in the right; or, to speak more exactly, to indicate the directions in which, as it seems to me, the boundaries of his work may profitably be widened.

Freud was, and is, above all things, a man to whom the exact methods of natural science were very dear, as, in his estimation, the only reliable means of investigation even in matters of personal motive and conduct. In this respect he belongs, of course, to that large class of persons whose labors are absolutely indispensable to the evolution of human knowledge; and Dr. Frink's expressions of opinion make it clear that he would wish to be classified in the same group. But there are also many men, whose voices never have been, and never can be, silenced, who feel convinced that the dicta of the natural scientists,—that is, of those who would eventually refer everything back to the laws of chemistry and physics,—are not to be allowed to have the last word. There are, indeed, many members of the scientific group itself, who have testified to their belief in this fact. Such persons not only feel it clear that these natural laws do not explain all the phenomena of life; they feel also that one of the most interesting outcomes of scientific, and still more of logical inquiry, is the fact that these sciences seem to prove not only that the laws which they recognize as valid are not only themselves limited in their application, but also that they actually point to the existence of forms of energy which they are powerless to describe.

The fact that Freud was so devoted to the scientific method, and, from the same standpoint, so devoted to the belief that mental phenomena are just as much subject to inflexible laws of causation as physical phenomena, and, in fact, that the causation in the two cases is virtually of the same sort, would perhaps have done no harm had it spent itself (as it did to a considerable extent) in leading him to measure and define the degree to which this doctrine represents the truth. But,—unfortunately, as it seems to me,—he went further than this, and in spite of disclaiming, as he has always done, any obligation to adopt a general attitude toward the "ultimate nature of things," in a philosophical sense, he does nevertheless do this very thing in his claim that we live, body and soul, in a deterministic world,[1] a world in which the last word belongs to physical science.

No one could, of course, deny him the right to this opinion; but if it is held, it should be justified through the presentation of evidence, on his part, of having taken all the arguments of both sides into account; and this evidence Freud has not given.

Dr. Frink brings the matter to a clear issue in his thesis (which is quite in accord with Freud's doctrine) that every individual when looked at from the standpoint of his childhood must be recognized as following two, and only two, tendencies,—those namely of self preservation and of race preservation. This is the accepted formula among perhaps the majority of biologists. But unless the word "preservation" is interpreted in such a way as to include far more than the simple preservation of life,—that is, unless it is admitted that from first to last the highest attributes of the human being are thought of as virtually present, (as in the form of what is vaguely described as "free will," existing as a partially guiding influence),—I should not feel at liberty to grant the claim.

The antithesis is between those who look on

[1] E. g. see statements of this sort in his paper entitled *Totem und Tabu.* Translation Totem and Taboo, N. Y., 1918.

what (for want of a better term) one must call the higher, more spiritual manifestations of life, as definable in terms of chemistry and physics, as ordinarily conceived of, and those who believe that chemistry and physics are to be defined in terms of these higher manifestations of life. The significance for therapeutics of the problem here involved is very clear.

The next point which seems to me important has reference to the scope of psychoanalytic work. Freud, with his keen sense of the difficulties and dangers lying in the path of the psychoanalytic movement, has strongly maintained that psychoanalysts would never do their best in the direction of keeping the movement free from degradation, or of helping their patients to make their memories and power of reasoning penetrate into the depths of their repressed experiences, unless they made these outcomes virtually the sole object of their treatments and resisted the temptation to act as mentors and advisors with reference to specific social difficulties of the hours. In spite of the apparent insistence and importance of the patient's immediately present problems, Freud held that the problems which they were really thinking of and needed most of all to solve, were those related to their repressed complexes.

On similar grounds he has strenuously objected to the introduction of ethical considerations, or aiming for ethical results. While believing that a psychoanalytic treatment was in a high degree a form of education, he has felt that the physician's part was only that of Vergil, in Dante's celebrated journey through Hell, Purgatory, and Paradise; not at all that of Beatrice. The patient comes to the physician, let us say, skilled in the art of self-deception, and suffering under a self-wielded lash. The physician's task is to see that he becomes undeceived, by helping him to bridge the wide chasm between his logical consciousness and his unlogical phantasies. When this task is accomplished, and thus a better understanding of himself is brought about, and when his fears or compulsions, or such other symptoms as he may have presented, have been dissipated by a thoroughgoing psychoanalysis, the physician's task, so Freud would say, is ended. The physician is under no obligation to inquire what use the patient makes of his newly acquired freedom, or to lead him further on the path of sublimation.

As against this view of the duty of the psychoanalyst, which I trust is fairly stated, it is reasonable to urge that whatever the actual so-called "symptoms" are with which the patient comes to his physician, he brings inevitably the *virtual* symptom which consists in an incapacity to express through his life the recognition of his social obligations and possibilities as an integral portion of the social organism. Yet these obligations and possibilities are his by birthright. From this standpoint a psychoanalytic treatment is not logically complete until the patient so thor-

oughly understands himself that he is not only
able, but feels himself compelled to see himself
and his social obligations in the best form possible
to him. Looked at in this way the functions of
Vergil and Beatrice coalesce.

If this mode of looking at the matter is correct,
the psychoanalyst of the future must himself be
a person of broad and ethical outlook, and yet
must learn to see and avoid the danger that he
may lose sight of his psychoanalytic ideals and
forget the technique of psychoanalytic practice.
Is this possible? I think, Yes.

Finally it is well known to all those who have
followed the literature of this subject, that many
persons who have been students, (and some of
them well-wishers) of the psychoanalytic movement, claim that Freud has made too much of the
sexual motivation of men's conduct and of the
sexual content of their unconscious yet active mental life. A prominent representative of a view
akin to this is Alfred Adler of Vienna, who ap-
proaches the subject of conduct from a somewhat
special standpoint, though one that Freud himself
has never failed to recognize. He calls attention
to the striking difference between individuals as
they start on their course of life, in that some are
handicapped by defects, of which the most typical
are weaknesses in certain organs and their functions. In consequence of these defects the person's life is spent partly in an instinctive seeking
for compensation,—which may become ''over-

compensation,''—partly in an effort to escape responsibilities which he feels he cannot meet.

It is not my place or desire to enter here on any adequate discussion, or even statement, of the situation raised by Adler. I would only say that in my opinion it does represent a more biological mode of looking at the causes of men's conduct, which at times has its convenience, and which, to say the least, is not incompatible with Freud's doctrines. It is unfortunate that his emphasis— which is a valuable one—could not have been given without his having found it necessary to attack Freud's fundamental doctrines, which have been of such immeasurable value. But behind both of these modes of approach, there lies the immensely important fact that man is a social animal and that he has, *of necessity,* ideals of life and conduct and the good, which, in a sense, transcend his recognition of weakness, temptation and defect.

JAMES J. PUTNAM.

AUTHOR'S NOTE

There are three classes of readers to whom a book on psychoanalysis might be of interest. In the first, would be those entirely unfamiliar with Freudian psychology and who wish to make a first acquaintance with the subject; in the second, those who already know something about psychoanalysis and are desirous of learning more, with the intention in some instances of using it in practice. The third, and by far the smallest class, would be made up of those having considerable training and experience in psychoanalytic work and whose interest therefore would be in the finer details of theory and technique and in the more elaborate reports of analyzed cases. It is to the second class of these readers that this book will be most likely to appeal.

That such is the case is not entirely in accordance with the plans I had in mind on beginning to write the book. The chapters that are presented here were intended, according to the original scheme, to serve a semi-introductory function in preparation for two final and more highly technical chapters wherein an elaborately analysed case and the more intricate details of theory and practice would be considered. But partly because I found unexpected difficulties in the way of compressing the case report sufficiently to conform to the physical limits set for this book, and partly from the reflection that such matter would have its interest for a different and smaller audience than the one to which the present chapters might appeal, I eventually decided to use this clinical material as the basis for a second volume, supplementary to this one, and in which also the question of analytic technique could be more suitably considered.

I am not greatly in sympathy with the theoretical and technical innovations in psychoanalysis introduced rather recently by the schools of Jung and of Adler, and the views set forth in this book are intended to represent the purely Freudian doctrines in so far as I am able to understand and interpret them. In some of the more highly theoretical parts of the present volume I have followed Freud's writings very closely, not hesitating at times even to borrow his words. Believing, however, that one may get a clearer view of involved material by looking at it from more than one angle, I have ventured to introduce, in some portions of the book, what amounts to a hybrid behaviorism. In doing this I have felt some misgivings, for behaviorism is a field in which I have little reason for feeling sure of myself, and I am aware that my efforts to produce clarity may perhaps result in confusion.

Some of the material utilized in this book I have published before. That which constitutes Chapter VI is, except for some minor changes and omissions, as it originally appeared in the *Psychoanalytic Review,* under the title, "A Psychoanalytic Study of a Severe Case of Compulsion Neurosis." A large part of the chapter on dreams is taken from two papers entitled, "Dream and Neurosis," and, "On Freud's Theory of Dreams," which were published in the *Interstate Medical Journal,* and *American Medicine,* respectively. The two analyses of name-forgetting are taken from "Three Examples of Name-Forgetting," and "Some Analyses in the Psychopathology of Everyday Life," which appeared in the *Journal of Abnormal Psychology.* I wish to express my indebtedness to these journals for permission to reprint this material. I owe a similar acknowledgment to the *New York Times,* the *New York Tribune,* and the *Louisville Times,* by whose courtesy the cartoons used in Chapter III are reproduced.

In reporting clinical material throughout this book I have made such minor changes or omissions as seemed to me necessary to conceal the identity of the patients in question, but none of these alterations are serious enough to affect the scientific value of the reports.

The bibliographies for the various chapters in this book are intended to serve as general references and to indicate lines for collateral reading. They are not intended to be at all exhaustive. For more complete lists of psychoanalytic literature the reader is referred to those given in the *Jahrbuch der Psychoanalyse,* Bd. VI., 1914. Specific references are given in some parts of this book but omitted in other parts, as for instance, in the Second Chapter, where to give them would involve referring almost every paragraph to the same small list of authoritative works.

In conclusion I wish to express my great indebtedness to Mr. Wilfrid Lay for his assistance in the preparation of this book.

H. W. FRINK.

CONTENTS

CHAPTER I

CONTENTS

CHAPTER II

CHAPTER III

CONTENTS

patient who identified himself with a patient of Dr.
Brill's. *Rationalization.* Neurotics rather more intelligent than the average. Few even normal people really
know the causes of their actions. Patient who declared
he would marry a rich girl gives wrong reason for
marrying a poor girl. Rationalization in another patient's arguments in favor of woman suffrage, of election of Wilson, against Wilson's election. A married
woman rationalizes her wearing of black clothes. *Defense and Distortion Mechanisms.* Patient with unconscious wish for mother's death distorted to remorse at death of another. Patient who dissuaded his
prospects from buying advertising space, on account
of not giving full return for value received. Patient who
would not bathe in cold water on account of "small-
penis complex." Washing compulsions; religious and
charitable work. The physician who blames the patient
for lack of understanding. *Transference* or objective-
identification. Examples. The "conditioned reflex" and
the "sensory pattern." Reaction patterns formed before
the end of sixth year, e. g., the Œdipus and Electra complexes. Freud's "Interpretation of Dreams" quoted.
Warning against misunderstanding Freud's statements.
The "Imago," not necessarily an accurate picture. Patient transfers to physician feelings she has had for
father. Resemblance of this process to psychical processes of certain primitive races. Case of young man
infatuated with divorcee older than he, to whom he had
transferred his mother imago. Reactions from father
complex; and from mother complex in man who could
have intercourse only with servants. Transference to
physician occurs . in every analysis, both positive and
negative; and is uncovered, but not created by it.

CHAPTER V

Neurosis at time of its appearance seems something
unprecedented in the individual, but is really not dis-
continuous with patient's former life. Continuity everywhere complete. Neurosis conditioned by a failure of
repression, which is, however, never complete. Neurotic
symptoms, like dreams, are manifestations of the Unconscious, which can only wish. Each symptom an attempted realization of one or more unconscious wishes,
chiefly sexual or holophilic. Question *why* this is so not
relevant. Sexual factor, present in all reported cases,
even when not seen or admitted by the writers. Physician with unsolved complexes unable to remove his own
and patients' resistances against sex confessions. Neurosis the negative of the sexual perversion; both repre-

CONTENTS xxv

senting a partial arrest of development. Fixation and inhibition of instincts by habit. Fixation of holophilic impulse not merely upon an *object* but upon an *aim* or type of action. Holophilic impulses not specific in aim, a condition which alone renders sublimation possible. Libido fixed on type of action becomes specific. Second object selection occurring after puberty influenced in normals by the unconscious portion of the libido, and *dominated* in neurotics. The love specifications of the neurotic more numerous. Early fixed libido can only exceptionally be satisfied in reality and wishes must remain in the Unconscious. Fundamental difference between neurotic and normal person is that neurotic has *learned to love and hate too soon*. Fixation points are weak points in the holophilic synthesis. Regression of libido to earlier lines of discharge paralleled by a regression to more internal paths of imagination, producing Introversion. Masturbation and phantasies later giving way to a real sexual object, a process reversed in neurosis. Regression a preliminary to neurosis. The neurotic uses his illness as a means to attain various ends. The neurosis a defense against the pain of non-realization of narcissistic wishes. Neurotics neither immoral nor unmoral. Immediate cause of outbreak of neurosis is deprivation of some love gratification; sexual abstinence. Freud quoted. Morbid fear or anxiety a result of damming up of libido. Difference between morbid and normal fear is that former is a relatively excessive one, and is a difference of origin. Normal fear originates from external world, morbid from the Unconscious. Nature of emotion—a deed yet retained within the organism. Sexual emotion physiologically like any other, but psychically less dependent on external stimulation than other kinds. Anxiety neurosis as described by Freud. Biological significance of fear. Source of morbid fear within the organism nothing novel as the distinction between external and internal is comparatively late in ontogenetic development. That which causes pain is regarded as external. Morbid fear causes subject to act toward a part of himself as if it were hostile. Morbid fear in one sense not morbid but a normal reaction to an abnormal condition. Anxiety neurosis a variety of anxiety hysteria. Warning against taking word sexual too narrowly.

CHAPTER VI

PSYCHOLOGY OF THE COMPULSION NEUROSIS . . . 270

Neurasthenia a misnomer. Phobias and panics. Examples of compulsions showing *mesalliance* between affect and idea content, both qualitative and quantitative.

CONTENTS

Source of affects entirely in the Unconscious, and affects are attached to wrong ideas. Necessity of admitting unconscious psychic activities. Repressed wishes just as dynamic as the unrepressed. Compulsion in the drug-taking case shows wish entering consciousness as a wish but attached to new idea. In compulsive fears the wish energy is transformed into anxiety. Case of young man buying a straw hat, showing overcompensation. Rôle of sadism in compulsion neuroses. Love and hate for same object. Weakness of will, in matters of love, spreading to other situations. Compulsions represent effort to compensate for doubt in love life. Compulsions are substitute activities. Two-sided compulsive acts, opposite impulses being discharged separately. Ambivalence. Regression of libido in compulsion neurosis which is the negative of the sadistic perversion. The curiosity impulse causes morbid pondering. Superstition in compulsion neurotics concerning the death of others. Omnipotence of wishes. Difference between compulsion neurosis and hysteria. Case of prostitute showing failure to see connection between her neurosis and her life.

CHAPTER VII

Introduction. Historical. Results of previous treatment. Analytic data. Father complex. Separation complex. Assault obsession. Resistance against marriage. Analysis of the assault obsession. Rôle of the tuberculosis complex in the love choice. Analysis of the Kishef obsession. Further details. Conclusion.

CHAPTER VIII

Most common in women, the compulsion neurosis in men. Chief manifestation of anxiety hysteria is morbid fear. Phobia and panic. Three examples. Ideational element. Story of the farmer getting drunk. Genesis of the anxiety through displacement of wish energy to substitute idea of dangerous man. Fears cannot be reasoned away. Revolver no protection against thirst. Morbid fear an expression of essentially feminine traits. Anxiety neurosis the negative of the masochistic perversion. Stella's fear of "dead souls" displaced from anal-erotic wishes.

CHAPTER IX

MORBID FEARS AND COMPULSIONS

CHAPTER I

THE SEXUAL SYNTHESIS

HIPPOCRATES, the Father of Medicine, taught that the malady known as hysteria arose when the unsatisfied womb, longing for the seed of the male, broke loose from its fastenings and restlessly wandered about the interior of the body. In accordance with this theory he applied sweet perfumes to the vulva of the patient and evil-smelling substances to her nostrils, with the idea that by such means the mutinous organ might be induced to return to its proper locus. Remnants from this theory are handed down to present day medicine as the name we apply to the disease (hysteria, from ὑστέρα, the womb) and the practice of administering to neurotic patients certain ill-smelling drugs such as asafœtida and valerian.

Since the days of Hippocrates the theories advanced to explain hysteria and the other psychoneuroses have been both numerous and varied, some of them being no less fantastic than his. But throughout there has been noticeable a persistent,

1

if ill-defined, tendency to locate the cause of the trouble in the organs of generation. The constant search for malpositions of the uterus, cervical or perineal lacerations or other pelvic disturbances in neurotic women, and the multitude of operations that have been undertaken with the idea of curing the neurosis by removing these conditions are but a few of the manifestations of this tendency.

It remained for Freud to show that this inclination to regard the reproductive organs as the site of the causal factors of the functional neuroses had, in a way, its justification, and really amounted to a dim, imperfect intuition of what actually is the truth. We know now, thanks to his genius, that in these cases the trouble really resides not in the sexual *organs* of the patient but in the sexual *instinct*.

The violent and bitter prejudice which arose against this doctrine of Freud's could in large measure be ascribed to the peculiar feeling prevalent among Caucasian peoples that there is something inherently shameful and indecent about sex, in consequence of which they are quick to resent whatever implies directly or indirectly that the erotic impulses are of much consequence to them.

Another important factor which interfered with Freud's teachings was that people failed to understand just what he meant by the term sexual, and thus saw in his writings meanings that he never intended, and derived impressions totally different from those he wished to convey. These false notions caused many to reject his teachings who, had they understood him, might have investigated further and readily accepted his views. What in many instances excited prejudice was really something quite different from what Freud had tried to teach.

In view of this, I think it well to begin by an attempt to make clear what is meant by the term *sexual* when used in the Freudian sense, and what we shall understand the sexual instinct to be.

Each individual leads a double existence; on the one hand he is an entity in himself, on the other an insignificant component of that larger entity, his race or species.

Corresponding to these two rôles he has two great groups of impulses or instinctive tendencies, the one wholly egoistic or self-preservative, the other essentially altruistic and preservative of the race. Of the first group hunger is the chief sensational representative, of the second the desire for sexual congress.

If one studies some simple organism, for instance the amœba, it is easily apparent that *all* its processes fall readily into one or the other of the two groups, self-preservative and reproductive. If comparative studies are then made with other organisms higher in the phylogenetic scale, it will be found that there is nothing, not excepting even the most complicated mental processes of civilized man, that is not represented in some simple and rudimentary way in the lower organisms, even to the amœba. Thus every item of human behavior whether it be "explicit" (action) or "implicit" (thought or feeling) [1] is revealed, either to

[1] J. B. Watson, "Behavior," Henry Holt & Co.

direct observation or by tracing it back through
phylogenetic history, as belonging either in the
self-preservative or in the race-preservative group
of reactions.

Now suppose we name these two great groups
each according to its chief representative. All
processes belonging to the self-preservative group
would then be called hunger processes, all those
of the other would be termed sexual processes.
Thus our desire to have warm clothes in winter
and cool ones in summer would be called a hunger
phenomenon, while a wish that these clothes might
look well would be considered to belong to the
sphere of sex. *It is exactly in this broad and inclusive sense that Freud uses the term sexual.*
With him it embraces all those reactions that are
race-preservative in purpose or effect according
to their phylogenetic or ontogenetic history. His
use of the word would be exactly paralleled by
including all the self-preservative processes under
the term hunger. The word sexual in the Freudian sense is thus most nearly synonymous with the
Greek Ἔρως (Eros) or the English word Love,
though having an even broader meaning than
either of them. The phenomena popularly termed
sexual represent only a comparatively small portion of the group which are sexual in Freud's
sense.[1]

[1] It may be conceded that Freud's selection of this term to
denote the large group of phenomena to which he applies it was
not particularly happy, for apparently it has led to much misunderstanding. Also it has been complained that he stretched
the meaning of the word beyond all reason. The situation was,
of course, that since there is no term current that expressed the

Corresponding to the two great groups of processes or reactions into which the phenomena of the individual life may be divided, there are assumed two great groups of impulses or tendencies, the self-preservative or ego-instinct, and the sexual or holophilic instinct as the source from which each group of processes gets its primal push and drive. For our reactions to the stimuli we receive usually if not invariably represent out-puts of energy entirely out of proportion to the amounts of energy impinging on our sense organs as the stimuli themselves. If for instance a photographic plate in a camera is exposed to the light rays coming from a grizzly bear, an impression is made on the plate which is directly proportional to the amount of light and the length of time of exposure. But

exact meaning he wanted, he had either to invent a new word or else broaden the meaning of the one already in use. That he chose the latter course instead of the former would have been all right, could people have been made to understand, as they did not, that it was in this new and broad sense that the word was generally used. As a matter of fact, in a good deal of psychoanalytic writing the word sexual is used now in the broad sense and now in the narrow sense, without the authors' always taking the trouble to state in which sense it is to be construed. It has occurred to me that the word holophilic, from ὅλος, whole, and φιλέω, love, thus meaning all kinds of sexual or love phenomena, might be a convenient synonym for the word sexual in Freud's sense, and that its judicious use would serve to avoid some possible misunderstanding. I do not wish to replace the word *sexual* entirely, for that, too, might lead to misunderstanding. In this book, therefore, I propose to use the two words interchangeably and as synonymous with one another, hoping by so doing to emphasize the broad way in which the word sexual should be construed without tiring the reader with repeated statements about it. I shall attempt particularly to use the word holophilic in such connections where the word sexual would be most apt to be erroneously taken in its narrow sense.

if these same rays impinge on another sort of sensitized plate, the retina of a human being or of an animal, there results an effect in the shape of fear and flight, the energy output of which bears no definite ratio to the energy-content of the incoming rays, and is of infinitely greater magnitude.   The rôle of the stimulus in this and practically all other cases is that of releasing into kinetic expression energy that is latent within the organism.   To express this notion of latent energy we require the term instinct which we conceive to be the source of the energy which is released as the responses to various external or internal stimuli.   To the energy itself which is thus released we give in the case of the holophilic group of phenomena the name *Libido*.[1]

Just as everything in the lives of the higher organisms can be found represented in some simple or rudimentary way in the lives of the lower, so practically everything in the adult has some sort of representation in the child.   However trite this statement may appear, its application in the psychosexual sphere was hardly recognized at all until the work of Freud.   The sexual instinct was popularly supposed to appear at the time of puberty; the child was tacitly assumed to be practically asexual before that period.   Whether the instinct

[1] Like the word sexual the word libido must be construed in psychoanalytic writing in a broad sense while popularly it is used in a narrow one, and hence the same objections apply to it that arise against the former. For this reason Jung has suggested that it be replaced by the Greek ὁρμή (Hormé). "On Psychological Understanding," *Journal of Abnormal Psychology*, Vol. IX, No. 6.

has any prepubertal representation or in what this representation might consist hardly anybody stopped to enquire. One of Freud's great achievements was the demonstration that the sexual instinct as first manifested at the time of puberty is not new but so to speak a synthetic product, formed by uniting certain of a number of holophilic trends or impulses which were present throughout childhood and thus that the germs of sexuality are present in the individual from his very birth.

That this discovery of Freud's should have given rise to astonishment and incredulity is from one point of view very surprising. All the receptor surfaces, all the complicated systems of voluntary, sympathetic and autonomic arcs and end-organs involved in the reactions represented by the love life of the adult are present in practically their fully developed form long before the beginning of puberty. Apparently the change which takes place at puberty results not from new arcs being introduced or in old ones suddenly becoming permeable, but rather in the maturing of certain glands which now begin to pour their internal secretions into the blood stream and, in the male, furnish a new substance for external discharge. It would be hard to believe all this complicated machinery waited silent and idle, or was responsive only to non-sexual stimuli and capable only of non-sexual reactions during all the years preceding puberty and this glandular activity. On the contrary it would be logical to expect the occurrence of many and complicated reactions,

lacking to be sure something possessed by the
sexual processes of the adult, but nevertheless
fully deserving to be called sexual. This doctrine
that adult sexuality develops by a sort of synthesis out of a preëxisting sexuality we should have
been prepared for by expecting that the effect of
the internal secretions appearing at puberty
would be merely that of adding further power
and emphasis to certain reactions of the complicated machinery already present and freely reacting before the attainment of sexual maturity.
We should have known that the psychosexual
phenomena of the adult could not have developed
de novo at puberty, but could only represent what
had been present much earlier, now brought into
high relief through the added effect of the new
secretions.

In the sexuality of the human being three phases
or periods of development may be distinguished:
(1) an infantile or pre-inhibitory period which
corresponds to the first three or four years of life;
(2) the childhood or latency period which succeeds
the first and ends with the onset of puberty, and
(3) the adult period, or phase of object-love.

The first period may be called the pre-inhibitory
period because it represents a stage in which
the so-called reaction-tendencies, (the inhibitory
trends such as shame, disgust, modesty, sympathy,
etc.) are not yet manifest. The child, during this
first period, is incapable of any of these feelings;
as soon as he becomes capable of them the period
comes to a close and the latency period has its beginning.

The holophilic phenomena of the first period consist chiefly in the pleasurable sensations which the infant derives from the stimulation of certain sensitive areas which are known as the erogenous zones. These zones are represented by the anal, oral, and urethral orifices, the penis in the male and the labia and clitoris in the female. The first pleasurable stimulations from them are incidental to the performing of the functions of alimentation. In the infant the pleasure derived from the taking of nourishment is not represented entirely by taste pleasures and the actual satisfaction of the craving for food; the tactile and kinesthetic sensations created during the act of sucking are distinctly agreeable and pleasurable in themselves. In the same way the voiding of excrement not only represents something more than simply the relief from the discomfort of not voiding, but also gives rise to tactile and muscular sensations that have a definite pleasure value in themselves.

Having experienced these pleasurable sensations as incidents to the performing of the alimentary functions, the infant soon seeks to re-experience them for their own sake. Thus, for instance, he develops the habit of sucking his thumb or some other available object, purely for the sensory pleasure the act of sucking affords and quite apart from any desire for nourishment. In the same way other children refuse to empty the bowel when placed upon the toilet, and hold back the feces until there is an accumulation of sufficient size and consistency to give the act of evacuation the greatest possible amount of pleasure.

It may be asked why such tricks of the infant as thumb-sucking and the holding back of the feces are classed in the sexual or holophilic group, and not as hunger phenomena. We may answer that the principal reason for so regarding them is because of their later history. By the study of the oral perversions or perversities (*fellatio, cunnilingus,* etc.,) the perverse action can be demonstrated as a direct descendant of the infantile pleasure-sucking which in most cases of such perversion had been indulged in with great fervor and continued for a long time. Then too the analysis of certain neurotic disturbances such as hysterical vomiting and some food idiosyncrasies reveals them as a reaction against similar oral-erotic longings and phantasies, now offensive to the controlling trends of the personality, but likewise easily traceable through the developmental history of the individual back to the pleasure-sucking of infancy. The oral erotism of the infant is represented in the normal adult as the pleasure in kissing. Of course the rudimentary sexual activities cannot be expected to be in every particular like those of the adult. Kissing in the adult excites the genital system while the sensations excited in pleasure-sucking remain local. But we must remember that the intercommunication of the various holophilic impulses (the sexual synthesis) has not yet been established, for the reason that the glands whose internal secretions are largely instrumental in its accomplishment have yet to mature. Nevertheless the infantile erotism as exemplified in pleasure-sucking is

not set off so sharply from adult sexuality as one
might perhaps expect.   In certain cases at least, it
proceeds to an orgastic climax succeeded by a period of complete passivity and relaxation, the
whole phenomenon bearing such a striking similarity to the sexual acme and immediately subsequent
relaxation in the adult that it could hardly escape
the observer.

The first stimulations of the penile and clitoris
zones appear to result either from irritations produced by discharged secretions or excretions in
contact with them, or from the manipulations involved in keeping the child clean.   These pleas-
urably experienced stimulations the infant then
seeks to repeat either by thigh rubbing or the use
of the hand.   The former appears to be more common in female infants, the latter in males.

All the erogenous zones in infancy have, at least
to start with, about the same degree of pleasure-
sensibility.   As time goes on the significance of
one zone may be accentuated over that of the
others through repeated stimulation, but there is
nothing corresponding to the primacy that in the
normal adult the genitals have over all other regions of the body.   Furthermore, the zones ordinarily remain perfectly independent of one another; excitement of one does not of itself produce
an excitement or heightened sensibility in any of
the others, as happens in the adult when for instance the oral zone is stimulated and the phenomena of sexual excitement occur in the genitals
without their being stimulated directly.

In addition to the zonal components of the holo-

philic instinct there appear a little later a set of
impulses which have at first no connection with the
erogenous areas. These so-called partial impulses
(Partial-triebe) go in pairs of which the one is active and the other passive. One of these pairs consists of the sadistic and masochistic impulse. The
former is an aggressive tendency, and is manifested as a desire to dominate, to use force, roughness or violence, and if it goes far enough, to inflict pain. [1] The masochistic tendency has just the
opposite nature, and is shown as a pleasure in obedience, submission, and the enduring of humiliation or pain.

A second pair consists of the impulse to showing and looking, the former passive and the latter
active. They refer not only to the genitals themselves, but to the entire body. Out of a union of
the looking impulse with a contribution from the
acquisitive trend of the self-preservative group
there develops the curiosity impulse, of which we
shall have a good deal to say in some of the later
portions of this book. The impulses to touch and
to be touched, etc., belong in the same group of
partial desires.

These partial desires of infancy are readily
identified as fore-runners of tendencies apparent
in the sex-life of the normal adult. The sadistic
impulse, for instance, corresponds to the normal
aggressiveness in courtship shown by the male in
comparison with the female, and his inclination to

[1] The wish to cause pain is not primary in the sadistic impulse, though early becoming associated with it. See Freud's
"Triebe und Triebschicksale," *Int. Zeitschrift für A. P.*, 1916.

master, and occasionally to be rough with the loved object. This inclination corresponds to an evolutionary period when the male had need of other means of overcoming the resistance of the female than those implied by the term courtship, (marriage by capture, etc.)

The disposition of the looking and showing impulses in adult life is well illustrated by the differences in the evening dress of the male and the female. As shown by this the female has a greater desire to be looked at than has the male, while in the male the pleasure in looking and the curiosity impulse (sexual curiosity) is stronger than in the female.

It must be pointed out that the partial impulses represent rudiments corresponding not only to tendencies normally present in adult life, but also to those of certain perversions, sadism, masochism, exhibitionism, etc. In fact there is a perversion corresponding to each one of the partial impulses of infancy. The same may be said with regard to the zonal components. In other words the perversions represent great exaggerations or over-developments of some one or other of the holophilic tendencies which are normally present in every child. This has led Freud to designate the infantile sexuality as ''polymorphous perverse.'' This is perhaps an unfortunate term for while it is true that the infant evinces holophilic pleasure in all these diverse ways there is nothing abnormal about it at that stage of development. The true perverseness results only when those trends experience a disproportionate development and fail to become subordinate to the genital zone at the time of the sexual synthesis of puberty.

The conspicuous feature of the sexuality of the infantile period (and for that matter of the childhood period also) is that it is predominantly autoerotic. By this is meant that the child for the most part gains his satisfaction from his own body; he is not dependent as is the adult, upon a second person for the satisfaction of holophilic needs. In the normal adult love life the sexual object (this second person) is indispensable; the sexuality of the infant is for the most part objectless.

Yet the predominance of autoerotism in childhood is not absolute. Often as early as the beginning of the second year one can see signs of the rudimentary object-love which foreshadows, and in a sense is the model for, that great factor in adult life. Before the end of the infantile period these indications are very clear and ordinarily bear the stamp of the normal heterosexual selection. The first extra-egoistic holophilic interests developed by the infant have as their objects the persons of the immediate environment, parents, nurses, etc., but the libido is distributed in unequal quantities to these individuals so that there is soon revealed (in normal children) a preference for the opposite sex. Thus the little boy loves the mother more than he does the father, while with the little girl it is the father who has the preference. Quite generally the parent of the same sex as the child is looked upon as an interferer and rival for the affections of the parent more greatly loved. The little boy, for instance, wishes that his father were out of the way so that he could have his mother all to himself.[1] This early object-selection forms the foundation of those important constellations, the Œdipus Complex (in the male) and the Electra Complex (in the female) which are of great significance not only in the later life of the neurotic but in normal people as well.

In these allerotic phenomena, as distinguished from the essentially autoerotic processes which constitute the major portion of the infantile holophilic reactions, the nearest approach is made to the phenomena of love in the adult. The essential difference is the lack of synthesis of the various impulses into any definite pattern or hierarchy such as exists in normal adult life. That is to say, all the impulses remain as separate and independent sources of pleasure; the significance of the genital zone is not, as in the normal adult, accentuated over that of all the others, and the partial impulses are not intimately connected with it. For instance, in the adult the gratification of one of the partial impulses, for example the desire to touch the loved object, though giving pleasure at the same time creates a desire for a greater pleasure, that of coitus. Thus the two stand to each other in the relation of fore-pleasure and end-pleasure. In infancy there is no differen-

[1] That this desire frequently takes the form of a wish that the father were dead need cause no astonishment, for at this period the idea of death means nothing more to the child than simply "gone away," and excites none of the horror that it has for the adult.

tiation into pleasures of different order. All the
holophilic pleasures are end-pleasures, and what
organization exists among the various impulses is
a pregenital organization. The sexual pleasures
of this period are for the most part lacking in the
genital component, unless the genitals are directly
stimulated.

It must not be understood from what I have said
about the Œdipus complex and the heterosexual
predominance in the infantile object-love that all
the child's holophilic interest or libido is distributed to the opposite sex. On the contrary a bisex-
ual or, to use Ferenczi's term, an *amphierotic* tendency is apparent. Thus some of the libido takes
a homosexual direction, being applied (in the boy)
to the father, brothers, or other males in the family. This homophilic application of the libido in
infancy corresponds to the normal friendships and
attachments for one's own sex in the normal adult,
and, in the abnormal, to the homosexual perversions.

The holophilic activities of the infantile period
reach a high point somewhere between the third
and the fifth years of life. There then begins a
period of latency, relatively complete in some individuals, but broken through in varying degrees
by expression of sexuality in others. The beginning of this period is marked by the first appearances of such reactions as shame, modesty, disgust, sympathy, etc. They are the foundation
and the forerunners of all those ethical and esthetic forces which play the rôle of inhibitions
upon the later sexual life and, like dikes or dams,

narrow the avenues of holophilic expression. The
first appearance of these inhibitory tendencies is
spontaneous and probably organically conditioned. But the further development of the inhibitory forces, which takes place all through the
latency period, is dependent in great measure for
its extent and direction upon the cultural and educational influences of the environment.[1] The
controlling forces which are thus shaped by educational influence and which eventuate in an apparent disappearance, more or less complete, of the
infantile sexuality as manifested in the first period
are in large measure developed at the expense of
the infantile sexuality itself and derive much of
their motive power from it. For instance, the
masochistic partial impulse furnishes the motive
for obedience, and leads the child to accept and to
embody into his own personality the codes or
standards of those about him. The exhibitionistic
impulse manifested at first in the desire to have the
body looked at, later expresses its energy in whatever actions may serve to win parental approba-
tion and praise. In other words the energy of
these impulses may eventually lead the child to

[1] Freud remarks that education remains properly within its
assigned realm only if it strictly follows the path sketched for it
by the spontaneously appearing inhibitory tendencies and limits
itself to emphasizing and developing them. The truth of this
statement will, I think, become clearly apparent at certain points
in the clinical portion of this book, where we shall become acquainted with instances where the well-meant educational and
corrective efforts of parents overstepped the limits indicated by
the spontaneous inhibitions and went too far in some directions,
thus producing an ultimate effect upon the child that was very
different from the beneficial one intended.

avoid the very acts by which he gratified them originally. In this manner the control and suppression of the primitive infantile sexuality is in large
part accomplished by motives derived from the infantile sexuality itself.

The measures of libido distributed to the members of the family or other persons of the environment tend more and more to be displaced from the
sexual aims of the first period and to depart from
manifestations coinciding with the popular meaning of the term sexual, taking on an aspect which
coincides with the meaning of love in its narrow
sense, that is to say, affection. The love for the
mother thus loses whatever crassly sexual appearance it might at first have possessed, while the infantile hostility and jealousy exhibited toward the
father may disappear from view entirely or be
represented only as a diffuse inclination to disobedience, dislike of authority, etc. In other words
the manifestations of the Œdipus complex undergo a profound amelioration.

This refining process, through which the energies of the primary components are divorced from
their original aims and applied to new aims and
activities of a higher and socially more valuable
order, is not limited to the formation of controlling
or inhibiting trends as just described and which in
large measure represent the basis for estheticism
and morality, but occurs in other connections.
The primitive sexual curiosity thus becomes a
desire for general knowledge, the sadistic impulse
finds expression as a desire to win or to excel in
games, sports or any other sort of competition,

etc. Such employment of the primitive energies for higher aims is known as sublimation. The extent to which it occurs in normally educable children is really enormous. We shall hear something more of it later. [1]

The latency period, as has been said, is by no means always complete and in many individuals is occasionally or even constantly broken through by some form or other of definitely sexual manifestation. In children with whom this occurs extensively it often may be interpreted as the foreshadowing of a later neurosis or sexual abnormality.

A wholly normal suspension of the latency occurs with the onset of puberty and with it the latent period is terminated. The holophilic instinct now changes from its infantile to its adult form. Hitherto its manifestations have been preponderantly autoerotic; now begins the predominance of object love. Hitherto the various partial impulses and zonal pleasure sources existed for the most part side by side in a sort of democratic equality; now they become organized into a hierarchy. The genital zone receives a primacy over all the other components of the holophilic impulse, and to this primacy everything else (normally) is subordinated. The partial impulses, looking, touching, sadistic aggression, etc., and their passive counterparts; the oral or other zones still susceptible to sexual stimulation, now fall into the subordinate rôle of fore-pleasure production, and the whole fore-pleasure machinery now serves the

[1] In Chapter IV on Mechanisms.

unified purpose of preparing for and urging toward the final holophilic act through which sexuality is articulated with the function of procrea-
tion, in the end-pleasure of coitus.   Autoerotism,
though in most cases holding its ground for a time
in the form of the masturbation that ordinarily appears about the time of puberty, is gradually replaced by the new régime of object-love.   The libido is eventually withdrawn from its affectionate
fixations upon members of the family or their surrogates, and, combining with the sensual libido
corresponding to the new glandular influences, is
at length transferred to extra-familial individuals
of the opposite sex with whom, as foreshadowed in
the masturbation phantasies of puberty, a complete love life can eventually be carried out.   Only
with the complete synthesis of puberty do the normal differences between the sexuality of the male
and the female come into high relief.   The active
or aggressive trends come to predominate in the
character of the male, the passive in the female.
Incidentally it may be remarked that the change
at puberty from infantile to adult sexuality is
more sharply marked and more sudden in the male
than in the female.   The love life of the female
retains in perhaps most cases a good deal of the
character of infantile sexuality all through adolescence and often well into, or even throughout, adult
life.

    This sketch of the ontogenetic development of
the holophilic impulses is intended (beyond making the reader familiar with the terminology I
shall need to use later) principally to indicate

what is the normal course of things. I shall not attempt to discuss the abnormalities or anomalies that may arise out of the many possibilities for aberration presented by the developmental changes taking place in a machinery so complicated. It will be sufficient at this point to say that every step in ontogenetic development, every transition that must be passed through, offers possibilities of morbid disturbance, through a persistence of this or that phase that should normally be passed, through the opening up of avenues for aberrant development, or through the formation of a *locus minoris resistentiae* at which the apparently normally accomplished sexual synthesis may give way under the strains and stresses of adult life. Later we shall gain some incidental familiarity with those particular types of imperfect synthesis known as the perversions and which correspond to an over-accentuation of some one or more of the normal components and to their consequent failure to become subordinated to the primacy of the genital zone and the end-aim of heterosexual coitus. Our particular study however concerns another sort of developmental aberration which we shall learn to know as the negative of the perversion, namely the psychoneurosis.

. . . .

Before closing this chapter I must mention a matter that really belongs under the heading of infantile sexuality: the formation of the so-called infantile sexual theories, which as we shall learn are often of much significance in the determination of the psychoneurotic symptoms in adult life.

Children of normal intelligence, about the age of four or five ordinarily pass through what is well named the period of sexual investigation. Previous to this period the small child is likely to take for granted the existence of himself, his family and his various neighbors and acquaintances, and displays no particular curiosity as to how he or they came to be. Then, partly through subjective and partly through objective influence, a new and burning desire for knowledge has its birth. In typical cases this interest appears as a reaction to the arrival of a new baby in the family. Such an event is not one which, by the average child of four or five, is looked upon with favor. On the contrary he is likely to regard the new-comer as an unattractive intruder with whom in future he will be compelled to share his cherished importance, his worldly possessions, and, worst of all, the parents' love.[1] Through the feelings of hostility born of such considerations the child is led to ask himself the important question: "Where do babies come from?" in many cases apparently in the hope that an answer thereto may place him in a position to prevent any repetition of the undesired occurrence.

Confronted with this problem the small investigator naturally turns first of all to his parents, a source of aid and information hitherto found reli-

[1] A child in whose family no birth takes place during his early years learns of the dreaded possibility from his acquaintance with other households. Older children are much less likely to be jealous of a newly arrived brother or sister than are younger ones, and in many cases they welcome their small relative with unmixed satisfaction.

able. But in most cases he gets little satisfaction; his questions meet with a laughing and evasive answer, an admonition not to speak of such matters, or some such interesting statement as "The stork brings the children," or "The doctor finds them in the woods." All such answers ordinarily affect children in much the same way. The stork or the doctor story is soon doubted, and, like admonition or evasion, merely serves to give the child the impression that the theme of birth is one to be avoided in the presence of adults. These stories, instead of removing his curiosity, simply cause him to conceal it and to pursue any further investigation in a less open and direct manner. At the same time the failure of his parents to aid and instruct him in a matter so serious to him gives rise to more or less distinct feelings of resentment, suspicion and distrust.

Finding that the parents will not explain birth for him, the child attempts to discover its explanation by himself. In secret he ponders the problem, and, from watching his elders, from seeing the sexual acts of animals, from the examination of his own body, from certain physical sensations, from vague impulses, inclinations and longings that begin to stir within him, he collects material, and from it constructs his own theories of reproduction, which, though grotesque and faulty, are on the whole surprisingly near the truth. The content of some of these theories we shall now consider.

Practically all children who form any theory whatever come to the right conclusion in the one important particular that the baby grows in the abdomen of the mother. It would seem at first thought, that if children are able to guess this much then the formation of correct conceptions of impregnation and birth would naturally follow. Yet such is not the case, for by certain faulty premises the infant theorist is led widely astray. The first of these erroneous premises is the theory, very commonly entertained, that every human being, female as well as male, possesses a penis. That among small boys who have never seen the female genitals such a belief should exist is of course not strange. But even those who have seen the genitals of some small female member of the family still cling to this notion, and reconcile their preconceived views with the actual evidence to the contrary by the reflection: "She is still little; when she gets older it will grow." Some little girls also have the penis theory, for after having seen the male organ, they conclude that they too are entitled to a like appendage. Misled by the faulty premises involved in the penis theory and by being ignorant both of the existence and of the functions of the vagina, the investigating child is prevented from guessing correctly the route by which the baby reaches the outer world. His most natural conclusion is that the baby must make its exit from the abdomen through the same opening as do the other solid products of bodily activity, in short that birth takes place *via* the rectum (the "cloaca theory").[1]

[1] In this connection it must be remembered that children of an age to form such theories would feel toward this hypothesis none

This theory, since it does not contain the concept of anatomical differences between the sexes, naturally results in the supposition that males can bear children as well as females.

When the child has answered to his own satisfaction the questions of where the baby develops and how it reaches the outer world, there remains another riddle to be solved. What starts the process? How does the baby get into the mother? The explanation most obvious to the child's mind is, that since the baby comes out like feces, it must go in like food. Therefore to start a pregnancy the mother must eat or drink something, a fruit or seed, or something furnished by the doctor, and from this substance the baby develops. This belief is strengthened if the child learns that rain and manure are required for the proper development of seeds planted in the ground. He reasons by analogy that urine and feces must be designed to favor in like manner the development of a "baby seed" within the abdomen.

Another fairly common theory, which was first described by Reitler, is that impregnation is accomplished by the parents placing the buttocks together and blowing flatus into one another.[1]

A notion somewhat different from these already described is formed by children who, through shar-

of the esthetic objections which could occur to an adult. "Then," as Freud says, "defecation was something that in the nursery could be spoken of without reserve; the child had not yet divorced himself from his constitutional coprophilic tendencies; it was no degradation to come into the world like a mass of excrement." —Ueber infantile Sexualtheorien.

[1] R. Reitler, "Zentralblatt für Psychoanalyse," Hft 2, 1912.

ing their parents' sleeping room or in some other
way, happen to overhear the act of sexual intercourse.   From such an experience they often derive the so-called "sadistic" conception of coitus.
"They see in it something that the stronger does,
by force, to the weaker; and they compare it (boys
especially) to a scuffle such as those with which
they are acquainted from their association with
other children." [1]   It seems probable that some
children recognize the true significance of coitus
and assume a connection between it and birth.
But a larger number apparently do not guess this
connection, and, therefore, look upon the act simply as one of violence.   The tendency of children
to regard coitus as a sort of assault and battery
committed by the male is strengthened if they see
the apparently hostile sexual activities of fowls,
cats and other animals, or if they find blood spots
in the bed or upon the linen of some woman in the
family.   Added to this is the fact that in certain
homes the entire married life presents to the ob-
servant child the spectacle of continuous strife,
expressing itself in loud words and hostile de-
meanor.   From this he takes it as a matter of
course that the quarrel is continued into the night,
and is decided by the same means that he is accustomed to employ with his brothers, sisters or
playmates.

   This early period of sexual investigation and
theory formation ordinarily comes to an end with
the beginning of the latency period.   The inhibitions that develop at that time against matters

   [1] Freud, l. c.

sexual soon cause these theories to fade from conscious memory, so that in adult life the individual is usually unable to recall ever having had any views upon or interest in sexual matters at this early period.

During the latency period, and consequent upon the quiescence of the investigating instinct, children often accept without any particular conscious doubt the stories that babies are brought by the stork or the doctor, or else they conclude that God makes some mysterious and supernatural arrangement by which infants appear in the homes of the married. These beliefs then remain in conscious memory and are recalled in after life as if they were the *only* ones that existed in childhood.

In most children, at the close of the latency period, the dormant sexual curiosity again appears, and a second period of sexual investigation begins. But the conditions are quite different from those of the first period. Children now discuss matters of sex with each other; the older and better informed share their knowledge with the younger, or, occasionally, more or less complete sex instruction is given by parents or teachers. Thus in some cases children learn the whole truth about reproduction. But more often the child is ignorant or misinformed concerning one or more important facts and so is prevented from drawing correct conclusions. Consequently the theories which are formed at this time are often extremely absurd and, because they are based upon such variable external conditions, of infinite variety. To be sure, a partial revival of the earlier theories

may occur and serve to color or modify later conclusions, but the uniformity of the primary and,
so to speak, endogenous theories no longer exists.

As these later theories are from the medical
standpoint much less important than the earlier
ones, I shall limit myself to making little more
than a brief mention of a few of them. One of the
most frequently found secondary theories is the
belief that birth takes place through the umbilicus,
through the linea alba, or through an artificial ab-
dominal opening made by a doctor. Even grown
women occasionally entertain some such view.
Such conceptions are really remnants of the cloaca
theory. When repression of the anal and coprophilic interests occurs the original cloaca theory
becomes objectionable and is excluded from consciousness. Then some less objectionable part
of the abdomen, such as the umbilicus, takes in the
new theory the place formerly occupied by the
perineal region.

One set of secondary theories depends upon the
fact that many children, though no longer in ignorance of the existence of the vagina, have not
yet learned of the seminal fluid. Hence, in some
cases, they conclude that the urine possesses the
power of fertilization; in others, that mere contact
of the male and female genitals (without penetra-
tion) is all that is necessary for impregnation.
According to my experience, the latter, or "con-
tagion" theory, is usually found only among
females. Other beliefs that may be mentioned
are the following: That impregnation results from
kissing, that coitus takes place by rectum, that

birth follows invariably or immediately after coitus, etc. One of my patients, apparently believing that some close analogy existed between human copulation and the incubation of eggs, concluded that intercourse had to take place every night for nine months in order to produce a child.

What significance these periods of theory formation may have in the later life of the neurotic we shall learn in some of the succeeding chapters of this volume.

CHAPTER II

IF you hold horizontally in your hand a sheet of stiff paper upon which some iron carpet tacks have been placed, and then move a magnet back and forth under the paper, the tacks will follow the magnet. To an ignorant person, not seeing what was beneath the paper, the behavior of the tacks would seem lawless and inexplicable.

The phenomena of mental life are quite as unaccountable as the movements of the tacks if we take into account in the former only the content of the individual's consciousness.

Not only in the psychically abnormal but in the normal as well there are many mental occurrences for the cause of which the individual's consciousness may be searched in vain. We are frequently surprised to find that we have dreamed of a person or event which we have not thought of for years. A tune starts running in our heads, or an unfamiliar verse, or we suddenly begin to hum or whistle some long-forgotten air. What evoked it? We have ideas, impulses, tastes or prejudices the causes of which we do not know; continually we find ourselves entertaining beliefs or arriving at conclusions the origin and basis for which we are entirely unacquainted with. There are sudden likes and dislikes, such as an unaccountable antipathy once felt by a young woman patient of the writer's for all men with light hair.[1] We feel sure of the guilt or the innocence of some one on trial for murder, though we cannot say exactly why we have that feeling. A man will suddenly in the middle of his busy day become sick of his business and want to give the whole thing up. Not only for our dreams but for our defective actions and, in neurotic individuals, for the various symptoms (anxieties, compulsions and the like) the content of the individual consciousness gives no adequate explanation. In short, if we attempt to explain every conscious psychic phenomenon by relating it to some other conscious phenomenon, we are utterly baffled and confused. The majority of mental happenings seem so entirely independent of any other mental happenings as to be entirely inexplicable on any causal basis that includes only conscious factors.

In psychology, just as in physics, we are compelled to assume that the law of cause and effect holds good. Every idea, impulse or feeling that appears in our consciousness, every action we perform, must have some adequate cause. None of the phenomena of either normal or abnormal mental life can be regarded as merely the result of accident or chance. Therefore, just as a thinking person who saw the tacks moving about a sheet of paper, as if they were themselves autonomous, would assume that they were actuated by some force the origin of which he could not see,

[1] See Chap. IV, p. 126.

so too we must assume the agency of unseen psychic forces if we are to regard the phenomena of mental life as having any law and order, or even continuity and connectedness. We are obliged to posit psychic acts and influences lying outside of the field of consciousness and inaccessible to ordinary introspection—which in other words are unconscious. Without this assumption it is absolutely impossible to reduce things psychic to any semblance of law, order, continuity or comprehensibility.

Another reason for assuming the existence of the non-conscious psychic factor is that the content of our consciousness comprises only an extremely small portion of what we are wont to call our conscious knowledge. I "know" the multiplication table, the date Columbus discovered America and an infinite number of other things varying from the names of the twelve apostles to the function of the cerebellum; but the greatest part of this information only occasionally occupies a place in my conscious thinking, and then only for a relatively short time. At all other times it is latent. I can recall any portion of it, if there is any occasion for so doing, but, unless attention is directed to them, all these memory impressions remain unconscious like an electric light bulb with the current turned off, inactive, unilluminated.

Yet even when they are inactive we must attribute to these memory residues some sort of psychic existence. I meet a man on the street and he speaks to me. I recall where I met him

and all the circumstances, but cannot remember
his name. What *is* his name? Is it Marshall?
No it's not Marshall. Is it Parsons? No it is
not Parsons, although it begins with a P. Several other names occur to me but I reject them.
An hour later I suddenly recall the name; it is
Pierson. But had I not some memory of the
man's name in the meantime, even though that
memory was not a conscious one? How can I tell
what a man's name *isn't*, unless I have some sort
of psychic record of what it *is?* And is not this
unconscious memory identical in every respect
with a conscious memory, save that it lacks that
quality which we know as awareness? Is it not a
part of the psyche, even when it is non-conscious?

It has been maintained, on the contrary, that
these memory impressions, when outside of consciousness, are not psychic states, do not belong
to mind but are physical and pertain to physiology; that in other words, they are correlates of
somatic processes in the brain cells, from which
the psychical emerges only in response to new
stimuli or with shifts of attention. To such an
objection one might, of course, reply that they are
equally entitled to be called the residues of psychic
processes, and that they are no more physical or
physiological than are conscious psychic activities, which of course must be assumed to have
their physical, chemical or physiological counterparts, although we do not know what they are.
This sort of argument is, however, rather sterile.
A refusal to call latent memories a part of the
psyche is either a begging of the question as to

whether only that which is conscious is mental, or else a matter of conventional nomenclature which arbitrarily defines the mind as that which is conscious.

This being the case, the question of whether we should adhere to the arbitrary and conventional definition of mind or abandon it in favor of a conception that includes non-conscious mental elements is really a pragmatic one and turns upon which one of the two ways of looking at the matter best accords with known facts and is the more useful. Once stated in these terms, the question becomes a very simple one. To define mind as only that which is conscious, and to remove from the field of psychology the latent memory impressions and other non-conscious elements of which we are obliged to infer the existence, is a procedure that cannot be defended from the point of view of utility. As Freud points out it separates phenomena that are actually continuous, plunges us into the insoluble problem of psycho-physical parallelism, and obliges us to narrow the field of psychological investigation without correspondingly widening any other field.[1] To accept such a way of looking at the psyche would be much the same as binding ourselves never to judge our fellows except on the basis of what they say, or refusing to employ any data for interpreting the behavior of our friends, acquaintances and people in public life except that furnished by what they choose to tell us. On the

[1] Das Unbewussten—"International Zeitschrift für Ärztliche Psychoanalyse," Vol. III, 1915.

other hand, a psychology which includes the non-conscious is extremely useful. This will, I feel, be so clearly shown in the following pages as to relieve me of the task of arguing the point just now.

If now we grant the right to posit an unconscious portion of the psyche, it is evident that latent, i. e., inactive, memory impressions and their like are not the only non-conscious mental elements which we must assume to exist. We have reason to infer the existence of other elements which are not simply latent but which, despite their not being conscious, are active and may exert an influence, even a profound one, on the individual's conscious thinking and behavior. In order to make this perfectly clear, let us suppose that I hypnotize a man and give him the suggestion that, fifteen minutes after he awakes, his arm will become completely paralyzed. He is roused and remembers nothing of what I have said to him during the trance. Nevertheless, when fifteen minutes have elapsed he is utterly unable to move his arm. He still has no recollection of what was said to him during the hypnotic sleep, nor does he realize what it was that caused his paralysis. In other words, my suggestions, the mental impressions causing his paralysis, though potent and active are at the same time unconscious. This proves conclusively that a mental element does not necessarily have to be in consciousness in order to be active or produce an effect.

A similar example we can take from the realm

of the abnormal.   A young woman, a patient of
the writer's, suffered from an uncontrollable impulse to take drugs.   But the case was not one of
a drug habit in the ordinary sense, for the drugs
she took were not as a rule of the habit forming
variety, and she showed no preference for any one
drug over any other.   She did not take them
for their taste, nor for any pleasing effect they
had upon her, for many of them were ill tasting or
had some action which she found very unpleasant.
Any substance so long as she could think it was
"medicine" suited her just as well as any other.
She had many times been questioned as to why
she had this peculiar impulse, and she had tried
very hard to find the explanation herself, but without any success.   The reason for her morbid
compulsion was as much a mystery to her as to
every one else, and was utterly inexplicable as far
as the data furnished by her consciousness were
concerned.

But while the compulsion could not be explained
by referring it to anything contained in the patient's consciousness, our conclusion should not be
that it had no cause, but rather that of its cause
she was unconscious; that it depended upon a
mental activity which lay outside the field of her
conscious introspection.   It was just as if some
one had hypnotized her and by suggestion given
her the impulse to take drugs, which upon awaking
she obeyed without remembering the suggestions
from which it originated.   In fact such an impulse
could be produced for a time at least, in that way.
In such a case we would know what caused the im-

pulse, even if the subject did not; in pathologically produced compulsion we lack such knowledge until after the case has been analyzed. We shall learn later, indeed, how it is possible to ascertain the causes even of these compulsions. In the case of this young woman, for instance, it will not only be shown that we are right in assuming some unconscious ideas and impulses as the real basis for her drug compulsion but also we shall learn what these unconscious ideas and impulses were.

It should be understood at the outset that we do not have to go into the field of psychopathology or to such unusual states as those induced by hypnosis to find examples of the influence of mental processes which are active though at the same time unconscious. Many are at hand in the phenomena of every day experience.

Thus a man's religion is rarely chosen by him only through conscious reflection. When a person is a Protestant, it is ordinarily supposed that he was caused to be so by what is popularly termed his "bringing up." That is, it is assumed that a large number of experiences which he has undergone, and of influences to which he has been subjected, have somehow prejudiced him in favor of the particular religion he has chosen and are really responsible for his choice. This does *not* mean, however, that he *remembers* all these experiences or is clearly conscious that they are influencing him. On the contrary the impressions having perhaps the greatest influence are usually the ones that relate to the moral and religious instruction he received in childhood, and these can be recalled only imperfectly, and many of them not at all. It is obvious therefore that to explain *why* a person has accepted a given religion we have ordinarily to assume that there exists a non-conscious biasing agent which is probably the most important factor in determining his choice.

If we now attempt to formulate some conception of this biasing agent (of this unconscious cause of belief) our result will be somewhat as follows: We shall expect it to be a very large group of memory traces, ideas and feelings connected in various ways with the central theme of religion. Some of these presumably had their origin in the various incidents of early moral instruction from the parents, of intimate family life, of childhood visits to church and Sunday-school, or in different vague perceptions of things wonderful and mysterious. Others resulted from various allied experiences occurring throughout the person's later years. Some of the elements of the group are doubtless recalled frequently, others seldom, a great many others never. That is, the biasing agent consists very largely of unconscious ideas.[1]

Such a system of connected ideas, having a strong emotional tone, and displaying a tendency to produce or influence conscious thought and action in a definite and predetermined direction, is called a complex.

A great part of our conscious activities is determined by such groups of thoughts, only a few

[1] Frink—"What Is a Complex?" *Journal of the American Medical Association,*" Vol. LXII, p. 897, 1914.

members of which are ever in consciousness. We have complexes concerning the different members of our families; complexes relating to each one of our important loves, hates, ambitions and recreations, and complexes concerning our politics, patriotism, pride, morality.

A statement like this will not be instantly accepted by every one. According to most people our thinking is determined by external facts, by our logical and reasoned judgment of them, by what we know and perceive, not by that of which we are unconscious. But though we do not underestimate the part played by logic and reason in mental life, it must be admitted that such forces have not by any means the wholly dominant rôle that is often unthinkingly attributed to them. "When the emotions are sitting as judges, facts make poor witnesses" will hardly be disputed by anyone who stops to think. We all have prejudices and are subject to their influence. "The wish is father to the thought" applies to all of us at times. But, common as the phenomena are, how seldom do we hear a person admit that he is biased in his thinking, or see him give any evidence of a realization that such is the case! Ask a German if he approves of Zeppelin raids and he says: "Certainly." Ask an Englishman and he answers: "Barbarism!" Then ask either one of them to give the reasons of his opinion, and you will get a more or less logical explanation. But is this explanation correct? Is it not more likely that the reason that the German believes in Zeppelin raids is that he is a German, and the

Englishman condemns them because he is an Englishman? Is it not practically certain that in nine cases out of ten the person is incapable of thinking without bias on a question so intimately affecting his mother country and himself, and that his complexes even more than the actual merits of the question are the main determinants of his opinions? But does the person himself realize and admit this? In most instances certainly not. On the contrary he is sincere in believing that the reasons he gives for his opinion are the actual cause of his entertaining it.

It is an extremely common occurrence that ideas, beliefs, actions, really having their origin in some one of the individual's complexes, and being at least partly determined by ideas and impressions of which at the time he is not conscious, he represents to himself and to others as being the result of a logical train of conscious thought. He manufactures *ex post facto* a plausible explanation of his belief or action which he unquestioningly accepts as its cause. This process of supplying the place of the missing (unconscious) link in the chain of reasoning with another (conscious) link has been named by Ernest Jones *rationalization*.[1] It is because we all rationalize very extensively that we greatly overestimate the rôle played by logical and reasonable judgment in determining the trend of our conscious thought and conduct, and, to the same or even a greater degree, underestimate the influence and potency of those factors which are not in consciousness.

[1] "Papers on Psychoanalysis," Chapter I.

(b) *The Unconscious and the Foreconscious*

Non-conscious mental elements may be roughly divided into two classes. For instance, it comes to my mind as I am writing, that the dose of phosphorus is one hundredth of a grain. I am sure that at any time since I first studied materia medica I could have remembered the quantity of the dose, if any one had asked me. But I am almost as sure that this is the first time I have thought of it since I left college. Though this particular memory was in the Unconscious all that time it could have been brought into my consciousness at any time if I had wished to recall it. On the other hand, the hypnotic subject may be entirely unable to recall the hypnotist's suggestions, the neurotic young woman was absolutely unable to bring to her consciousness the ideas which operated to form her drug compulsion, nor can the German through any effort of voluntary introspection, become aware of any but a relatively small portion of all those past impressions, going even back to his childhood, which make up his complex concerning the Fatherland. Some unconscious mental elements, then, can be brought into consciousness at the will of the individual; others can not, but remain in the Unconscious in spite of any ordinary effort of the individual to recall them.

Mental impressions or processes of the first class above mentioned are spoken of as foreconscious and are said to belong to a region or system in the psychic apparatus which is named the Fore-

conscious.[1] Those of the second class are known
as unconscious and are said to belong to a system
or region called the Unconscious. The word Unconscious is often used to embrace both systems—
all the non-conscious impressions and processes,
those of the Foreconscious as well as those of the
Unconscious proper. The mind, then, in Freudian psychology, is conceived as having three
levels, the superficial one or Consciousness, em-
bracing all those mental processes which at any
given moment possess the quality which we call
awareness. The next, the Foreconscious system
or level, contains those elements which could be
reached by voluntary introspection, and are capable of being brought to consciousness, but at the
time lack awareness. The third and deepest level,
the Unconscious Proper, embraces all those impressions or processes which not only lack awareness but also cannot, by any unassisted effort of
the individual, have it conferred upon them. Obviously the boundaries between the three systems
are not sharp or absolute. An idea that is conscious at one moment may be foreconscious the
next, and perhaps eventually unconscious. But
the interchange between the foreconscious and
consciousness is much more free than that between the foreconscious and the unconscious or
between the unconscious and consciousness.

What is it that prevents ideas or processes of
the unconscious proper from being accessible to
consciousness? Processes belonging to the unconscious system may be active, and capable of

[1] Called preconscious by some writers.

exerting a strong influence in and through consciousness—may, in fact, as I hope to show eventually, possess nearly every quality or attribute of conscious mental processes save that of awareness. What is it then that keeps them from gaining entrance into consciousness?

In the case of foreconscious processes the lack of awareness seems easy to explain. I walk along the street with my mind absorbed in some engrossing problem. I have no true consciousness of what is going on about me. Nevertheless I turn the proper corners, avoid collision with other pedestrians, and stop at the right house. All the processes necessary for doing these things are carried on without exciting awareness or diverting my conscious attention from the problem which absorbs it. These processes are carried on in the foreconscious. Not enough attention, or better, interest is distributed to them to give them the quality of awareness. Yet at any time they could come into consciousness and acquire awareness if my interest or attention were directed to them. In the same way my memory impression of what is the dose of phosphorus remained latent and in the foreconscious until attention and interest were distributed to it. When, however, it was thus energized or activated, it came into consciousness, only to return to the foreconscious state as soon as the activation-energy was withdrawn.[1] Foreconscious memories or processes seem, then, to be those which either are prac-

[1] I have preferred to use the terms "activation" and "activation-energy" instead of "occupation" and "occupation-energy"

tically unactivated or else carried on with such a
low pressure of activation-energy that they fail
to rise above the threshold of consciousness.

The lack of awareness of those processes belonging to the unconscious proper cannot be explained in any such manner. When, for instance,
they produce such an imperative and powerful
compulsion as that exemplified by the young
woman who was impelled to take drugs, we cannot believe that they possess only a low degree of
activation. On the contrary, their activation must
be very high. We must therefore find some other
explanation of their not being conscious than that
of a withdrawal of activation such as would account for our lack of awareness of the content of
the foreconscious.

Of the little outlays of money I make during the
day, for carfare, lunch, telephone calls, etc., I
have no conscious recollection at night. If there
were any occasion to do so, I could perhaps recall
how much I had spent and for what I had spent it,
but ordinarily these minor outlays have not sufficient importance to keep their mental records long
before my consciousness. They promptly lose
their activation; its withdrawal is a passive and
negative process.

Suppose, on the other hand, I pay a high price
for a piece of furniture under the impression that
it is a genuine antique. Hardly do I get it home
when a friend, who is an authority on such matters, demonstrates to me that it is not genuine, but

which Brill, the translator of Freud's works, has employed as the
equivalent of the German "Besetzung" and "Besetzungs-Energie."

a relatively valueless imitation. I investigate and find that the conditions under which I bought it are such that I cannot make the dealer take it back and return my money. Now the memory of this expenditure does not quietly and passively fade from my consciousness like the recollection of the nickel I spent for carfare. Instead it continually intrudes upon me, causes me to berate myself for the credulity that allowed me to be taken in so easily, and keeps me in a state of exasperation and annoyance. But finally I say to myself that there is no use crying over spilt milk. "If I am a fool, I am, and that's all there is to it. I will put the matter out of mind and forget it. I refuse to think or worry about it any longer." With an effort of will I extrude the incident from my consciousness. It returns again after an interval but I again extrude it. Soon the extrusion becomes easier. Eventually it is automatic, and the memory of the annoying incident either entirely ceases to be reproduced in my consciousness or else appears only at long intervals.

Now it is obvious that the process by which *this* memory is eventually rendered unconscious is quite different from the quiet and passive loss of activation which causes the fading of the memory impressions of insignificant matters. There is no passive withdrawal of activation from my memory impression of the disagreeable incident, at least not at first. On the contrary it is highly activated, and insists upon forcing its way into my consciousness even when I am trying to give my attention to other things. How then do I get rid of it? Apparently by attempting a forcible withdrawal of conscious activation and by initiating through a conscious act of will a *counter-activation* which is shortly taken over by the foreconscious and becomes automatic, serving to protect me from the displeasure of having the recollection of the disagreeable incident reproduced in my consciousness, and apparently persisting at least until the activation of the memory itself in the course of time is eventually withdrawn. [1]

This gives us the key for an understanding of why it is that certain processes of the Unconscious, in spite of their high activation, fail to gain entrance to consciousness. The reason is that *their reproduction is opposed by a counter-activation* located for the most part in the foreconscious, which automatically and without involving the participation of consciousness, keeps them submerged. The non-consciousness of the elements belonging to the unconscious system is not then something passively conditioned, but the result of a positive and active counter-force.

The process which consists of the withdrawal of conscious or foreconscious activation from a mental element and which consists also of the establishment of a foreconscious counter-activation, which confines it to the Unconscious, is called *repression*. The mental element so relegated to the unconscious and unable to return therefrom is

[1] Strictly speaking, the counter-activation is not initiated by a "conscious act of will"; in fact, the act of will might be more accurately said to be initiated by it. The counter-activation is really represented by my wish to forget the incident.

said to be *repressed*. The repressing force impeding the return of the repressed element to consciousness is often spoken of as a *resistance*.

The unconscious consists in large part of repressed material, though not everything in the unconscious is repressed or is there by virtue of repression. The facts are as follows: the psychic apparatus is to be thought of after the model of a reflex arc. Thus it has its sensory, or afferent, side, which receives the stimuli coming from the external world or from the internal end-organs excited by changes within the body. It has also its efferent side through which discharges take place to the voluntary muscular apparatus as motility, or to the involuntary muscular and glandular systems as feeling or emotion. The Unconscious is toward the afferent side, the Foreconscious next to the efferent. All excitations of the psychic apparatus (all mental processes) begin at the sensory end of the system and are thus, to start with, unconscious. [1] Some of them remain unconscious, while others pass through to the foreconscious and to consciousness to discharge ultimately as emotion or motility. Whether a given process remains unconscious or is allowed to gain access to the foreconscious or to conscious-

[1] This is not strictly true unless we make the assumption that sensations or sense perceptions coming from the end organs applied to the external world pass through an unconscious phase. Freud regards consciousness as, functionally, a sensory organ for perceiving psychic qualities. He speaks of it as having two surfaces, one which is excited by the stimuli entering through the sense organs applied to the external world, the other by changes or processes within the psychic apparatus itself.

ness and so to efferent discharge, depends on
whether or not it meets on its way with a resistance.   For at the border line between the unconscious and the foreconscious the repressing forces
or resistances exert a certain censor-like action.
Mental processes beginning in the unconscious
have, as it were, to undergo an examination before
they are admitted to the higher psychic degrees
or systems.   Depending on their character or
qualities (a matter of which we shall hear more
later) [1] some of them are rejected, and remain repressed and in the unconscious; others are allowed
to pass to the foreconscious system from which
they may or may not enter consciousness.   In
normal conditions the foreconscious system must
be traversed before an excitation gains discharge
as affectivity or motility.   The most important
function of this system is that of opening or closing the avenues to such discharge.   The content
of the unconscious is, then, made up of latent (unactivated) psychic formations, mental processes
that are *in statu nascendi,* and other processes or
activated impressions which are not allowed to
pass the censor and are thus repressed.   We shall
consider the content of the unconscious from a
different point of view later.[2]   At present we
must devote ourselves to gaining a clearer understanding of repression, its function and the motive
for it.

A repressed element, as I have indicated, is one
from which conscious and foreconscious activation is withdrawn (if the element ever possessed

[1] Page 57.   [2] Page 62.

such activation) and against which a counter-activation exists in the foreconscious. Its activation, if it has any, belongs entirely to the unconscious system. What is the purpose of this process? Why is anything ever repressed? We get a hint of the answer to this question from the example I have given. I repressed the recollection of my being taken in by the furniture dealer because this memory was annoying me, and giving me displeasure, for the most part apparently because it showed me in such a light as to injure my self-esteem. That is to say, we get the suggestion that repression is a protective mechanism, that its motive is the avoidance of pain, or a painful feeling. This is, in fact, the correct explanation. The function of repression is that of defending the ego against those ideas or processes which are incompatible with, and painful from the point of view of, the main trends of the individual's conscious thought and feeling. This means in general that the elements in question depend, for their power to cause pleasure or pain, upon their being out of accord with his individual ethico-esthetic ideals and impulses and upon their militating against his self-satisfaction and self-esteem.

(c) *Repression and the Psychology of Conscience*

Since the concept of repression is one of the most vital in psychoanalysis we must consider it in greater detail. But to get a fuller appreciation of it, we have to depart from the somewhat meta-psychological point of view which we have been occupying and approach the subject from another angle. This will involve what may seem a considerable digression, though on the whole our course will be one of progress.

In the first years of childhood there is nothing resembling that which in the adult we call self-control. The infant fulfills every wish he has, if it is physically possible for him to do so. There is no subjective restraint, no inhibition arising from within, to oppose or interfere with anything he wants to do. He knows no shame, no disgust, nothing resembling morality. He has no motives save those of getting immediate pleasure or avoiding immediate pain. Of pains and pleasures temporally and spatially remote he takes no cognizance; they mean nothing to him. His behavior consists solely of simple responses to the stimuli of his environment, and of expressions of the various tendencies of the hereditary instincts, the self-preservative, and the rudimentary sexual.

As we have seen, [1] a different state of affairs is initiated with the beginning of the period of latency, somewhere about the third year. There then appear certain inhibitory impulses or reaction-tendencies: shame, disgust, sympathy and a rudimentary morality. [2] These new tendencies to some extent oppose and limit the freedom of·expression previously enjoyed by the primary in-

[1] Chapter I.

[2] These reactions which appear spontaneously do not for the most part bring with them their object. That is to say: they are first represented by a *capacity* for such responses. The type of situation or condition which provokes the actual response is determined in large part by education and environment.

stinctive impulses. Situations and reactions that formerly were wholly pleasure-giving now become, to a varying extent, sources of displeasure. Thus acts, like running around naked, so much enjoyed by young children, which gave pure pleasure through gratification of the exhibitionistic impulse now provoke the displeasure of shame or embarrassment; those acts which, like torturing animals and teasing, gratified the sadistic impulse now give rise to feelings of sympathy or moral repugnance, etc. The possibility of internal conflict has been introduced into the psychic life.

In this way comes about the first repression. An impulse, when opposed by one of the newly developed counter impulses in such a way that expression of it gives a greater amount of displeasure than pleasure, shortly disappears from view. In other words, it is repressed. The activation energy which it originally possessed (its *libido,* if it is a question of a psycho-sexual impulse) is withdrawn; a counter-activation, corresponding to the inhibiting trend, appears in place of it.

The beginning of repression is the beginning of the Unconscious, as such. In early infancy there is no differentiation into systems, just as there is no repression. The first repressed elements form the nucleus of the unconscious. To them is added all that which later succumbs to repression in the course of the psychic development of the individual.

But the process of repression is not all so simple as that which we have described as the first

repression. Though the avoidance of pain or displeasure is throughout the immediate motive for
repression (whether the element repressed be a
wish-presentation or a memory) the sources of
such displeasure are not to be found solely in the
hereditary and spontaneously arising inhibitory
reactions, as we shall presently see.

There is in childhood a certain phase of development, (the existence of which is better demonstrated by some of the pathological conditions of
adult life than by direct observation of the child)
which is known as the phase of Narcissism. It is
a transitional phase interposed between the pre-
dominant autoerotism of infancy and the later
state of object love, and partakes of the nature of
each. It is distinguished by the fact that the
individual's holophilic impulses and interests
are for the time being directed toward himself,
in much the same manner that in the adult they
are directed toward another person. That is to
say, the child is for a time his own sexual object;
he loves or is in love with himself.

Subsequent to this transitional phase in the psycho-sexual development, the main streams of
libido are withdrawn from the self and applied to
sex interests and objects of the external world.
But not all the libido is so employed. Some of it
remains directed selfward, though not now to the
real self primarily, but rather to an ideal. The
complete self-satisfaction which the child enjoys
during the phase of primary narcissism, when he
is his own ideal, he can not long retain. Admoni-

tions and criticisms from the parents, his observation of the people about him and the comparisons he makes of himself with them soon give him a sense of imperfection and disturb his self-contentment. Thus he begins to desire to be, in certain respects, what actually he is not; to have qualities which actually he lacks; to be rid of traits which in fact he possesses. He forms, in other words, an ideal for himself, of what he would like to be, and to this ideal that portion of the libido remaining in selfward distribution is now transferred. In so far as he can bring his real self into correspondence with this ideal of self, his narcissistic libido is gratified, and in a measure he regains the self-satisfaction he formerly enjoyed. On the other hand, to whatever extent a disparity is perceived between the real self and the ego-ideal, to that extent the narcissistic libido fails of gratification and remains free, as some form of self-dissatisfaction or discontent.

What later becomes an ego-ideal was at first an external critique. The control which the child primarily exercises through fear of his parents' disapproval (or punishment) he eventually maintains through fear of his own disapproval. Such terms as right and wrong, proper and improper, at first mean nothing to him in and for themselves. He would just as soon do a thing labeled "wrong" as one labeled "right," if it were equally pleasurable. But with one group of terms he learns to associate displeasure in the shape of disapprobation or punishment from the parents; with the other, pleasure in the form of rewards and praise; and he begins to avoid actions belonging to the first category and to cultivate those of the second purely because of the extrinsic consequences of so doing. But gradually the external standards are assimilated. To do "wrong" begins to mean not only to be less loved but to be less lovable. "Right," "proper" and "nice" connote not simply praise but to be praiseworthy.

Just as the first specifications of the ideal are founded on considerations of what would win or lose parental approval and love, so later contributions to it have their origin in the desire to be thought well of by one's teachers, by admired or respected persons, by one's fellows and by the general public. Thus the essentially homosexual libido, originally (in the boy) the desire for the approval of his father, contributes largely to the formation of the ego-ideal.

The narcissistic libido, and that portion of the homosexual libido directed toward the self, find their satisfaction through the individual's bringing (or thinking he brings) his real self into correspondence with the ideal he has made for himself. This gratification is what we know as self-satisfaction, self-esteem and self-content, the pleasures of self-respect, of moral or esthetic self-satisfaction. If, however, a disparity is perceived between the real self and the specifications of the ego-ideal, a portion of the selfward directed libido fails of satisfaction, remains a free tension or yearning, and is felt as shame, guilt, humiliation or a sense of inferiority. The free homosexual libido is converted into anxiety [1] and is perceived as a fear of the public (shyness, diffidence, self-consciousness) or a fear of "the father" (self-consciousness, etc., before men who are older or distinguished or in positions of authority and who are therefore unconsciously identified with the father).

We perceive at this point that what we have really been talking about is the psychology of conscience. Conscience is nothing other than a censorial function or "instance" of the psyche which performs the task of watching over and insuring the gratification of our narcissistic libido by warning us of any disparity existing between an impulse or contemplated action and the specification of the ego-ideal. The inner voice which torments us with "You must" and "You must not" was primarily the voice of the parents, later of our teachers and those about us, from whose verbally conveyed praise or dispraise we built up the structure of our personal moral and esthetic ideals.

In the symptoms of certain pathological states, notably paranoia, the developmental history of conscience is seen regressively reproduced. The patient complains that some one knows all his thoughts, and watches and foresees all his actions. He hears the voice of this person continually commenting and criticising. At times it reviles him, accuses him of foul thoughts, of abnormal practices. In some cases the voice seems to be that of some particular man, especially an elderly man.

[1] See Chapter VII for the relation between free desire and anxiety.

Other patients complain that all people watch them when they appear in public, pass unfavorable comments upon them, call them bad names, etc.

That "something," however, which knows the patient's thoughts, foresees and criticizes all his actions, is merely an externalization of conscience, which with all of us was once external, and now for paranoiacs has become external once more. The voice which these patients hear is the same voice to which all of us have to listen; only it is perceived by them not as an inner but as an outer voice as it once was with everybody.

We see much the same thing in neurotics and even in so-called normal people. The speaker who trembles in stage fright before his audience, which, despite all his reason may tell him to the contrary, seems to him hostilely critical, the over-conscientious clerk who lives in constant anxious expectation of a "call down" from his employer, which however never comes,—these and similar people are suffering from symptoms produced in much the same way as are the paranoid delusions of critical observation. For the sense of impending hostile criticism, referred in one case to the audience, in the other to the employer, really has origin in the criticizing instance or element of the individual's own psyche—his conscience.

In some connection (one, however, that has nothing to do primarily with either the audience or the employer) a disparity between the real self and the ideal is felt by the individual; a certain measure of the narcissistic homosexual libido thus fails of satisfaction, and regresses in the direction of those earlier points of attachment whence the ideal came, thus becoming an anxious concern over the opinion of the public (the audience) or of the person *in loco parentis,* the employer. The paranoiac who thinks he is watched and unfavorably commented on by the public, or who hears himself reproached and accused by the voice of some elderly man, is showing regressive phenomena of essentially similar significance.

Our consideration of the psychology of conscience is really but a preliminary to the statement we now wish to make that *the formation of an ego-ideal is one of the chief conditions for repression.* Those wish-presentations (impulses, desires, cravings, etc.) which of themselves or because of the sort of action to which they impel us, run counter to, and are incompatible with, the specifications of the ego-ideal, tend to succumb to repression. Thus if they are in consciousness, the conscious or foreconscious activation energy (their *libido* if it is a case of psychosexual wishes) is withdrawn and a counter-activation is established against them. Or if they are unconscious to start with, they are prevented by the counter-activation from gaining activation in the conscious and foreconscious systems. Not only wishes are repressed but also ideas, memory impressions or any mental element which is sufficiently incompatible with the ideal. A considerable amount of psychic material is also repressed which, though in itself eligible for consciousness, meets with repression because it has close associative connection with what is ineligible and already repressed.

Let us again point out that the purpose of repression is in every case the avoidance of displeasure or pain. Those elements, whether they be wishes, memories or ideas, are repressed which, if admitted to or retained in consciousness, would create a sense of disparity between the real self and the ideal, and deprive some of the narcissistic libido of its gratification, would in other words lower the individual in his own eyes, and subject him to the displeasure of a loss of self-respect or the tortures of a guilty conscience.

The term conscience, as it is ordinarily used, implies an endopsychic censorship which deals with moral matters almost exclusively. But the ego-ideal contains many other specifications than merely moral ones, and self-satisfaction has other components than simply moral self-content. Our self-satisfaction is disturbed quite as much by non-moral disparities between the ego and the ideal as by strictly moral ones, and in either case the narcissistic libido is freed in just the same way, and the type of displeasure experienced has essentially the same quality. To use the wrong fork at a formal dinner, to pass flatus in public accidentally, to make a serious mistake in diagnosis, or to have on dirty underwear, are not matters that can be classed as sins, though in certain circumstances they can produce a sense of shame and humiliation which has no essential qualitative difference from that produced by actions which the individual does regard as sinful or immoral. We are apprised of incompatibility between a wish or contemplated action and the esthetic, ambitious or grandiose specifications of the ego-ideal apparently in just the same way and by just the same function as that which applies in matters ethical. It would seem then not only convenient but justifiable to broaden the term conscience to include not only that which measures the self according to the purely ethical terms of the ideal, but also that which does all such self-measurings whether they be according to moral, esthetic, ambitious, patriotic or any other variety of ego-ideal specifications. [1]

If we ask a person (or ourselves, for that matter): What is your ego-ideal? What are the standards and specifications that you try to live up to? we are not likely to get a satisfying answer. Some would say frankly that they could not answer such a question. Others might attempt to formulate their standards for us, and perhaps feel that they had succeeded in doing so. But in such a case, if we had a chance to observe the person further, we would see that he does things that are entirely contrary to the standards he stated, yet without displaying any sign of unpleasant emotion or appearing to suffer any loss of self-esteem; while certain other acts which are per-

[1] Perhaps it should be pointed out that the specifications of the ego-ideal are not necessarily consistent with each other. Thus, one of my patients, who in company with a friend "picked up" a couple of prostitutes, felt ashamed to go to a hotel to spend the night with them, yet almost as much ashamed to back out. A man who would be ashamed to appear irreligious may also feel ashamed to say his evening prayers in the presence of another man who occupies a room with him.

fectly in accord with any standards he mentioned
seem nevertheless to cause him acute shame and
humiliation and seriously to injure his self-content.

Observations like this, if carried far enough,
teach us two important things: first that a mere
intellectual acceptance of a given action as right
or as wrong does not constitute an incorporation
of that judgment into the specifications of the individual's ego-ideal.   A person may say and really
believe that we ought to return good for evil and
yet not feel the slightest compunction or self-reproach when he fails to do so.   Nor does an intellectual rejection of a given moral code mean that
it has ceased to exist as one of the stipulations of
that individual's ego-ideal.   Thus one of my patients, an ardent feminist, railed against marriage
and advocated free love, asserting that as soon as
she became entirely self-supporting, she would
enter such a relationship.   Nevertheless when at
length she came to the point of actually putting
her long contemplated plan into execution, she was
overcome by a spasm of moral repugnance and
broke out with a neurosis.

Thus for a given code or standard to be a part
of the ideal means not an intellectual but an emotional, not a descriptive but a dynamic acceptance
of it; it means, on the other hand, that considerable libido is attached to it and that it has experienced an incorporation into the individual's personality.   Observation shows that impressions received in early childhood are the most potent in
determining what sort of an ideal the individual

fashions. Later experiences which contribute to the ideal or modify its specifications as a rule gain their power to do so through some similarity or associative connection with the earlier impressions or the persons making them.

The second important fact that is brought out by questioning people as to the nature of the ego-ideal they possess is that the ideal is not consciously formulated. They can give some of its specifications very readily, but are unable to draw a definite word picture of it. The ego-ideal is not a conscious formation. For the most part it belongs to the foreconscious system. Nobody is continuously or completely conscious of what his ego-ideal is, though perhaps the major portion of it (even if not definitely formulated) is accessible to consciousness in accordance with the demands of any given immediate situation.

It should be added that the foreconscious system is the seat not only of the ego-ideal but of all the rest of the controlling trends which distinguish civilized man from the savage and the constitutional criminal, and adapt his thinking and behavior to the demands of civilized life. It is the system which in the main brings about and maintains repression.

I have spoken of the existence of a censor between the unconscious and the foreconscious, which determined the eventual admissibility or inadmissibility to consciousness of the mental processes starting in the unconscious. By the term censor was not meant any separate psychic entity but rather the effect exercised by the trends of the foreconscious upon the unconscious activities impinging upon their lower surface. [1] The action of this censor we can now identify with the action of conscience (I am here using the word in the broad sense in which I earlier defined it). At the same time I recognize that the censoring, rejecting and repressing action which conscience exercises upon wishes and ideals that press toward conscious representation and expression does not have to be deferred until the elements in question have already entered consciousness, and is not limited to ejecting and expelling them therefrom after they have entered, but may be, and extensively is, exercised still earlier, and may entirely prevent the presentations from reaching consciousness. Consciousness does not participate in any but relatively a small number of the acts of rejection and repression.

(d) *The Content of the Unconscious*

From what has been said about the development of conscience and of the rôle of the foreconscious as a controlling and repressing system, we get the suggestion that the unconscious or the nucleus of it must represent something existing in the psychic apparatus from the beginning, while the foreconscious must develop gradually in the course of life. This is found to be the fact. The unconscious is the primitive both phylogenetically and ontogenetically. It represents that which is uncontrolled in the savage but controlled in the civi-

[1] I hope to be excused for using such mechanistic phraseology in the discussion of such intangible matters.

lized; what is uncontrolled in the child but controlled in the adult. The foreconscious represents all that is introduced in the higher stages of
the evolution of civilized man out of the savage,
and of the adult out of the infant. This is true
not only in the sense that the content of the unconscious consists largely of trends or tendencies to
action that are more primitive than those of the
higher psychic systems, but in the sense that the
mental processes themselves, the ways of thinking,
are also more primitive. [1]

The content or nature of the unconscious as
compared to the higher systems will be made
clearer by the consideration of the following example. A friend once came to me to ask advice
about a neurotic young woman in whom he was
much interested. The girl was an only child of a
widowed mother who was not in the best of health
or of financial circumstances. The mother
showed the utmost devotion to the girl, thought
only of her, and never hesitated to make any sacrifice, no matter how great, if her daughter demanded it, or if it promised in any way to contribute to the girl's health or happiness. The daughter, my friend said, was equally as fond of the
mother. She was always praising her mother,
worrying about her health, and bemoaning the
fact that she had been the cause of so much
anxiety, and could make so little return for her
mother's sacrifices in her behalf.

Yet strangely enough all the many attempts
she was continually making to relieve her mother

---

[1] See Chapter III—The Two Kinds of Thinking.

of some of her burdens, and be a help and comfort to her, invariably came to naught, and in many instances had just the reverse of the happy effect for which they seemed to be intended. For instance the girl at one time had a physical illness which left her in a very much incapacitated condition and required her to go to the country to regain her strength. The mother succeeded in finding a satisfactory place for the daughter where at a very small expense she could remain until her convalescence was complete. The girl seemed to improve quite rapidly, and the mother was delighted. Very shortly however the girl returned home. She could not bear, she said, to be away from her mother any longer. She felt she must be home to help her mother, to relieve her strain and to avoid expense. Compared to her mother's welfare her own health was nothing.

The fact is that this return home had upon the mother just the opposite effect to that for which it seemed to be intended. Instead of helping her mother and allowing her to rest, the girl caused more work and more worry by being home than by remaining away. She saved no expense by being home for it cost less to keep her away than at home; because when she was home she was so helpless that her mother had to hire an extra servant. And by delaying her convalescence she prolonged what was the immediate cause of her mother's anxiety. This is only a sample of many instances of a similar character where by attempting to make life easier for her mother she actually made it harder.

In commenting upon these things my friend said with exasperation: "The girl acts as if she *wanted* to make trouble for her mother, as if she hated her and was not satisfied to let her have a moment's peace or happiness. But to say such a thing is absurd, for I've told you how fond she really is of her mother."

Yet what my friend said was not as absurd as he thought it. In a way he had interpreted the girl's behavior correctly, only he took no account of the unconscious. The obvious fact of the girl's protestations of love for her mother made him reject this interpretation. His statement (that the girl acted *as if* she hated her mother; *as if* she wanted to make trouble), was right as far as it went. But where he said *as if* she hated, he should, to be entirely correct, have said *unconsciously*.

In the normal person, the foreconscious and conscious systems dominate the avenues to motor discharge—to affectivity or action. [1] Only those impulses or excitations which are in accord with the trends of the foreconscious, and which pass its censorship are given efferent expression. [2] But in cases such as that of this young woman the sway of the higher psychic systems is imperfect. Impulses which normally belong to the unconscious and are repressed perfectly are here not fully controlled but find their way to action. The effects of these actions indicate the quality of the uncon-

[1] Of this I shall have more to say later. Chapter VI.

[2] The higher psychic systems control only the form of the expression of the urge and not its quantity or continuousness.

scious processes which furnish their motivation. From these *"as if's"* of the girl's conscious life we learn the *Is* of the unconscious.

As far as the consciousness and foreconscious of the girl were concerned she had a real and great love for her mother. But unconsciously she hated her and did desire to make her unhappy. If we seek to learn how this strange state of affairs came to be so, we get a good deal of information about the unconscious. We see first that the unconscious is primitive.[1] The hostile, vindictive reactions constantly expressed in the girl's behavior are not what we expect from a cultured civilized woman under any normal circumstances but are more in keeping with the character of an American Indian or any other savage.

In the second place we see that the unconscious has no regard for reality. It was not to the girl's ultimate advantage to make her mother miserable. Nor was hate the appropriate emotion for the actual situation. The mother was devotion and kindness itself; so why should her daughter hate her? The ethical values of the situation were entirely ignored.

In the third place, if we go far back into the girl's psychic history (to her childhood, in fact), we find that there was a time when hostility toward the mother was an emotion not so entirely senseless as it seemed later. For as a little child the girl was greatly attached to her father and envied the position the mother occupied with him.

[1] I may say that what is true of the unconscious in the case of this girl is true of the unconscious generally.

The hate toward the mother was originally the hate of jealousy; the little girl wished the mother out of the way in order to have her father all to herself. But at the time I saw the patient the father had long been dead, and there was no present reason why the daughter should be jealous of her mother. Yet the old infantile jealousy and hate remained. Thus again we see not only that the processes of the unconscious are uninfluenced by reality but also that they are not oriented according to time. We get the further suggestion that the unconscious is infantile and that it has to do with the holophilic impulses; and that therefore its content is in large measure sexual.

To recapitulate then what has been indicated by this case (for in fact it gives a good indication of the qualities of the unconscious in general) we may say that the unconscious is instinctive, primitive, infantile and unoriented as to time and reality.

Perhaps it may not be entirely clear just what is meant by these statements. What, for instance, is meant when we say the unconscious is instinctive?

I say to a man: "Have you a sexual instinct?"

"Certainly," he replies. "Of course I have."

"But how do you know that?" I ask.

"How do I know it? How can I help knowing it? If I see a pretty girl, I want to kiss her. If I fondle her, I get an erection and desire intercourse. If I have intercourse, I enjoy it and for a time feel satisfied. And if I do not have it at regular intervals, I find myself thinking of sexual

things and craving sexual gratification even
though I might will to do otherwise."

"Yes," I say, "but what of the instinct itself?
These thoughts and feelings and actions of which
you speak are not your sexual instinct. The
most you can say is that they are some of its manifestations. What of the thing itself? Of that
you say nothing.

"As a matter of fact, have you not accepted the
assumption of a sexual instinct simply *as a way
of explaining* the phenomena you describe, very
much as a savage explains the growing of a tree
or the flowing of a river by assuming that a spirit
dwells within them? Is this instinct, as far as
you can say, anything more than a hypothesis?
Have you ever seen it? Or touched it, heard it
or smelt it? Have you, in short, any *direct* knowledge of it, any more than the savage has of the
spirit he believes to reside in the tree? Can
you know of it in any other way than inferentially,
or in terms of its manifestations?"

"No," he replies, "you are right. My sexual
instinct, as such, never is and never can be an
object of my consciousness."

Yet though we cannot have direct knowledge of
any of our instincts or instinctive tendencies, we
must assume their existence, just as we assume
the existence of ether waves which we know as
light, or the waves of air which we know as sound.
We do not doubt them though our knowledge of
them is purely inferential. At the same time we
recognize that what to-day we call instinct may
sometime in the future be translated by science

into terms of reflex arcs and glands, of nervous impulse and tensions, of chemistry and electricity, just as we replace the spirit with which the savage explains the flowing of a river by another (and equally hypothetical) something, the attraction of gravitation. Of the *reality* of that which we call instinct and of the reality of what the savage called spirit there can be doubt. There *is* a something which makes the tree grow or impels us to sexual actions. Only when we try to draw conclusions as to the *nature* of the force in question do we go wrong.

When we say the unconscious is instinctive we mean that we include within it all those primal urges and impulses which we must assume to belong to the nature of man, to be inherent rather than acquired from education or environment, but which we know indirectly only, as causes inferred from some of their effects, never as themselves.

Likewise we say the unconscious is infantile, because of certain phenomena, particularly apparent in abnormal states, which we must infer to be effects of the persistence of certain urges or tendencies which are normally present and quite manifest in the actions of the child, but which disappear under the refining influences of education and of which the consciousness of the adult gives no *direct* information.

We say further that the unconscious is, in large part, psychic material that has been repressed, for we assume that every person has nearly the same heritage of instincts, and possesses the same infantile tendencies. Those which are not represented in his consciousness or apparent from his behavior we do not assume to be necessarily non-existent but rather that they are inhibited and perfectly controlled. To our thinking, then, they exist as potential rather than as kinetic forces, and in this assumption we are confirmed by the observation that in certain individuals, in whom they are the least apparent, they may unexpectedly some day become manifest under the guise of neurotic compulsions or other psychopathological symptoms.

Inasmuch as the unconscious is largely made up of instinctive forces or of infantile tendencies which behave like instincts, the statement that it is not oriented with regard to time and reality is not difficult to accept. An instinct represents a measure of energy which urges toward a certain more or less specific type of action, and may therefore be called a creator of tensions. These tensions remain until they are released in the acts which satisfy the instinct or, possibly, dissolved by some change within the organism. Obviously these tensions occur without regard for time or for reality. Thus we may feel hungry irrespective of whether or not it is the logical time to eat or whether eating is at the moment convenient or food accessible. The inhibition and control of the instinctive urge, the deferment of its gratification according to the demands of time and reality, belong neither to anything in the instinct itself nor to anything in the unconscious, but rather to forces of the foreconscious and conscious systems. In the unconscious there is no inhibition, no negation, no conflict. Its energy is all wish-energy, continuously urging and pressing for outlet like steam within a boiler. It is all tension. There are no counter-tensions, a phenomenon which occurs only in the conscious and foreconscious systems. "The unconscious can only wish."

We have said that the unconscious, as far as its energic content is concerned, is all wish, urge or tension, pushing for discharge. All inhibition, denial, conflict, control, moral or esthetic; all adaptation to the demands of reason, logic and reality come not from the unconscious but from the higher pyschic systems, consciousness and the foreconscious, especially the latter. Thus the foreconscious stands like a screen, to use Freud's metaphor, between the unconscious and consciousness. It controls, directs, inhibits or modifies the energy outflowing from the unconscious, decides the eligibility or ineligibility for consciousness possessed by the presentations coming from the unconscious and admits only those compatible with its trends and which pass its censorship. All people are practically alike in the content of the unconscious. The differences between people, between personalities, depend upon differences in the foreconscious. For in the foreconscious reside all the controlling forces derived from education, culture, morality, judgment and reason. The unconscious comprises all that belongs to primitive man and to the child; the foreconscious, that belonging to civilization.

I believe that the comparison of the foreconscious to a screen between the conscious and the unconscious is somewhat unsuitable because of its implication that the foreconscious is passive. Really the foreconscious is active and in other ways than merely that of admitting or obstructing presentations that press forward to it from the unconscious. Another figure perhaps more appropriate to represent the psychic processes of the foreconscious would be that which compared it to the managerial staff of a theater. We may compare the whole mind to all the persons in a given city engaged, or desiring to engage, in theatrical production, whether they be actors, would-be actors or those constituting the machinery of management. The persons actually occupying the stage at any given instant would correspond to a moment of consciousness. Like our thoughts, they appear, occupy our attention for a limited time, and retire to be succeeded by others, or to reappear after an interval. When off the stage and waiting in the wings for their cue they are like thoughts in the foreconscious, latent memories, such as that of the multiplication table. They are not dead and non-existent, but merely out of sight for the time being, though ready and waiting to play their respective parts as soon as the cue is given. These are the thought-processes passed by the censor and eligible for consciousness but not actually in consciousness.

To the unconscious correspond the great mass of people with histrionic aspirations who have not theatrical engagements. It is from this horde that those actually on the stage originally came and to it some of them will at length return. They represent the primal urge toward the stage, the force back of it which makes it possible, in a way its *fons et origo*. Those actually occupying a place before the audience are but end-effects, epiphenomena from that great lift and urge represented by the whole mass of the theatrically aspirant populace.

As our conscious thoughts correspond to those persons actually playing in the glare of the footlights, and the unconscious to the horde of aspirants from which these players came, the foreconscious in its censoring action corresponds to the managerial machinery of the theater, the unseen forces which sift from the mass of aspirants those worthy to play a part upon the stage. Just as the management stands between those who aspire and the longed-for place upon the boards, the foreconscious stands between the urge and drive of the unconscious and the opportunity for expression in the lime-light of consciousness. The actors whom we see and the thoughts of which we are conscious are thus resultants from the action of two systems of forces both of which are unseen, the one being a lifting force which strives for expression, the other a sifting force which examines, inhibits and directs, and allows expression to only a relatively small proportion of the aspirants that present themselves to it.

We come now to the point which this figure was selected to emphasize. The action of the foreconscious is not limited to merely letting through or refusing to let through the presentations submitted to it. Those let through do not as a rule enter consciousness in exactly their original form. The foreconscious adds something to them, or forces them to conform to qualities of its content. Its action is therefore more accurately described by comparing it to the managerial system of the theater than to a screen or sieve. Those aspirants who are accepted by the management to play parts upon the stage are not ordinarily free to choose their parts. The would-be Hamlet may have to appear as a coal heaver; the aspirant for show-girl honors may be compelled to play the part of a hag. So it is with the relationship between the foreconscious and the unconscious. An unconscious idea, in order to become eligible for consciousness or to enter consciousness must gain activation from the foreconscious system in addition to its activation from the unconscious system. It must unite with, and conform to, something already existing in the foreconscious system, or else remain in the unconscious, just as an actor must accept the rôle provided for him by the theatrical management or else be resigned to remaining unheard and unseen.

The foreconscious system not only determines the admissibility or inadmissibility of ideas to consciousness, but also controls the outflow of energy toward a motor discharge, whether to the voluntary system, as motility (conduct and behavior) or to the involuntary as affectivity (feeling, emotion). If those excitations or tensions, belonging to the unconscious and called wishes, are out of accord with the trends of the foreconscious, they are denied efferent expression. The ideas representing them are not admitted to consciousness; their energic quota develop no affects.[1]

(e) *Failure of Repression, and Descendants of the Repressed*

The control exercised by the foreconscious (repression) is none too stable, even in normal persons. This is particularly noticeable in respect to discharge into affectivity. Even in the most normal, the unconscious at times forces its way to emotional expression in defiance of the controlling tendencies. The periods of unreasonable irritation or worry, the seemingly inexplicable prejudices and antipathies and the transitory feelings of discouragement and depression to which all healthy people are at times subject are instances of imperfect control by the foreconscious over the avenues to affective outflow, and thus represent slight failures of repression.

In the psychoneuroses are represented the more serious failures in the control exercised by the foreconscious. Tensions and wishes, arising in the unconscious, and of a nature really incompatible with the trends of the foreconscious, force their way to discharge as emotions in spite of its inhibiting tendency, and become manifest as neurotic symptoms. Only in the major psychoses, however, do such massive failures of repression

---

[1] Strictly speaking there are no unconscious affects, the affect being a sensory report of a bodily state. See Chapter IV, also cf. Freud: "Das Unbewusste." To speak of unconscious affects (love, hate, etc.), is a clinical inaccuracy so current as to be legitimate.

occur as to allow the unconscious free access to motility.

The purpose of repression, as we said, is the avoidance of pain or of the development of painful affects. This is accomplished by withdrawing or withholding from objectionable ideas any foreconscious activation and by maintaining against them a counter-activation. Repressed ideas are thus activated only by the energies of the unconscious system. The activation-energy of the unconscious (and generally this means holophilic energy or libido) can never of itself be an object of consciousness. The libido-strivings, or as we say, "wishes," can gain representation in consciousness only when attached to, and activating some idea. But this idea must be of a kind that will be passed by the censor. Otherwise neither affectivity nor movement is developed from the unconscious wish or striving, no matter how intense it may be.

Though the idea representing or activated by an unconscious wish is rejected, the wish may in certain circumstances gain representation in consciousness or in efferent discharge by transferring itself to some new idea which is not inacceptable to the censor nor incompatible with the trends of the foreconscious or with the specifications of the ego-ideal. In this way impulses of the unconscious which are qualitatively at variance with the ruling forces of the personality do at times evade the repression by hiding behind an apparently unobjectionable idea. Thus the protective purpose of repression is defeated, for repressed tensions develop affects, or, less often, produce action. The repression is in part a failure for it keeps unconscious only the ideational and not the energic content of the unconscious presentation.

This matter of the transfer of the activating libido from a rejected idea to one that will pass the censor can perhaps be made clearer by means of a concrete example from a case where it has taken place. I choose one with which we already have some acquaintance, namely the case of the young woman mentioned in the early part of this chapter who suffered from a morbid impulse to take medicine.

This drug-taking compulsion was obviously an example of an effect produced by unconscious forces, for the young woman was entirely unable to explain what its motivation was, by any effort of voluntary introspection. It is clear that the wish-energy which reached her consciousness in the shape of the powerful compulsion to take medicines must have belonged in the unconscious to some other idea than that of taking drugs, but this idea we should suppose was repressed by the censor. The idea of taking medicine, against which the foreconscious interposed no resistance, thus played the part of a substitute for the first one and took on the activating libido belonging to it.[1] The energy of the compulsion thus presumably belonged to some wish of the unconscious in-

[1] Such a substitute idea is ordinarily found to have some close associative connection with the first one.

compatible with the trends of the foreconscious, a
wish which escaped repression only by means of
displacement.

We find confirmation for these theoretical ex-
pectations in viewing the ascertained facts of the
case. The young woman in question was a de-
vout Catholic. To be a good Catholic involves
more repression than is required of the adher-
ents of most other faiths. This girl was unmarried, and the church not only puts a strict prohibition on a single woman *doing* anything of a
specifically sexual nature, but it also teaches that
thinking sensual things and entertaining lustful
wishes is wrong and must be vigorously combated.
Thus the foreconscious of a Catholic girl (assuming that she seriously accepts these teachings)
would contain strong resistances against any
ideas, or wishes of a sensuously erotic character.
Counter-activations would exist against such
ideas; they would be denied activation in the foreconscious or the conscious, and their activation
which is derived from the sex impulse and from
the unconscious would be likely to find expression
in feeling or action only if it succeeded in attach-
ing itself to some apparently non-sexual ideas
which would not meet with counter-activations or
resistances.

The young woman of whom I speak was in most
robust physical health, and, as might naturally be
expected, had an equally vigorous sexual impulse.
She had a strong instinctive (one might say organic) yearning for sexual experience and to bear
children. For these longings no legitimate outlet

was provided, since she was not married, while her conscience and reason withheld her from any actions that might gratify them in illegitimate ways. In addition the religious and family teachings incorporated in her ego-ideal and in the trends of the foreconscious created counter-activations and resistances against her admitting to herself the whole reality of these wishes or indulging in any phantasies corresponding to their fulfillment. Had her repression, in accordance with the teachings of her religion, been perfect (as it was not), practically no sensuously erotic ideas would have been allowed access to her consciousness and no affects would have been developed from her sexual longings.

Complete repression of such powerful forces is by no means easy of achievement and we need not be surprised that this patient failed to accomplish it. She was fairly successful, to be sure, in excluding from her consciousness the *ideas* corresponding to her sexual wishes, but she did not succeed in keeping their *energy* confined to the unconscious.

In the course of my analytic work with her she at length recalled that as a little child she had been much interested in the question of where babies come from. She had asked her parents to answer it and had received the very unsatisfying statement that they grew on trees in the garden. Thereafter she pondered the question in private and came to some conclusions of her own that seemed more acceptable. She had made the observation that the arrival of a new baby in the family invariably coincided with an apparently severe illness on the part of her mother. She soon concluded that a causal relation existed between the two phenomena. Then arose the question as to what caused these illnesses of her mother which gave rise to such remarkable sequelæ. It must be, she at length decided, that her mother made herself sick by means of some drug or medicine obtained from the doctor. Little girls, then, if they only knew what this medicine was and could get some of it, could have babies just as well as the mother and would not have to play with dolls.

We realize at this point what was the meaning of the patient's compulsion. It is clear that in carrying out her impulse to take medicine she was acting just as she might have acted in her childhood if she had been desperately anxious to have children. At the time of her childish meditation she never did decide what drug the doctor gave her mother, and thus, as far as she knew, *any* drug might have been the one to produce a baby. By virtue of her infantile sexual theory the taking of any kind of medicine could be a symbolic equivalent for the act of fertilization. Though an innocent and harmless idea in itself, it served to represent in consciousness the libido really belonging to the idea of coitus and reproduction,—wishes, which, because of her moral resistances, were denied either free entrance to her consciousness or discharge as feeling or action of obviously sexual quality. Now that we know from what source this compulsion derived its motive power, we need not be astonished that the patient was unable to resist it.

It may be pointed out that the substitute idea of taking drugs not only bears a close associative relation to the repressed ideas, but also that it must once have formed a part of the same sexual complex which, at the time of the patient's illness, was subject to repression. In short we may say that it was a descendant of the repressed. It should here be mentioned that the foreconscious is in large measure made up of what in one sense must be regarded as descendants of the repressed, and thus of the unconscious. This is true not only of ideas and memories which have associative connection with unconscious ones, or were at some time a part of the repressed, but likewise of trends or activations some of which, from the point of view of function, are directly opposite to the repressed. Some of the inhibiting impulses, some of the specifications of the ego-ideal, really had a common origin with certain trends of the unconscious which in their nature would be regarded as the least ideal and most fully deserving of repression. Repressed and repressing forces in many instances really developed out of the same primitive instinctive tendencies. This is a fact which we have mentioned in Chapter I in discussing the latency period.

I have brought up the matter of foreconscious descendants of the unconscious in order at this point to correct the impression which was permitted to be made in the early part of this chapter, that all of the content of the foreconscious is eligible for consciousness and thus within the reach of voluntary introspection. Such, as a matter of fact, is not the case. Though a large part of the foreconscious is passed by the censor and thus is eligible for consciousness and within the reach of introspection, some of it, represented by certain descendants of the unconscious cannot be brought into consciousness by any ordinary introspective effort. These are the descendants of the repressed which possess close associative connection and qualitative similarity with it. In consequence of their quite readily demonstrable existence in the foreconscious we have to assume a second censor which stands at the border between the foreconscious and conscious systems just as the other censor stands between the foreconscious and the unconscious. This superficial censor operates against certain descendants of the unconscious which exist in the foreconscious but which bear the closest association with the unconscious and with the original repressed. Whether such descendants are rejected by the superficial censor or whether they are admitted to consciousness not only depends on their quality and their close association with the unconscious but often on the intensity of their activation. Ideas or phantasies, which through their content, might be deemed deserving of repression may be admitted to consciousness provided they have a relatively weak desire content. For instance a married woman may not object to being attracted by a man not her husband, or to having a few erotic day dreams about him as long as she feels that the attraction for him is not strong or that the happenings depicted in the day dreams do not indicate an intense wish that they might take place in reality. But if, for any reason, her feeling for the man threatened to become stronger, her resistances would be brought into action, the ideas and phantasies might be repressed completely, and she would soon cease to be conscious of any interest in him whatever.

To illustrate what has been said about the existence in the foreconscious of numerous descendants of the repressed, a concrete example may well be in order, even though the introduction of it may involve anticipating certain matters the full discussion of which is reserved for later chapters.

A friend once asked me if I knew of a firm dealing in a certain commodity he desired, and no sooner had I replied that I did than I found that I had forgotten the name of the firm. I did remember the location of their place of business, a large down-town office building, and, as I happened to be passing there a few days later, I stepped in and found that the missing name was Pond.

This forgetting is to be explained as follows: We should assume that in my mind there must have existed some resistance against the word *Pond*, in other words that I was unable to recall this name, which really is very familiar to me, because of the action of the censor which refused to pass it. We should also expect that the resistance which prevented the word from coming to my consciousness arose not so much against the word itself as against some group of ideas of which the word formed a part or with which it was associated. The word, presumably, was repressed not because it was offensive in itself, but because of its association with the offensive and repressed. At the time I was unable to recall it we should suppose it existed in the foreconscious as one of the descendants of the repressed to which the superficial censor denies entrance into consciousness.

The essential procedures of psychoanalytic technique rest upon the assumption that many descendants of any repressed trend or complex exist in the foreconscious, and one seeks to learn of the repressed by bringing into the patient's consciousness some of these descendants. The patient is therefore instructed to give up any goal-idea in his thinking and to tell all the thoughts that come to his mind, carefully resisting every tendency to ignore or reject any of them. This really means that he is to combat as far as possible the rejective action of the superficial censor and so to allow some of the descendants of the repressed to enter his consciousness, for this is just what these seemingly random and meaningless associations really are.

In seeking then to discover why I could not recall the name Pond, or rather with what group of ideas painful to me it had become associated, I applied the technique above described with the results that are here recorded.

Upon fixing my mind on the word Pond it occurred to me that a certain Dr. Pond used to be a pitcher on the old Baltimore baseball team. Next I thought of Indian Pond, where I used to go fishing as a small boy, and I had a memory picture of myself throwing into the water the large stone used as an anchor for the boat. Then I thought of a man named Fischer who is at present a pitcher for the New York Americans.

Continuing, I thought of Pond's Extract and of the fact that it contains witch hazel. This reminded me that I used witch hazel to rub my arm when in my school days I was pitcher on a baseball team. I also thought of a certain fat boy who was a member of the same team and recalled with amusement that in sliding to a base this boy once went head first into a mud puddle, so that as he lifted his face plastered with dirt, this, combined with his marked rotundity, had given him an extremely laughable and pig-like appearance. I further recalled that at that time I knew a boy nicknamed "Piggy" and that at a later time I had been nicknamed "Pig."

At this thought I was interrupted for a few moments, and when I returned to the analysis the word Pond brought the associations: Ponder—think—"sicklied o'er with the pale cast of thought"—Hamlet—the memory of my having referred to a certain village as a hamlet—the recollection that a farmer in this village once told me that a neighbor, out of spite, killed two pigs and threw them into his (the farmer's) well.

Then there suddenly occurred to me the follow-

in incident from my seventh year which appears
to have been the cause of my forgetting the word
Pond.

At the time I refer to I had a dog to which I
was greatly attached. My brother and I were
playing one day on the edge of a small pond near
our house, and this dog was in the water swimming. We began to throw small stones into the
water in front of the dog, and as each stone struck
the surface he would jump for the splash, try to
bite it, and bark in joyous excitement. Finally,
I was seized with the malicious desire to scare
the dog and, picking up a stone weighing three or
four pounds, I threw it, intending it to strike
just in front of him and frighten him by its enormous splash. Unfortunately, my aim was bad.
The big stone struck the dog squarely upon the
nose and stunned him, so that he sank beneath the
surface and was drowned.

My grief over this incident was without question the greatest that I experienced in my childhood. For days I was utterly inconsolable, and
for a long time there were frequent occasions
when I would be so overcome with sorrow and remorse as to cry myself to sleep at night. I suppose, however, that my grief seemed greater than
it actually was. That is to say, it was exaggerated to serve as a compensation and penance for
the painful perception that a cruel impulse on
my part was responsible for the dog's untimely
end.

At any rate, as is plain, the memory of the incident was a very painful one, and, in consequence,

I had good reason to wish to forget not only the incident itself but also any word (such as Pond) which might serve to bring it before my consciousness.

The matter to which I wish particularly to call attention is the relevancy of my seemingly irrelevant associations. For instance, my first association—that of the pitcher, Dr. Pond—contains three ideas connected with the repressed memory; viz., *Doctor* (myself), *Pond* (the place of the incident), and *pitcher* (one who throws). My second association—concerning Indian Pond and my throwing into the water the big stone used as anchor—is equally relevant. Indian Pond is in the same town as the other pond in which the dog was drowned; my memory of throwing overboard the anchor is connected with the memory of throwing into the water the other big stone which caused the dog's death.

The association *pig* which came up several times in the latter part of the analysis seems at first glance to have no connection with the concealed memory. A connection does exist, however. The letters P-I-G reversed are G-I-P, which spells the name of the dog. Thus the association concerning the pig-like boy and the mud puddle—which contains the elements *P-I-G*, baseball (*i. e., throwing*), and *water*—or that of the farmer and the pigs—*P-I-G, death, throwing*, and *water*—is seen to be perfectly relevant.[1]

Thus it may readily be seen that every idea that

[1] Frink—"Some Analysis in the Psychopathology of Everyday Life," *Journal of Abnormal Psychology*, Vol. XII, No. 1, 1917.

came to my mind was in some way associated with the repressed memory, either directly, as are those I have mentioned, or through some intermediate idea, such as the drowning of Ophelia, which connects Hamlet and the quotation therefrom with the drowning of the dog.

This little analysis gives a miniature view of what takes place in analyzing a case of psychoneurosis. The associations the patient produces in the therapeutic analysis are relevant to, and suggestive of, the repressed material on which the symptoms depend just as in this analysis all the associations bore a certain similarity to the repressed memory, so that, even if it had not come up to consciousness, one could have, from these associations, drawn some conclusions as to its probable content.

Thus we may close this chapter with the statement that our knowledge of the content of the unconscious is derived chiefly from the study of the descendants of the repressed which exist in the foreconscious and which, by abandoning any goal-idea in one's thinking and resisting the action of the superficial censoring tendencies, may be reproduced quite freely in consciousness.[1]

---

[1] The repressed painful memory which caused me to forget the word Pond, though an entity in itself, is at the same time a part of a larger entity, the whole sadistic complex. The facility with which it was repressed (I do not suppose I had thought of it in many years until I attempted to analyze my forgetting) was doubtless in part dependent upon its association with other repressed material belonging to this complex.

IT is readily apparent upon a moment's reflection that there are two distinct types of mental processes going on in our minds, and obeying two entirely different general laws or principles. The one type of thinking, which is represented in its most highly developed form by reasonings, judgments and various sorts of intellectual work, takes place in accordance with what Freud calls the Reality Principle. The other, most familiarly exemplified by day-dreaming, is governed by what he has termed the Principle of Pain and Pleasure, or, more briefly, the Pleasure Principle.

Thinking of the first mentioned type, or Reality Thinking, concerns itself mainly with actualities, with the answering of questions and the solving of problems, and serves to bring us into closer touch with the world as it is, and to assure and perfect our adaptations to it. Thinking of this type is for the most part done in words, it is directed in accordance with some goal-idea, and it tends to produce fatigue.

The second type of thought activity, or Pleasure Thinking takes place in pictures, in images rather than in words. It is not directed by any goal-idea, but wanders in apparent aimlessness from one theme to another, and does not tire us.

Its only concern is with that which is pleasant, and instead of bringing us into closer touch with reality, tends rather to withdraw us from it, particularly when reality is unpleasant. The gain or pleasure in this type of thinking comes from what is thought rather than from the result of thought, as is mainly the case with reality thinking. Reality thinking seeks to achieve the fulfillment of our wishes by things actual, and leads to the making of such changes in the external world as are required for that result. But in pleasure thinking the wishes are fulfilled in an hallucinatory manner, by imagination, and in total disregard of time, space and reality. Thus no amount of reality thinking can restore the past or awake the dead, yet in pleasure thinking I can, for example, become a general under Alexander the Great, fight in his armies, hold converse with him or for that matter, be Alexander himself; and if I want more worlds to conquer, find them and conquer them, in total disregard of time or space and every law of nature. Thus in day dreaming we have pleasure thinking exemplified in its most familiar form.

In a measure, though not accurately, the two types of thinking correspond to the differentiation of the unconscious from the higher psychic systems. While processes of the pleasure thinking type may occur in the conscious or foreconscious systems, reality thinking belongs to them exclusively and all the processes of the unconscious are of the pleasure thinking type. This is in accord with the statements made in the preceding chapter to the effect that the processes of the Unconscious are unoriented with regard to time, space and external reality, and that the Unconscious can only wish.

Obviously those processes governed solely by the pain and pleasure principle and disregarding reality are the more primitive and the older in the history of the mind. They correspond to phylogenetic and ontogenetic phases antedating the use of words, but in a sense are even more primitive than is implied by that statement. One can conceive of a period in the history of the psychic apparatus when they were the only type of mental process.

Against this assumption the objection of course arises that an organism which merely hallucinates its inner needs and disregards reality could not maintain itself for even a short time and hence never could have existed save as a fiction. But the employment of such a fiction is, as Freud explains, justified by the observation that the suckling infant almost realizes such a state of affairs through the aid of the nursing by the mother. "He apparently hallucinates the fulfillment of his innermost needs, displaying meanwhile through the motor discharge of crying and kicking, the displeasure arising through the increasing tension and failed satisfaction, and thereupon he experiences the satisfaction hallucinated.[1] Only later does he learn to use these discharge expressions purposely as a means of communication." At first he has no appreciation of what

[1] "Jahrbuch für Psychoanalytische und Psychopathologische Forschungen," Bd. III, Hft I, 1912.

intervenes between a wish and its fulfillment; for anything he may sense to the contrary a wish fulfills itself. His crying, etc., is at first simply an epiphenomenon of unsatisfied wish-tensions; that it informs another person of his desires and that the satisfaction shortly experienced comes only through the instrumentality of another being he does not at first know.

The attempt to realize all satisfactions by the hallucinatory method is abandoned with the first disappointments. The psychic apparatus is compelled to image what is actual, not simply what is wished for; it must depict the real, even if reality be unpleasant, and must strive for real changes, not simply imaginary ones. From these necessities reality thinking, so important in its results, begins.

In his paper *Formulierung über die zwei Prinzipien des Psychischen Geschehens*,[1] Freud gives a schematic outline of the development of the psychic functions a portion of which is somewhat as follows. The progressively increasing significance of external reality which begins as soon as the purely hallucinatory method of wish fulfillment commences to decline, correspondingly increases the significance of the sense organs receiving impressions from the external world and of that part of consciousness connected with them. The individual now becomes interested in *sense* qualities in addition to the qualities of pain and pleasure with which he was exclusively concerned

[1] "Jahrbuch für Psychoanalytische und Psychopathologische Forschungen," Bd. III, Hft I, 1912.

at first. A special function, that of *attention,* is
then arranged which examines the external world
in order that data concerning it may be on hand
at any time an urgent need arises. Instead of
merely waiting for the coming of sense impressions, this activity goes out to meet them. At the
same time a system of records is devised in which
the results of this examination are preserved and
which constitutes a part of what we call the
memory.

Instead of repressing everything painful, instead of denying activation to all those presentations tending to create displeasure, of ignoring
everything unwished for, the psychic apparatus
begins to exercise the function of judgment which
seeks to decide whether the incoming presentations are true or false, that is to say in harmony
with reality, accepting that which so harmonizes
even if it be unpleasant, and determining what
shall be accepted as true by comparing the presentations in question with the memory records
of reality.

The motor discharges which during the reign
of the pleasure principle simply served the function of relieving the apparatus from the tensions
produced by incoming stimuli, by draining off
these tensions as affective phenomena, motor restlessness, etc., now become employed in a new function, that of producing desirable changes in the
external world. They now become purposeful
actions, the forerunners of work.

The stimulus no longer results immediately in a
complete motor discharge. Between the receipt

of the stimulus and the motor discharge as action now intervenes the process of thinking which was originally represented by, and is formed from, the act of imaging. Originally thinking as a process distinct from mere imaging, and applied to the relations between impressions of objects, was probably unconscious. Only through connections with verbal residues does it gain such qualities as render it perceptible to consciousness. The psychic apparatus learns to tolerate the greater degrees of tension necessitated through the deferment of motor discharge, and thinking, that is to say reality thinking, really represents a sort of experimental paying out of these accumulated tensions in small quantities.

While those processes dominated exclusively by the pleasure principle represent nothing but *wish*, and strive for nothing but the securing of immediate pleasure or the avoidance of immediate pain, the goal of reality thinking is essentially that of *utility*. Thus the replacement of the pleasure principle by reality thinking in the consciousness of the individual is never complete, as we know. From the beginning of the influence of the reality principle in the mental life there remains split off a certain amount of thought activity dominated by the old laws and absolved from being tested or evaluated in accordance with the impressions of reality. It is represented in the play and "make believes" of children and by the phantasies and day dreams of the adult, where real objects are dispensed with throughout. The processes of the unconscious remain always under the domination

of the old principle of pleasure. It is the only
law they know, and of this fact, we shall, in the
following pages meet with numerous examples.[1]
The general tendency to satisfy with pictures

[1] "The release from the principle of pleasure by means of the
reality principle, with the psychical results which proceed from
it (the release) which here in a schematic exposition is restricted
to a single proposition, really is completed neither at once nor
simultaneously on the whole line. But while this development
takes place in the ego-impulses, the sexual impulses are released
from it in a very significant manner. The sexual impulses at first
behave autoerotically; they find their satisfaction in the individual's own body, and do not reach the situation of denial which compelled the installation of the reality principle. When later the
individual begins the process of finding an object, he waits a long
time because of the period of latency, which prolongs the sexual
development up to the time of puberty. These two elements—
autoerotism and the period of latency—have the result that the
sexual impulse is retarded in its psychic development and remains
a great deal longer under the dominance of the pleasure principle, from which many persons can never free themselves.
"Because of these relations there is a closer connection between
sexual impulse and phantasying on the one hand and the ego-
impulses and the activities of consciousness on the other. We
find this connection, in normal persons as well as in neurotics,
a very intimate one, although, by means of these considerations
from genetic psychology, it is recognized as a *secondary* one.
The continually operating autoerotism makes it possible that the
easier momentary and phantastic satisfaction on the sexual object
is retained so long in the place of the real one which however
requires trouble and delay. In the realm of phantasy repression
remains all-powerful. It makes possible the inhibition of ideas
(Vorstellungen) *in statu nascendi* before they can enter consciousness, if their activation can occasion a release of pain. This
is the weak spot of our psychic organization, which may be employed to bring under the dominance of the pleasure principle
again those thought processes which have already become rational.
An essential bit of the psychic disposition toward neurosis is
accordingly produced by the delayed education of the sexual impulse to regard reality through the conditions which render possible this delay."—Freud, l.c.

of the imagination (images of any sense quality)
the desires that reality leaves ungratified, as most
familiarly exemplified in our day dreams is not
limited in its operation to our waking hours. The
tensions represented by various ungratified wishes
of the day persist in some measure after we go to
sleep and, if of sufficient intensity, serve to disturb our rest. Then pleasure thinking comes to
our aid and, as in the suckling period, an attempt
is made to still and satisfy these longings by the
hallucinatory route—by pictures of the imagination—and upon awaking we say that we have
dreamed.

In short, the night dream and the day dream are
really analogous. We may define either one as
the imaginary fulfillment of a wish. Nevertheless, the truth of this statement is by no means
self-evident. That the day dream is a phantasied
wish-fulfillment is perfectly obvious. But that
the night dream invariably fulfills a wish seems
on first thought impossible. Over fifty per cent.
of dreams seem to the dreamer distinctly disagreeable, while many others, though not actively
unpleasant, nevertheless apparently fail to represent anything for which a sane person might
be supposed to wish.

Yet the apparent unlikeness between the night
dream and the day dream is not due to any lapse
of the principle of wish fulfillment but rather to
a difference in the way the desired things are represented. The representation in the day dream
is direct; the thing or occurrence desired is pictured as actual and present without any ambigu-

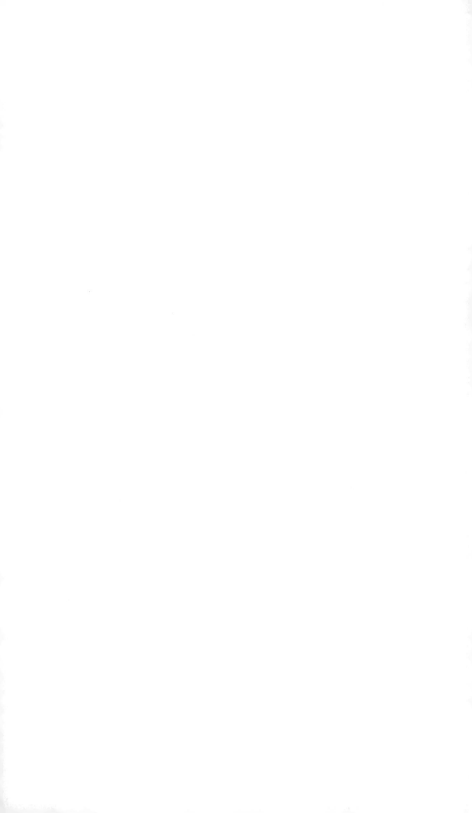

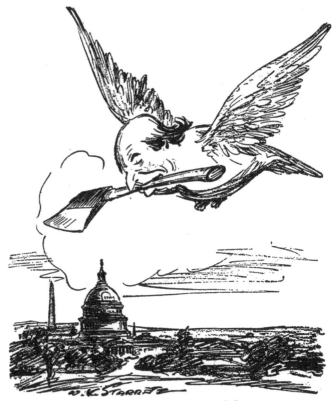

Courtesy of the New York Tribune

ity or vagueness. But in the night dream the representation is indirect. What is desired, instead of being pictured in its true form, is represented by implications, innuendoes, symbols, allegorical figures, etc. Thus while the day dream may be taken more or less at its face value, the meaning of the night dream is not to be found on its surface. The night dream, like a rebus or an allegory, has to be interpreted if we wish to know its meaning. Only in this way can we learn what wish it fulfills. That our night dreams seem to be senseless and absurd is not due to their actually lacking meaning but for the most part to the fact that indirect rather than direct representation has been employed.

In order to make perfectly clear the difference between direct and indirect representation, and how readily an appearance of absurdity is created by the use of the latter, I will introduce an example of indirect representation in the shape of the picture, Figure 1.

This is a copy of a cartoon which appeared in the New York *Tribune*, March 6th, 1916, just after Mr. Bryan had made a trip to Washington, ostensibly in the interests of pacifism. It expresses the artist's opinion that this trip did not spring from entirely altruistic motives—that, in figurative language, the Great Commoner, in appearing in the rôle of the dove of peace, really had an ax to grind.

A direct expression of the ideas represented by the cartoon would be the simple statement that Mr. Bryan's visit to Washington was primarily

intended not so much to further the interests of
pacifism as those of Mr. Bryan himself. But the
cartoon, which expresses the same thought in an
indirect manner, if taken merely at its face value
would seem to refer to something entirely different. If, for instance we were in the position of an
Icelander, and unfamiliar with American politics
and the figures of English speech, the cartoon
would seem just as senseless, bizarre and fantastic
as do most of our dreams, and precisely for the
same reason, for it would then be a case of indirect representation which we had not interpreted.
To us the cartoon has a meaning only because of
our ability to interpret it. To be able to make
the interpretation we need to possess certain information which is not given by the cartoon itself.
Thus we have to know the setting—what was going on in the political world at the time the cartoon
was drawn. We must be able to recognize the
features of Mr. Bryan, and must be familiar with
the symbolic figure, the dove of peace, and the col-
loquialism "to have an ax to grind." If we do
not have this information we can take the cartoon
only at its face value and then it seems utterly
senseless. What is true of indirect representation as exemplified in this cartoon also applies
everywhere else. In order to see any sense or
meaning in it, one has to have certain information not given in the representation itself, and to
use this as a means of interpretation. When we
have the required information and use it, the appearance of senselessness vanishes at once.

I will now relate a real dream and I think it

will be apparent that the means by which ideas are represented in it are almost identical with those of the cartoon. To see what it means, the same sort of extra information and interpretation is required as in the case of the cartoon, and, when the interpretation is made, what seemed nonsense suddenly appears as sense.

An acquaintance of mine once dreamed that he was kicking a skunk but that animal, instead of emitting its usual odor, gave off a strong smell of Palmer's perfume.

This dream of course seems absolutely absurd and meaningless. But we must remember that as yet we know nothing of the dreamer, nor of the setting in which the dream occurred. In short we are in about the same position as would be an Icelander in attempting to interpret the cartoon. When, however, the setting is known the dream is not at all difficult to interpret.

In discussing his dream with me the dreamer, whom we may call Taylor, was reminded by the idea of Palmer's perfume that he had been employed as clerk in a drug store at the time the dream occurred. This brought to his mind the following episode which, as will readily be seen, was what gave rise to the dream.

There had come to the drug store one day a man who demanded ten cents' worth of oil of wormseed (Chenopodium), and, as this drug is not classed as a poison, Taylor sold it to him without asking him any questions. The man then went home and administered a teaspoonful of the oil to his six months baby. The child vomited the first dose, a second was given and thereupon the child died.   Then, instead of taking the responsibility upon his own shoulders, the father sought to blame Taylor for the child's death.   The town in which the occurrence took place was a small one and in a day or so most of the inhabitants had heard his very untrue account of the affair.   Then Taylor, who was naturally very unwilling to be thus exposed to public censure, sought to defend himself by setting forth *his* version of the matter to every customer that entered the drug store.   In a few days the proprietor, annoyed by this constant reiteration, said to him: "Look here, Taylor, I want you to stop talking about this affair. It does no good.   The more you kick a skunk, the worse it stinks."

That night Taylor had the dream I have related. It is not difficult to see why it occurred and what it meant.   By the proprietor's command Taylor had been robbed of the only means at his disposal for squaring himself with the public, and in consequence he went to bed that night very much worried and disturbed.   Though he dropped off to sleep, these tensions persisted sufficiently to disturb his rest.   He therefore dreams that he is still kicking the skunk but without any unpleasant results, for it has a sweet smell instead of an evil one.   In other words the meaning of the dream is that he continued to defend himself and that good rather than ill came of it.   The way these thoughts are expressed in the dream is obviously almost identical with that employed by the artist in the cartoon.   For instance the dream

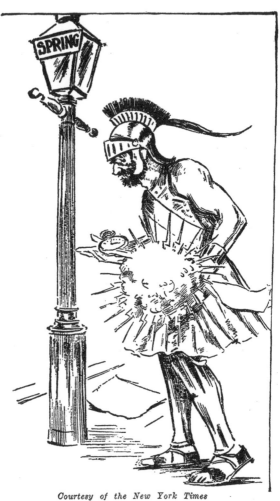

Courtesy of the New York Times

uses the proverb of the proprietor in just the same manner that the artist employed the phrase "to have an ax to grind." One might easily imagine a cartoonist for the local paper in Taylor's town (if all the circumstances were known to the public) drawing a cartoon with the title "What Taylor would like to do" which would be identical with the dream.

We may now consider another instance of indirect representation as exemplified by the newspaper cartoon. (Fig. 2.) We behold a picture of a man who, judging from the armor he wears, would seem to belong to the time of Julius Cæsar. Nevertheless, he stands near a very modern lamp post on a curb of what one would suppose to be Spring Street. He holds in one hand a watch of remarkable size and in the other a bouquet apparently composed of flowers and bayonets. In short the picture gives about the same impression of fantastic absurdity as do most of our dreams, and like a dream it requires interpretation.

This cartoon is not, however, as easy to interpret as was the first one. In fact, as it stands, it absolutely defies interpretation. We assume that indirect representation, some sort of symbolism, was used in forming it, but in order to interpret it we must know the meaning of these symbols and something of the setting or of what the artist had in mind when he drew the picture. As we look at the picture now, we are just as ignorant of the meaning of its symbols as we are of the dream symbols of another person.

This picture appeared in the New York *Times* in the spring of 1915, with the title "This is the Place, but Where's the Girl?" In the original the symbols employed by the artist were labeled. On the sheet of paper which lies on the sidewalk in front of the man was inscribed the phrase "Italy to go to war in the Spring" and the tag attached to the bouquet he carried bore the words "For Miss Italy." At the time the picture was published, Italy, in spite of numerous predictions, had not yet joined in the European war.

By the aid of these hints the picture is very readily interpreted. The meaning is something like this: "Italy is behaving like a fickle girl. No reliance can be placed upon her." The artist has used as symbols a man, a bouquet and a lamp post to express a thought *about something entirely different,* namely the attitude of that country toward the great conflict.

In this cartoon, as in the first one, the same method of indirect representation is employed that is used in dreams, with one difference however. The artist has labeled his symbols. The symbols in the dream are not labeled as they were in the original of this picture. The dream is like the picture as I have displayed it—that is, without the hints to interpretation that appeared in the original. Hence if we wish to interpret a dream we must get the dreamer to label his symbols in the waking state and after the dream is finished. This is accomplished by the "method of free association" with which we already have some slight acquaintance from the analysis of my forgetting of the word *Pond*. The dreamer is asked to fix his mind upon each part of the dream in turn and to relate, without exerting any critique, all his incoming thoughts. For, as will be explained shortly, the dream is really a product of the unconscious and of the repressed, and we learn what it means by getting the dreamer to reproduce by free association various descendants of the unconscious. These descendants, or associations, play in dream analysis about the same rôle as the words the artist painted in his cartoon; they represent labels for the dream symbols. By means of them we may learn of the hidden meaning of the dream.[1]

The following simple examples in the form of parts of two dreams show anew the way thoughts are expressed through indirect representation, and also the relation of the free associations to the thoughts represented, or in other words how dream symbols may be labeled.

A woman received a visit from one of her old lovers who now lives in Massachusetts. A few nights later she had a dream in which she found herself standing in an open window. The grass all about her was of a very fresh brilliant green. Close by was a tiny stream of water which seemed to have its source at the base of a rocky ledge a short distance away.

---

[1] It may be remarked at this point that not much can be accomplished unless there exists a certain trust or *rapport* on the part of the dreamer toward the person analyzing his dream. Without this, so much censorship is exercised over the incoming thoughts that the reproduced associations are superficial and it is difficult to deduce much from them.

This, it will be remembered, was indirect representation. We cannot interpret it without the dreamer's associations; we must get her to label her symbols. Her associations were as follows: The bright fresh color of the grass reminded her that she had seen just this color when as a girl she lived in the country and went out to gather cowslips early in the spring. The little stream of water coming from the ledge of rocks she recognized as a memory picture of an actual stream which rose from a spring in a meadow near where she lived in her childhood. This particular meadow was spoken of in her family as the "spring lot."

Her associations, then, were *a field in the spring* and *a field with a spring in it,* which, furthermore, was known as the *spring lot.* I may therefore, state, without more ado, that the field in which she found herself in the dream represented the city of *Springfield* in Massachusetts. This is the town in which her former lover lives. The dream fulfills a wish to be there with him.

A second example of indirect representation is the following. A man who was much annoyed with himself for having done something very foolish had a dream in the first part of which he found himself in the center of an oval sheet of paper. The sheet of paper had a hole in the middle and his body was thrust through this hole so that the paper stuck out horizontally from his waist on all sides. When he was asked for associations, the sheet of paper brought to his mind the fact that he always carries with him sheets of tissue paper with a hole in the center which he uses to cover the closet seat when he has occasion to use a public toilet. A sheet of paper of this sort he is accustomed to refer to humorously as a "peri-anus." In the dream then he finds himself in the center of a "peri-anus." But the thing one might expect to find in the center of a "peri-anus" is an anus itself. This fact the dream utilizes to make reference to the foolish act I have spoken; that is, the dream, by representing the dream in the center of a "peri-anus," expresses his annoyed conviction that he is an ass.

I hope that these examples have made it clear that in a way there are two parts to every dream. These are the actual text of the dream (the collection of pictures which the dreamer remembers on awaking) and the hidden thought which these pictures represent, and which can be obtained only by analysis. Those who read the New York *Evening Mail* may realize that the way in which the thoughts are expressed in the examples of dream symbolism I have given is very similar to that employed in the "Book Lovers' Contest" which used to appear in that newspaper. The *Mail* used to print a series of pictures, each one of which was supposed to represent the title of some book, and the reader sought to guess from the picture what particular book was represented. Now the dream as we remember it upon awaking, corresponds to the picture representing the title of a book. This part of the dream is known as its *manifest content*. The hidden part of the dream (the part which we obtain only by analysis) corresponds to the actual title of the book in the newspaper contest. This part is known as the *latent* dream content. It is not the manifest but the latent content of the dream which in each dream corresponds to the thing or occurrence wished for. The manifest content simply *represents* what is wished for, in the same way that the pictures in the newspaper *represented* the title of some book but *were not* the actual title.

This distinction between the manifest and the latent content of the dream has been repeatedly emphasized by all psychoanalytic writers, but their readers with almost unbelievable regularity have failed to comprehend and appreciate it. Again and again one hears the objection that the dream cannot represent a wish fulfillment because all people have unpleasant dreams. Such an objection is possibly only through misunderstanding. The manifest content is not what is wished for any more than the United States Ambassador to England *is* the United States. The manifest content, like an ambassador, merely *represents* something, and what fulfills the wish is not the representative but the thing represented. The fact, then, that the manifest content or representative may appear unpleasant does not imply that the thoughts represented must be unpleasant.

In the clinical chapters of this book we shall become acquainted with dreams which, from the point of view of the manifest content, were very unpleasant but which were revealed upon analysis to represent wish fulfillments, nevertheless (e. g. the case of Miss Sunderland, pages 451, 452).

Through what has been brought out by the examples of dreams already given, we are now prepared for the statement that while the night dream and the day dream are both phenomena of pleasure thinking and both represent an effort to attain satisfaction by the old hallucinatory route, the night dream ordinarily differs from the day dream in that its wish fulfillment is *disguised*. The explanation of this fact takes us to a point with which we are already familiar, namely, the inhibiting power and censoring influence exerted by the foreconscious over wishes and ideas coming from the Unconscious. The chief reason why the hallucinated wish fulfillment in the night dream occurs as an indirect and distorted presentation is that disguise is required to evade the censorship. For the wishes fulfilled in night dreams are either those directly repressed or else those closely associated with the repressed; are, in other words, those of such a nature that a phantasy depicting frankly and directly what is wished for would be rejected by the censor. The disguise really has the purpose of protecting the dreamer from realizing what it is he is dreaming about. As a matter of fact it is only because of the relaxation of censorship that occurs with sleep that many of the dream wishes are able to find any representation at all in consciousness. During the day repression is so strong that their exclusion would be practically perfect; in sleep the inhibition by the foreconscious is relaxed, and the wish tensions of the Unconscious are then able to secure hallucinatory fulfillment provided always that it is so disguised and distorted as to appear unobjectionable.

The dream then represents a compromise between two opposed psychic streams or forces, the repressing force from the foreconscious which would repudiate the wish, and the repressed trend of the Unconscious which seeks wish fulfillment. In the dream both are satisfied in a measure.   On the one hand the repressing stream can tolerate the repressed ideas corresponding to the wish fulfillment because their meaning is so veiled as to be unrecognized and the wish is not perceived by consciousness *as* a wish.   On the other hand the wish in the repressed stream finds representation in consciousness but is forced to secure its hallucinatory gratification in a modified form.   Further conflict is thus avoided and the dreamer continues to sleep.

The amount of distortion and censoring which the latent dream content is made to undergo varies directly with the amount of repression.   In young children there is little or no repression, and so there is little difference between the manifest and latent content of their dreams.   The dream of a child can be recognized, often without analysis, as a direct fulfillment of an unfulfilled wish of the preceding day.   In some dreams of adults that result from desires arising during sleep, such as the desire for micturition, there is little or no repression and hence little or no distortion.   Whatever distortion appears in such dreams comes from their wishes being associated with others that are repressed.

I will now relate a dream with its analysis and

after this take up some of the special processes in dream formation.

A young woman, a patient at Cornell Dispensary, told me a dream as follows: "I dreamed last night that I walked up Fifth Avenue with a girl friend. We stopped at a millinery store and looked at some hats in the window. I think that I finally went in and bought one." The analysis is as follows: When the patient was asked what was suggested to her by a walk with the girl of her dream, she immediately thought of an occurrence of the preceding day. On this day she had really walked up the same avenue with the same girl, and looked at hats in the same store window that she saw in the dream. In real life she bought no hat, however. Asked what more came to her mind, the following occurred to her: On the day of the dream her husband was in bed with some slight illness and, though she knew it was nothing serious, she had been terribly worried and could not rid herself of the fear that he might die. On this account, when the friend of the dream happened in, the husband suggested that a walk with this girl might help her. After telling me this it also occurred to the patient that, during the walk, some mention had been made of a man she knew before her marriage. When urged to continue, she hesitated but finally said that she believed that at one time she had been in love with him. Asked why, then, she did not marry him, the patient laughed and replied that she had never had a chance, and then explained that the man was so well off and so far above her socially that she had always considered him out of her reach. After this, in spite of my urging, she could not be induced to pursue the subject further, and persisted in saying that it had been merely a silly, girlish affair which amounted to absolutely nothing.

I then asked her to think of buying a hat and relate everything this suggested to her. She then told me that she had very much liked the hats she had seen in the store window and she wished that she could buy one of them, though she knew this was out of the question as her husband was a poor man. Evidently this wish is fulfilled in the dream, however, for in it she does buy a hat. But this is not all. She suddenly remembered that the hat she bought in the dream was a black hat, a *mourning hat*, in fact!

This little detail, hitherto concealed, when considered with the associations previously brought out, immediately gives the key to the interpretation of the dream. On the day of the dream the patient had been fearful that her husband might die. She dreams that she buys mourning, thereby implying the phantasy that his death has occurred. In real life she had been prevented from buying a hat by the fact that her husband was poor. In the dream she is able to buy one and this certainly suggests a husband who is not poor. To answer the question of who this rich husband might be, we need only turn to the associations of the first part of the dream, i. e., the man of whom she refused to talk and with whom she might have been in love. He, as she said, is well off and as his wife she could

buy hats as she wanted them. One may therefore
conclude that this patient was dissatisfied with
her husband, that she unconsciously wished to be
free from him even at the cost of his life, and that
she longed to marry another man who would be
better able to supply her wants.

When the patient was informed of this interpretation of her dream, she not only admitted the
truth of my conclusions but, as her resistance was
then broken, gave a number of other facts in corroboration. The most important of these was
that, after her marriage, she learned that the man
whom she had considered above her was by no
means as indifferent to her as she had supposed.
This, as she acknowledged, tended to rouse her old
love for him and make her regret her hasty marriage, for she felt that if she had waited only a little longer, she might have fared better.

Let us now consider some of the processes at
work in the formation of dreams. In the example
given, the manifest content is the dream story as
related by the patient. This as we have seen,
gives expression in consciousness to certain unconscious ideas, the latent dream content, which
may be stated about as follows: "I am tired of
poverty. I do not care for my husband. He dies
and frees me. I marry the man I prefer and so
am no longer poor." In this dream, as is generally the case, the material forming the manifest
content (the representatives for the unconscious
dream thoughts) is taken from the thoughts of the
day before. However, in some dreams, older material, often from early childhood, is employed.

As in this dream, the dream material usually appears to concern matters which seem very trivial.

The conversion of the latent dream thoughts into the manifest content is called the dream work (Traumarbeit) and is accomplished by the coöperation of four different processes or "mechanisms." The first of these is called *Condensation* (Verdichtung). This mechanism accomplishes just what its name implies. It forms a conscious surrogate by abbreviating, symbolizing, fusing and condensing the unconscious ideas of the latent dream content. The manifest content of the dream is therefore laconic. It is always much less in extent than the latent content. Hence, it follows that quite generally one element in the manifest dream represents several in the latent. Such an element is then said to be "overdetermined." This overdetermination is well shown in the example given. The purchase of a mourning hat expresses both escape from poverty, the death of a husband and a new and better marriage. Condensation may also produce a fusion of the memories of different scenes or objects into new scenes or objects, different persons into one composite person or different words and sentences into seemingly senseless phrases or neologisms. Thus one of my patients dreamed that he received a letter signed "Helva." This word, upon analysis, resolved itself into the two words "Helen" and "Elva," names which belonged to two young women with whom he was anxious to correspond.

An example of condensation exactly like that which occurs in dreams is afforded by the first cartoon given above. Essentially it is a composite formed by the fusion of the three images into a single one, namely that of Mr. Bryan, the dove of peace and a man with an ax. Similar examples of condensation in dreams will be found in the clinical chapters, for instance the dog in the dream of Miss Sunderland (Chapter IX). Many of the most fantastic dream figures, such as strange looking animals, persons half human and half beast, are condensation products whose absurdity disappears as soon as they are resolved into their constituent elements.[1]

The second dream mechanism operating to form the manifest content from the latent is called *Displacement* (Verschiebung). Through displacement important ideas in the latent content are made to seem unimportant in the manifest,

[1] Condensation, a phenomenon of comparatively infrequent occurrence in the thought processes of the foreconscious and conscious systems, is not a peculiarity of dream thinking *per se* but of unconscious processes generally. The same may be said of displacement, the mechanism we are next to take up. The existence of these peculiarities of the unconscious processes bears witness to the high importance of the primitive activation energies being readily mobile and facile of discharge. The fact that we find these processes frequently occurring in the foreconscious and conscious systems only in pathological cases does not indicate that they are abnormal in themselves. The fact is they are primary in the psychic apparatus; they occur wherever thoughts abandoned by foreconscious activation are left to themselves and can fill themselves with uninhibited energy striving for discharge from the Unconscious. They are, in short, natural modes of activity of the psychic apparatus when freed from foreconscious inhibition. Compare Chapter VII of Freud's "Interpretation of Dreams," and his later paper, "Das Unbewusste." When such activities do reach consciousness they give rise to a feeling of comicality.

while some minor thought in the latent content
may be represented as the central feature in the
manifest part of the dream. This mechanism is
well shown in the dream just given. In it, the
walk up the avenue is the most prominent portion
of the manifest content, though in reality it is the
least significant part of the dream. At the same
time, the most important part of the dream, the
purchase of the hat, was given a minor place and
mentioned by the patient almost as an after-
thought. Thus the manifest content of the dream
may said to be eccentric. Its central idea is not
directly in line with the central idea of the latent
dream thoughts.

The following cartoon is also an example of
displacement. The central thought in its latent
content is one of impatience over the delay in set-
tling the *Lusitania* matter. This is expressed by
a mere detail of the manifest content of the cartoon, namely the long beards and the aged appearance of the men represented. There is nothing in
the cartoon itself save the word "Lusitania" to
indicate that it has to do with the sinking of a
great ship and an international controversy.

Equally important is the displacement of affects. In the second chapter we learned that an
unconscious wish whose idea content would be refused passage by the censor might gain representation in consciousness and access to affective
discharge by transferring its activation energy
to an associated and more acceptable idea. Many
such displacements occur in the formation of
dreams. Thus one finds in a dream some emo-

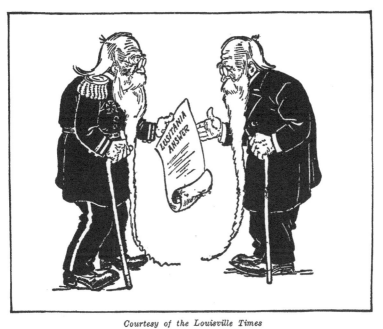

Von Bernstorff Presents Lansing with Germany's Revised
Answer

tion such as anger, love or fear referring to an image of some logically indifferent object, or vice versa. This mechanism is responsible for the fact that so many dreams are made up of trivial and hardly noticed impressions of the day preceding. Such impressions are used in the dream to represent more significant ideas whose affects have been transferred to them. One should not judge that a dream deals only with trivialities if its manifest content seems trivial. The following dream is an example of this fact.

A young woman suffering from a compulsion neurosis, dreamed that there was at her house some person (whose identity in the dream was very vague) toward whom she felt herself indebted for many attentions. Wishing to reciprocate in some way, she offered her hair comb for this person's use. This is all there was of her dream. Judging from its manifest content one would hardly expect that it dealt with anything of great importance.

As an introduction to the understanding of this dream I should state that the patient is a Jewess and that about a year before this dream occurred a young man, a Protestant, fell violently in love with her and besought her to marry him. She liked him very much, and, as she explained to me, had it not been for the difference in race, she could easily have reciprocated his feeling. But not only did she regard the question of race and religion as important in itself but even more so as applied to the matter of children. Marriages between Jews and Gentiles turned out well enough, according to her observation, so long as there were no children, but as soon as children came and the question arose as to whether they should be brought up as Jews or Christians, the situation at once became complicated, and, it seemed to her, trouble and unhappiness invariably resulted. In view of this she had schooled herself, she stated, not to care for her Christian admirer.

The dream which I have related occurred one night after she had had a violent quarrel with her mother, as a result of which (when she retired for the night) she reproached herself for the trouble she was continually causing, and decided that it would be better for both herself and her family if she did not live at home. She fell asleep thinking of ways and means to get away from home and to support herself without calling upon her family for assistance. Once asleep, she had the dream just related. In the light of these facts as to the setting the interpretation of the dream is very easy.

Without going into details, I may say that the person in the dream to whom she felt indebted for many attentions represented her Gentile lover, for whom, as I have said, she had schooled herself not to care because of the question of children. The offer of her comb in the dream refers to this question, for in telling what she associated with the comb she mentioned that when one person is about to use another's comb or brush the remark is sometimes made: "Don't do that; you will mix the breed." In the dream the offer of the comb for another's use represents an *intention to mix the breed* in the sense of marrying a Gentile and having children by him. The dream thus expresses as fulfilled her wish to accept her Christian lover and corresponds to a reflection that, in view of the trouble she has at home, a marriage with him in spite of the disadvantages of mixing the breed might be better than remaining with her family. Thus the affective content of a matter of great importance, namely her very real and strong repressed interest in the Protestant lover and her wish to give herself to him, finds expression in the dream by displacing itself to ideas apparently most trivial.

The third dream-forming mechanism is known as *Dramatization* (Rücksicht auf Darstellbarkeit, regard for presentability). It concerns the *means* by which the thoughts of the latent content of the dream are represented in consciousness. In the manifest content of a dream there is no intellectual activity. All the thinking is done in the Unconscious. [1] The manifest content consists merely of various ideas that have been sifted from the unconscious dream thoughts by the action of the censor. These ideas are then rendered objective in the form of pictures (images) mostly visual, though tactile, auditory or other sensory impressions do occur, and they are comprehended by the

---

[1] The fact that in some dreams intellectual operations do appear (both the forming of judgments and the drawing of conclusions) is an apparent but not a real contradiction to this statement. These processes originate not in the manifest content but in the underlying dream thoughts. They may be reproductions of actual intellectual operations that had taken place previously, i.e. memories.

dreamer as something outside of himself. This mechanism thus presents to the dreamer the representatives of the latent dream thoughts by dramatizing them, so that they are expressed as in a pantomime or by moving pictures. This is shown by some of the examples I have given. This kind of representation, however, has its limitations. For instance, as in a play, events which really extend over a long period of time have to be represented in a few moments. Logical relations often can not be represented at all. Thus ideas such as "if," "when," "either," "because," etc., cannot be pictured and usually no attempt is made to represent them. Occasionally such relations between the various latent dream thoughts are expressed by special devices. Thus thoughts corresponding to a subordinate clause are represented in an introductory dream while the ideas corresponding to the principal clause follow as the main dream.

Identity or similarity between two ideas or things or persons is expressed by combining their representing images (Condensation). Many of the dreams in the clinical chapters show this mechanism. It is the same as that employed in the following cartoon from the New York *Tribune,* November 26, 1915 (an excellent example of condensation) which expresses through a fusion of images the idea that this country *is like* the statue of Venus, or in other words, is lacking in *arms.*

In connection with dramatization I desire to mention two special points. The first is that the dreamer is always represented in the dream and is

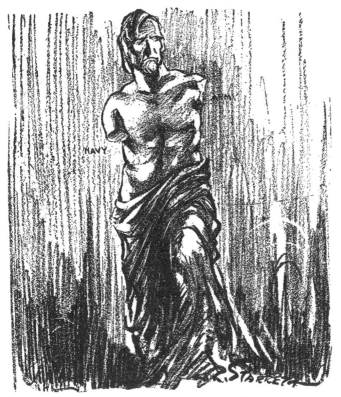

Courtesy of the New York Tribune

Preparedness

usually the chief actor therein. The following is an example. A young lady dreamed that a man was trying to ride a very frisky small brown horse. He made three attempts but each time was thrown off. At the fourth attempt he was successful, however, and began to ride the horse up and down. Apparently the dreamer is not represented in this dream. Yet we know that she must be there, masquerading as the man or as the horse. This is shown in the analysis as follows. When the patient was asked what *horse* suggested to her, she suddenly recalled that, when she was a little girl, her father told her that her surname, Cheval, was the French word for horse. The patient is small, dark and lively. In similar words she had described the horse of her dream. We suspect therefore that this horse represents herself. The man of the dream she recognized to be one of her most intimate friends. When she was asked to relate what came to her mind about this man she finally confessed that she had been carrying on a very ardent flirtation with him. He attracted her very strongly and on three occasions she had betrayed so much sexual excitement that the man tried to have intercourse with her. Each time her moral feelings came to her rescue, however, and at the last moment she repulsed him. All this is symbolized in the dream by the three efforts of the man to mount the horse. But in sleep the inhibitions that saved her while awake were less active. Her repression was relaxed and she dreamed that she received the sexual gratification for which she really longed. This is shown by the man's finally mounting the horse and riding it up and down.

This brings me to the second point which I wish to mention. Any one familiar with dream analysis would know in a general way, the meaning of the dream just related without having to ask the patient any questions or collect any associations. That is, in some dreams, of which the foregoing is an example, the latent content is expressed by means of symbols which nearly always mean the same and, if we are familiar with this symbolism, we can often read these dreams without depending on the lengthy process of free association. This symbolism is not only to be found in the dreams of all people, no matter what their language or environment, but also it may be detected in folk lore, myths, proverbs, and ancient ceremonies of all nations. This is explained by the assumption that, deep down in the minds of even the most cultured people, there still goes on the same kind of primitive thinking that, in our prehistoric ancestors, gave rise to the legends and customs that have been handed down to us.

The symbolism in the preceding dream, an animal for a person, riding for coitus, is very common, and is no doubt familiar to many readers. Others of the many common dream symbolisms that might be mentioned are the dream of losing a tooth, which, in women, sometimes means a fancied fulfillment of a wish to have a baby, and in men usually signifies masturbation; dreams of sword, spear or snake, all of which usually symbolize the male genitals, or of fighting, dancing or climbing stairs which signify coitus.

The fourth dream mechanism is known as *Secondary Elaboration*. It comes into play after the dreamer wakes. For the waking mind tends to alter the recollection of the dream by smoothing out its inconsistencies and forming it into a story with some semblance of logical sequence. The portions of the dream most likely to be affected in this way are those points at which the disguise of the latent thoughts is weakest, and the changes in general serve to strengthen this disguise. In perhaps the majority of dreams the rôle played by this mechanism is an insignificant one. Examples are not required.

The function of the dream is that of satisfying, in so far as is possible, those unfulfilled wishes of the day having a combined tension sufficient to disturb the sleeper and to tend to wake him up. The dream is thus the guardian of sleep. The first dream is a good illustration of this function. What was disturbing the sleeper was the fact that he would no longer be permitted to defend himself in the matter of the child's death. But in the dream he imagines himself continuing his defense and with good results. The dream phantasy was thus a direct antidote to the reality which caused the concern menacing his rest. We often hear people complaining that they rested poorly because dreams disturbed their sleep. The real situation is the reverse, however; what disturbed their rest is the tensions of unsatisfied or conflicting wishes; but for the dreams they might have slept even less.

In one notable class of dreams, the nightmares, the sleep-preserving function of the dream fails and the dreamer awakes in fear. The origin of the fear dream is as follows. Due either to unusual relaxation of repression or to unusual strength of a repressed desire, the fancy corresponding to a wish fulfillment has begun to be represented in consciousness with inadequate disguise. Just as the dreamer is about to become aware of what he is really thinking, the feeling of fear takes the place of the censorship and awakens him before his dream is complete. The fear is really converted desire (libido) escaping from repression, the same desire that the dream phantasy attempts to satisfy. Of the relationship between fear and desire we shall learn in detail in the clinical chapters.

The significance of the dream for psychoanalysis grows out of the fact that, as Freud says, the dream is the *via regia* to the understanding of the Unconscious. As we shall shortly learn in detail, the neuroses represent a breaking through of wishes of the Unconscious despite the control of the foreconscious, in other words a partial failure of repression. The symptoms, like the dream, thus correspond to a compromise between two psychic streams, the repressed and the repressing. But the wishes fulfilled in the dream are, as we have said, repressed wishes, and thus arise from the same part of the personality as do those forces which in predisposed individuals represent the motive force of the neuroses. Hence by studying and analyzing a patient's dreams one gets direct information regarding those trends responsible for the symptoms of his neurosis. And since, as we shall shortly see, the analytic treatment largely consists in the physician's gaining and imparting to the patient a full knowledge of the impulses or wishes from which the symptoms derive their motive power, dream analysis is of infinite importance. This will be so amply illustrated in the clinical chapters as to make examples unnecessary here.

CHAPTER IV

IN the preceding chapter we learned that the manifest content of the dream is formed from the unconscious dream-thoughts by the operation of certain techniques or processes which were designated by the not altogether satisfactory name of "Mechanisms." Now, the same or similar mechanisms participate in like manner in the formation of still other phenomena which occur in consciousness but have origin in the unconscious processes. Chief among these are the neurotic symptoms. These mechanisms likewise play a rôle in the mental activities of even the most normal people, on the one hand, and in the abnormal productions of the insane, on the other. They are not in themselves abnormal though they take part in the formation of all sorts of psychopathological manifestations.

We have to have knowledge of these mechanisms in order to interpret or explain any given neurotic symptom for one or more of them is sure to have participated in its formation. In addition a knowledge of them is required for the interpretation of the material which comes up in the daily work of an analysis—those "descendants of the repressed" through the study of which we at last

124

gain insight into the basic trends from which are derived the symptoms themselves. For this reason I shall devote considerable space to describing and illustrating these mechanisms and allied matters even though their bearing on the question of fears and compulsions as such is not entirely an immediate one. Unless we are thoroughly familiar with them the report of an analysis could not readily be understood or appreciated.

Not all the examples to be given are in themselves abnormal or taken from abnormal persons. The interpretations are in no case exhaustive, for that would require a fuller description of the details of the person's life than is practicable in this connection.

(a) COMPENSATION

At the close of the chapter on the unconscious we considered an example of the forgetting of a name and learned that this forgetting was really a phenomenon of repression and signified a protective effort against the reproduction in consciousness of the painful group of ideas with which this name happened to be associated. We may now consider another example of name forgetting and we shall immediately be introduced to a new form of defense phenomena.

Some time ago I was for a few days the guest of a certain married couple with whom I am intimately acquainted. One evening while my hostess, her husband and I sat reading, she suddenly looked up from her book and asked: "Who was it that wrote 'Paradise Lost'? Was it Dante?"

Her husband replied that she had confused the
authors of "Paradise Lost" and of the "In-
ferno," and nothing more was said at the time.
A little while later her husband left the room, and,
just as I was about to speak of her forgetting,
she herself brought up the subject of psychoanalysis by asking me to explain a very annoying
feeling which she had for some time experienced.
This feeling consisted in a sense of aversion or
repugnance toward all young men with light hair
and blue eyes. She had been caused much discomfort by this singular antipathy as a number
of her husband's friends belonged to this type,
and their frequent visits to her house always
made her uneasy and unhappy. She realized perfectly that there was nothing in the character or
behavior of these men to justify her peculiar feeling, but all her efforts to reason it away had been
of no avail. There, obviously enough, was an
affective reaction the source of which must have
been in the Unconscious. No introspective effort
on her part had furnished conscious data sufficient to explain it.

Pursuing the technique of free association,
with which we have already become familiar, I
asked her to fix her mind on the particular type
of man she had described, and to relate all her
incoming thoughts, expecting that in this manner
she would produce descendants of the unconscious
trends causing her strange aversion and sufficient
to give some insight as to its nature. In response,
she reported that she found herself thinking of a
certain blond man, with whom we are both slightly

acquainted, next of another of much the same appearance whom also she knew only slightly. Then, after a short pause, she suddenly laughed, blushed and said with some confusion, "I just now thought of some one else." Having had from the start some rather definite suspicions as to the general significance of her antipathy to blond men, I asked at this point: "And towards this man you felt no aversion?" She at once admitted that I had guessed correctly, and then went on to relate what follows, which, as may be seen, affords an explanation both of her dislike of light haired men and also of her failure to remember who wrote "Paradise Lost."

The man she had thought of was her first cousin. He is a very handsome specimen of the blond, blue-eyed type that later inspired feelings of repulsion. When she was about sixteen years of age she had seen a good deal of this man and had found herself falling seriously in love with him. But because of their close relationship and the fact that he was nearly ten years her senior, she had decided that it was very wrong in her to entertain any amorous regard for him. She had therefore resisted his attractions and endeavored to banish from her mind all sentimental thoughts concerning him. These efforts at repression were apparently successful for, as far as she was aware, he had ceased to be of any particular significance in her emotional life. But this complex, though it had become in great part unconscious, was by no means entirely deprived of expression. For instance, when, just before her marriage, she destroyed her collection of photographs of former admirers, she "forgot" to destroy the only picture she had of her cousin.

This forgetting we can hardly regard in any other way than as purposeful. Unconsciously she desired to keep the photograph. This little item, small as it is, has no mean significance. From it we are easily led to suppose that, in the Unconscious at least, more of her holophilic interest remained attached to the memory of her cousin than she was consciously aware of or ready to admit. In other words, her efforts to forget him, instead of annihilating this interest, had merely accomplished its repression. But no sooner have we made this statement than we notice that her aversion toward all light haired men is a trend diametrically opposite to that which we have just assumed to exist in the Unconscious. Are we therefore to suppose that because of this aversion we must have been wrong in assuming that toward that particular light haired young man, her cousin, she had feelings just the opposite of aversion? Hardly. We can better explain the conditions by assuming that this aversion toward all light haired young men was rather an overdevelopment of those trends or counter-activations which produced the original repression, and that the reason for this overdevelopment was that the repression was threatening to fail and required an increase of activity on the part of the repressing forces in order to prevent this. In other words this over-activity on the part of these trends from the fore-conscious served as a correction or antidote for what existed in her Unconscious. Thus consciously she wished to forget her cousin and was unwilling to care for him; unconsciously she still retained some love interest in him and wished to remember him. Her forgetting to destroy his photograph is an expression of the love trend. Her failure to recall who wrote "Paradise Lost" was an effect of the repressing trend. For it so happens that her cousin's name was Milton.

We have thus been introduced to a new form of manifestation of unconscious processes, in addition to the dream and the forgetting of names— the two with which we are most familiar—that is to say, an exaggeration or overdevelopment of conscious and foreconscious trends serving as a defense against unconscious wishes of an opposite character, which threaten to break into consciousness. This may recall to us the phenomenon known in pathology as compensatory hypertrophy. A defect or deficiency in some organ is made up for by an overdevelopment and increase of functional activity on the part of the same organ or of its mate. Thus the effect of a leaky heart valve is discounted by an increase in size and strength of the heart muscle, or an increase in the frequency of the heart's action; disease or removal of one kidney results in an increase in size and functional capacity on the part of the other kidney, etc.

The somewhat analogous phenomenon which occurs in the psychic sphere, as has just been exemplified, goes by the same name, compensation. Thus when a given trend succumbs to repression, there usually appears what amounts to a compensatory hypertrophy on the part of the repressing forces, the counter-activations of the foreconscious. When the repressed trend is a particularly strong one and the repression maintained with difficulty, the counteractivity on the part of the repressing trends is then correspondingly exaggerated and the phenomenon is known as *over-compensation*. It may be added incidentally that some of the energy manifested in the form of the compensatory activities is probably derived from the same instinctive sources as the tendencies they serve to repress.

One of the most commonly observed over-compensations is represented by the exaggerated anxiety so often displayed by neurotics over the health of some person close to them. Thus for example a neurotic girl is continually in a state of alarm concerning her mother. If her mother complains of being over tired the girl thinks this presages an apoplexy. If the telephone rings while her mother is out, she thinks this is a message from the police saying her mother has dropped dead on the street. If she hears a noise during the night, she interprets it as her mother choking in a death agony.

Or again a married woman shows a similar concern about her children. As soon as they are out of her sight she begins to worry about something happening to them. If a fire engine goes by the house, she has a vision of it crushing their bodies. If they are late in coming home from school, she goes out to search for them fearing they have

been killed or kidnapped. If they cough or
sneeze, she is in terror lest this be a sign of impending pneumonia.

Such exaggerated concern, which ostensibly indicates an affection of unusual strength, is hardly
that in either of these cases but rather an over-
compensation for repressed wishes of a hostile
character. The married woman referred to was
unhappy and dissatisfied with her husband. On
more than one occasion she had allowed herself to
think that had she no children she would leave
him. Her exaggerated concern over their welfare
thus serves to compensate for the wish that they
might die and allow her to be free. In the case of
the daughter who worried about her mother a
similar state of affairs prevailed. As a little girl
she had wished her mother might die so she could
have her father all to herself. Later as a young
woman she fell in love with a man and would have
married him had it not been for her mother's opposition. Thus her unreasonable worries about
her mother really conceal and compensate for the
instinctive wish that her mother would die and
leave her to the man of her choice.

In these and all other examples of over-compensation it is to be seen that the compensating motives belong essentially to the cultural, ethical and
acquired group of reactions and so to the foreconscious. The repressed trends which are com-
pensated for are in the main more primitive, and
are derived from instinct and the unconscious.

A not uncommon form of compensation for repressed sexual trends that are conceived by the

subject to be base or sinful is represented by an
effort to divert the thoughts to some theme of an
opposite character as for instance religious work,
philosophical or metaphysical studies, the ascetic
pursuit of music or art. An excellent example is
afforded by the case of a young woman who in a
sudden and apparently inexplicable way developed
a profound interest in Christian Science. After
studying for a short time she announced herself
entirely convinced of the truth of its tenets, and
soon after became a healer. Then she alternated
between preaching its doctrines and railing at
doctors in a quite fanatical manner, until at last
she broke out with neurosis.

The analysis revealed the following facts. Previous to the beginning of her interest in
Christian Science she had suffered from an organic illness which required the constant attention of a physician for a long period of time. Not
unnaturally she became much attached to her
medical attendant and, though he happened to be
a married man, she got into the habit of having
certain romantic phantasies about him. He in
turn soon began to display more interest in her
than is demanded by an ordinary professional relationship and shortly a little rather furtive love-
making began. Then, without further warning,
the doctor made what was practically an attempt
to rape her, and before she had time fully to recover from the shock of this experience (which
was not lessened by her discovery that something
within her strongly impelled her to let him have
his way) she learned of his having made a similar

attempt with another of his female patients who happened to be one of her acquaintances. Her suddenly born interest in Christian Science was a reaction to her romance with the doctor and served as a compensation for that stream of her libido which was applied to him. Thus in place of her love for the doctor there appeared mockery and hate of all medical men. In place of sexual interests, which to her mind were of the flesh and degrading, there appeared interests in the spirit, in God, in religion. Instead of being absorbed in what she had felt to be bad she was now steeped in the good.[1]

[1] I have often wondered if some considerable number of Christian Scientists are not perhaps cases parallel to this one; but my experience in this direction is too limited to allow me to venture any positive statements. I am inclined to think, however, that there is a good deal to be said on this point. The image of the doctor has a most intimate relation with the sex life. The child is early impressed with the fact that the doctor sees what nobody else sees, hears what nobody else hears, and knows what nobody else knows. He could, if he would, answer all questions and satisfy all sexual curiosity. In connection with "playing doctor" many children have their first gross sexual experiences. Partly through early impressions of the family doctor along these lines, and partly through the objectively conditioned rôle of guide, philosopher and friend to which the doctor accedes by reason of the necessary intimacies of later life, it is extremely common for women to develop strong, even though unconscious, erotic attachments for their medical attendants. It seems to me highly probable that no small number of the cases of sudden conversion to Christian Science represent reactions to trends of this sort which were developing such strength as to break through foreconscious control. I can also trace one or two cases to the masturbation complex. The patient could not bear to undergo examination and treatment at the hands of a medical man. She feared that the secret guilt would be revealed by such means. She therefore sought other means of healing her ills where there would be no danger of such a revelation.

An interesting example of compensation is afforded by the case of an unusually intelligent young woman who, from about the age of eighteen had been a most ardent and militant feminist. On all such questions as woman suffrage, equal pay for teachers, marital reform, etc., she had talked, written and fought with the enthusiasm of a fanatic. Her dream was of a time when woman should be on the same plane with man in all particulars, doing the same work, enjoying the same rights, having, in short, complete equality. Aside from problems such as these there was very little in life that seemed to interest her.

There were certain features of the case, however, which, even before she broke out with a definite neurosis, might well have indicated that her absorption in these matters was not entirely a normal one. In the first place, for any one possessed of such really unusual intelligence and knowledge of her subject, her methods were very ill-considered and her results surprisingly meager. Though a very industrious worker, she was an astonishingly inefficient one. In addition to this was the fact that her emotions on some of the questions of feminism were so markedly exaggerated as to be quite obviously abnormal. For instance, the slightest suggestion that women were in any way inferior to men, even in physical strength, would set her in a passion of the wildest anger and let loose a flood of vehement and for the most part unreasonable denials. For her to hear it mentioned that the first coitus is painful to the woman, or, for that matter, any statement that tended to associate the idea of pain with the performance of the sex functions, would have a similar maddening effect, as would a tale of a man's being brutal or domineering to a woman, compelling obedience from her, or treating her as an inferior.

Upon analysis this patient's violent warfare against all forms of subordination of women was revealed to be very largely a compensation for a strong but imperfectly repressed masochistic tendency. That is to say, the idea of a man's mastering, domineering over, and inflicting pain and violence upon a woman, particularly in an erotic way, strongly appealed to the patient's instincts and Unconscious, though in the main repellent to her conscious personality. Some of the very stories of brutality and suggestions of subordination which most excited her rage at the same time gave rise to intense sexual emotions and compelled her to masturbate. Her militance against the subordination of women was thus in essence an effort to do away with those sources of stimuli which, in her, inspired feelings she felt to be morbid and shameful.

I have reason to believe that this case of militant feminism is not entirely unique. A certain proportion of at least the most militant suffragists are neurotics who in some instances are compensating for masochistic trends, in others, are more or less successfully sublimating sadistic and homosexual ones (which usually are unconscious). I hope this statement may not be construed as an effort on my part to throw mud on woman suffrage, for on the whole I am very much in favor of it. As a matter of fact it is nothing to the discredit of any movement to say that perhaps many of its conspicuous supporters are neurotics, for as a matter of fact it is the neurotics that are pioneers in most reforms. The very normal people who have no trouble in adjusting themselves to their environment, are as a rule too sleek in their own contentment to fight hard for any radical changes, or even to take much interest in seeking such changes made. To lead and carry through successfully some new movement or reform, a person requires the constant stimulus of a chronic discontent (at least it often seems so) and this in a certain number of instances is surely of neurotic origin and signifies an imperfect adaptation of that individual to his environment. Genius and neurosis are perhaps never very far apart, and in many instances are expressions of the same tendency.

Compensation for an overdeveloped and imperfectly repressed sadistic tendency seems not infrequently to take the form of a passionate devotion to antivivisectionist activities. In certain cases that have come under my notice the patients, during early childhood, were exceptionally cruel to animals, and delighted in torturing them. This was succeeded by a period of relatively perfect repression. Then when the repression began to fail, the antivivisectionist interests became conspicuously manifest. That this interpretation of certain cases is correct will not, I think, be difficult to believe. One would expect a person really

lacking in cruelty and possessing a real sympathy
for children and animals to be slow to suspect and
accuse others of being cruel to them. In fact such
a person might readily underestimate the likelihood of such cruelty and refuse to believe in its
existence where actually it did occur. At any
rate he would welcome, and be relieved by, reasonable evidence tending to prove that where he had
feared cruelty existed, there was no cruelty at all.
But not so the antivivisectionists, if my experience
is worth anything. They see all kinds of outlandish cruelties and barbarities where in fact
there are none, evidence to prove that there is no
cruelty where they suspected it enrages rather
than soothes them, and in spite of their own professed tender-heartedness it is impossible to persuade them that the rest of the world is not extremely cruel. This seemingly paradoxical state
of affairs can be readily understood if we remember what has been said about the Unconscious.
Their tendency to see limitless and fiendish
cruelty where nothing of the sort exists is a product of the Unconscious and expresses their own
instinctive pleasure in that very sort of thing.
Their warfare on cruelty, real or phantastic, is
then a compensation for their own unconscious
sadism and represents an hypertrophy and over-
activity of the counter-activations of the foreconscious serving to maintain a repression which constantly threatens to fail.[1]

A not altogether dissimilar but more compli-

[1] The cruelty which such persons so readily believe others
capable of is really a projection of their own sadism, which by

cated form of compensation, which, however, serves a valuable adaptive purpose, is to be found exemplified so commonly in the character of men of our Southern states as to be a popular rather than an individual constellation.[1]

What I have reference to particularly is the attitude of the southern man to the opposite sex. Woman is idolized and adored in the South to a degree that is quite unique. Nowhere in the world is she treated with more courtesy, delicacy, respect and homage. Nowhere is she so consistently protected, honored, deferred to and waited upon. And nowhere is any act involving coarseness, meanness or brutality to a woman so little tolerated or so summarily punished. Chivalry toward women is one of the most conspicuous traits of the Southern character.

This attitude of exalted chivalry is really a by-product of the influence of the negro upon the character of the people of the South. It is in essence a compensatory development serving to correct some of the ill effects of this influence. The presence of an inferior race in the environment of the Southerner, toward the members of which the same limitations or inhibitions of conduct which govern the relations with the whites do not prevail, serves to develop or keep alive the inherent sadistic tendencies of man, or at least to

such means they escape from perceiving as an endogenous force. The mechanism of projection is discussed elsewhere. (Page 155.)

[1] Certain adaptive reactions characteristic of whole races or peoples Brill has discussed in a most masterly study, shortly to be published. His observations on the psychology of the Jews are particularly interesting.

prevent their fundamental repression. In his relations with the negro the Southerner is (and if we are to believe him, he has to be) somewhat barbaric. The negro apparently needs a master. He must be dominated. The resources of fear and pain cannot always be dispensed with in dealing with him. He cannot always be governed by the milder methods that serve well enough for laborers and servants who are white. Thus the environment of the Southerner has this peculiar feature, reminiscent of a barbaric age, which not only makes possible the relatively free exercise of more or less brutal or sadistic tendencies but even encourages and perhaps demands them. It is natural, therefore, that southern men should as a class be more sadistic than their northern neighbors. That they are so is clearly apparent. The Southerner is proverbially impetuous, hot headed and hot blooded. He is quick to resent an injury and quick to avenge it. In his anger he resorts to physical violence and to firearms with quite astonishing readiness. Call him a liar and he instantly responds with a blow. Injure him and he threatens to shoot you; injure him again and he keeps his promise.[1]

[1] An article in *The Spectator*, an insurance journal, on "The Homicide Record for 1915" says: "The homicide impulse is most strongly developed in the Southern and far Western States, and least so in the New England, Middle Atlantic and North Central States." Memphis, Tennessee, had the highest homicide rate for the country, 85.9 per 100,000 population. The rate for New York City was 4.7. Reading, Pennsylvania, had the lowest rate, 1.9.

Of the seventy-four lynchings which took place in the United States during 1915 nearly one-third were committed in Georgia.

But it is in the measures with which he punishes brutality that his own brutality, or as we prefer to call it, sadism, is most clearly apparent. Take, for example, the institution of lynching, an essentially southern one, though unfortunately by no means unknown in other parts of this country. Here we find sadistic tendencies plainly expressing themselves under the very transparent disguise of a horror of the sadistic. There is little room for doubt as to the real significance of these occurrences. Is it conceivable that without a strong sadistic tendency any man would choose to assist in lynching a fellow being when the punishment of the offender could just as well be left to properly constituted authorities? Would not a man lacking in brutality shrink, no matter how "public spirited" he might be, from participating in such an act as the burning of a negro at the stake? Would he not infinitely prefer to leave to the law the taking of lives, particularly in view of the fact that when one joins a lynching party, he can hardly escape some grave misgivings as to whether it will be the right negro who will be lynched? It is true that in many instances of lynching the provocation has been great, but this is by no means always so. A good many lynchings have occurred for some other and much less serious offense than the "usual crime" and in many instances the alleged malefaction has been so trivial as hardly to deserve being called an excuse. The cause of the lynching was not anything that particular negro had done, but rather the exuberance of Southern sadism, which southern environment has so successfully fostered.

The Southerner's chivalry, and, to a less extent, his generosity and warmheartedness, are very largely compensatory corrective reactions developed against his strong and imperfectly repressed sadism. His environment will not admit of any complete repression or sublimation of the sadistic tendencies. He has therefore to compensate for them and perfect his adaptations by over-developing some corresponding virtues.

The reason the compensations take the form of chivalry is this: Tendencies to brutality when fostered always tend to express themselves in the sexual life.. The sadistic instinct is a survival of those evolutionary periods when it was normal and necessary for men to take delight in the pursuit, capture, torture and killing of other men. An environment which fosters it by reproducing even on a milder scale these older conditions tends also to reproduce the attitude of primitive times towards women. The male in savage life courted the female with a club. Marriage began as a forcible abduction of the female and continued as a relationship more like that of slave and master rather than that of husband and wife in the modern sense. A regression to this sort of attitude is strikingly exemplified in cases of sadistic perversion, where the sadist is impelled to reduce the female of his choice to a state of slave-like subjection, to submit her to gross indignities, and to inflict upon her various degrees of violence and physical pain.

But an environment that fosters brutality in

one direction favors the growth of all tendencies of that character. A person can not be brutal or sadistic in one department of his life without fostering a tendency to the same in all departments of his life, and particularly in the sexual sphere—to specific sadism. But to be sadistic or barbaric to a white woman is very different to the mind of the Southerner from expressing such tendencies toward a negro. A tendency to barbarity of the latter sort he can permit to enter his consciousness. Even so flimsy an excuse as is afforded by some of the occasions for lynching is sufficient to reconcile with the foreconscious, sadism in one of the grossest forms. But sadism of the other sort (toward respected white women) must be firmly excluded from consciousness and withheld from action. And thus, as if to make assurance doubly sure against any manifestations of such impulses in the direction of his womankind, the Southerner compensates by going to the opposite extreme. Instead of making woman his slave he places her on a pedestal and professes to be a slave to her. Instead of inflicting pain upon her, he displays an exaggerated chivalry and is ready to defend and shield her against anything suggesting violence even at the cost of his life. His attitude of chivalry and gallantry is, in short, diametrically opposite to that of the sadist and savage. And the reason the Southerner has so consistently to maintain it, is that, as regards the Unconscious, he is to such a large extent one with the sadist and the savage. His chivalry performs the function of correcting

and compensating for this identity. It is to his
character what a blow-out patch is to an automobile tire. It covers a point where trouble threatens; it strengthens a weak spot.[1]

(b) DISPLACEMENT

As was indicated in the second chapter, the
control and inhibition which the Foreconscious exercises over the processes and trends of the Unconscious is none too stable and, even in normal
persons, is not perfectly complete. The material
just given, most of which either belongs to or
borders on the domain of the pathological, tends
to demonstrate the instability of repression. The
phenomena of compensation are, for the most part,
representative, so to say, of desperate efforts on
the part of the Foreconscious to maintain the repression of trends so strongly activated that the
repression constantly threatens to fail. In some
of our examples appears a partial failure of repression. A part of the energy of some compensatory measures comes from the repressed trends
themselves and in some instances retains their
qualities. In this way a sort of compromise is
formed between the repressed and the repressing

[1] It may be noted that the "Age of Chivalry," a period in
which this highly commendable quality was carried to extremes
far surpassing anything to be observed in the South, was one in
which, as in the Southern environment, sadistic tendencies were
on the one hand fostered (in wars, the customs of dueling, beating
servants, public whippings, beheadings, etc.) and on the other
required to be controlled and repressed. Thus similar conditions
in periods temporally remote from one another called forth
practically identical adaptive compensations.

forces so that they find simultaneous expression in a single form of activity. Lynching is an example of this. In it are expressed a sadistic tendency and a rage against the sadistic. The tendency of some of the anti vivisectionists to see unspeakable cruelties where none exist and at the same time vehemently to condemn them has a similar significance. So too the sense of discomfort and aversion experienced by the young married woman in the presence of young men with light hair and blue eyes. Some of the desire to get away from them came from the repressing forces. Yet a part of the unrest she felt in their presence was really love-desire for them, in a somewhat transformed state (or, more accurately, a desire for the person of whom they reminded her) and was thus a part of the repressed energies.

The processes by which the trends of the Unconscious find representation in consciousness we must now view more narrowly. Repression is a process that occurs at the border between the Unconscious and the Foreconscious, and I must now emphasize the fact that it has to do primarily with *ideas*. A wish presentation arising in the Unconscious remains there repressed unless its idea-representative secures activation in the foreconscious. This activation, according to some of Freud's most recent teachings,[1] appears to be a gaining of access to the word memories which are only of the Foreconscious. The processes of the Unconscious are in all probability wordless, just

[1] Das Unbewusste—Zeitsch. f. Arzt. Psychoanalyse—Vol. III.

as the thought processes of infancy are wordless, but nevertheless contain ideas of *things*.

Word ideas belong to the conscious and foreconscious systems and correspond to a higher developmental state of the psychic apparatus than the thought processes of the Unconscious. So that unless an unconscious excitation or wish succeeds in getting the thing-ideas representing it translated into word-ideas (but not necessarily into actual words), or, to express it differently, unless in the foreconscious the word-memory residues are activated which correspond to the unconscious ideational representatives of the wish, it remains an unconscious and repressed one. Its energy develops neither affects, nor movement.[1]

In the chapter on dreams we learned, however, that an unconscious wish could secure representation in consciousness by indirect means, provided that the ideas in the Unconscious corresponding to the wish were replaced by others more acceptable to the censor. One of these important distorting mechanisms, which consisted of a transposition of the wish energy or activation from its

[1] There are no unconscious affects. One often speaks, to be sure, of unconscious affects (love, hate, guilt, resentment, etc.) and this usage, though not strictly correct, is a legitimate clinical convenience. An affect is really a conscious sensory perception of a bodily state. Without consciousness it does not exist. When we speak of an unconscious affect we mean either that the affect is really developed and therefore conscious, though attached to some other ideas than those originally representing it, or else we mean merely a potentiality of its development—the tensions of the Unconscious that might develop as affects of hate, love, etc., if released from foreconscious inhibition.

unconscious ideas to new and associated ideas which would pass the censor, is familiar to us under the name of displacement. Displacement is a phenomenon occurring not only in dream formation. It has also very much to do with the formation of practically all the various kinds of psychoneurotic and psychotic symptoms and is likewise very frequently exemplified in the happenings of normal mental life.

Like all neurotic symptoms the manifestations included under displacement are compromises formed between repressed and repressing trends. The compromise consists in the fact that though the ideas which, in the unconscious, represent wishes or libido strivings remain repressed and withheld from translation into word-ideas, yet the wish-energies themselves are given access to consciousness and to the avenues of expression as feeling or action by transposing themselves to word ideas of the foreconscious which are apparently innocent and so passed by the censorship.

What in the first chapter we briefly referred to as sublimation is really a sort of displacement or at least allied thereto. By sublimation is meant the utilization of the energy really belonging to one of the primitive holophilic impulses or sexual components for some higher and non-sexual aim. The original crassly sexual aim of the impulse is abandoned and the libido displaced to find outlet in some useful and socially valuable form of activity.[1] Thus the exhibitionistic im-

[1] One of the most interesting contributions to the psychology

pulse finds outlet in histrionic activity; the sadistic is sublimated into an interest in surgery, military matters, business competition, etc.; the curiosity impulse leads to study, investigation, research or philosophical speculation. In many instances the early sexual curiosity later leads to an interest in the study of medicine. What in certain cases was originally rebellion against the authority of the father, later becomes a devotion to legal reform, to socialism, or to other movements designed to better the conditions of the wage-earning classes who have to submit to authority or to certain forms of oppression.

One of my patients who in his childhood was very fond of his aged grandfather who was very tender and indulgent with him, and to much the same degree hated his mother, a rather puritanical widow who was extremely and unreasonably strict and severe with him, was always seeking as a little boy to learn if there were not some medicine that would prevent his beloved grandfather from growing older and dying. Less openly he kept on seeking for some other medicine that would quietly put his mother out of the way. As a boy he took great interest in doctors, but finding them somewhat disappointing as regards knowledge of how to preserve and prolong existence, his early desire to possess the secret of a control of life and death eventually found a sublimated outlet in a passionate devotion to the study of chemistry, which became productive of

of sublimation is Brill's study of choice of avocation,.to be published shortly.

socially valuable and financially profitable results altogether different from the early homosexual and hostile aims from which these interests derived a large part of their motive power.

But we are more interested in the pathological forms of displacement than in that sort which is represented by normal sublimations. Some of the most interesting examples are afforded by the symptoms of the compulsion neurosis, a malady which we will consider in detail later. We are already acquainted with an example of such displacement in the drug-taking compulsion of the young woman mentioned in the second chapter. The energy driving this compulsion was specifically sexual wishes. The ideas corresponding to these wishes were refused passage by the censor, but their energic content was able to evade the censorship by means of displacement to the apparently innocent ideas of drugs, against which there were no serious resistances. This obsessive impulse, like many other compulsive phenomena, resembles in its formation certain examples of wit—"smutty" wit, particularly.[1] For instance, a man says, in mixed company, that though he was brought up to be religious, industrious and serious-minded yet there are periods when he forgets that it is better to watch, with the wise virgins, than to sleep with the foolish ones. His words, if taken at their face value, are perfectly innocent, yet they express, through the double meaning of the phrase "to sleep with," certain ideas which his hearers would not have tolerated

[1] Compare Freud's, "Wit and the Unconscious."

had he stated them directly. But the resistances
of his audience, operating as an inhibiting force
upon open expression, he circumvented by a special technique in much the same way the foreconscious resistances of the young woman just mentioned were circumvented and certain essentially
objectionable ideas and impulses allowed expression by the use of equivocal terms. In the case
of this patient, the word-idea, "to take medicine"
could represent *two* different thing-ideas. One
was the actual thing-idea of taking drugs, while
the other as the result of an infantile sexual
theory, the memory of which had long faded from
her consciousness corresponded to the thought
"Something one does to have a baby." Yet
by virtue of this double meaning the later thing-
ideas of what one does to have a baby—that
is to say, intercourse—and the strong corresponding impulses, had at their disposal a word-
idea to represent them in consciousness which
on the one hand seemed totally innocent, yet
on the other contained their true meaning. Hence
the patient could release into action a portion of
her sexual wish-tensions, which had they been
more plainly labeled would have been denied even
this imperfect outlet.

A business man, who had to do a fair amount
of traveling, had a peculiar habit about catching
trains. If he planned to go anywhere, he would
not look up a time table to find what time the
trains went or what would be a convenient one.
Instead he would take his time about attending
to what work he had to do at his office, and when

this was finished, would leisurely proceed to the station, where, if there was no train ready to depart when he got there, he would wait until it was time for one. Naturally this habit caused him to waste a good deal of time, a fact which he realized perfectly, but nevertheless he would not abandon it. He'd be damned, he said, if any railroad company could hurry him at his office and make him adjust his work according to the demands of a miserable time table. He would go to the station when he got ready and not before, and neither the railroad company nor anybody else might dictate when this should be.

This habit was really a displacement of impulses belonging to the father complex, and represented a rebellion against the father's authority. The patient's father was really an exceptionally fine man to whom he was greatly attached. Nevertheless the old gentleman had a certain tendency to dictatorialness, from which the patient had as a boy suffered considerably. It was characteristic of his father that when once he made up his mind he wanted a thing done, it must be done at once; he would brook no delay. Thus when he gave his son an order, it mattered not what the boy might be doing at the time, he would have to abandon it instantly and carry out his father's wish. Because of his very deep affection and respect for his father the patient very naturally repressed any resentment over this impatience, and had no consciousness of ever feeling rebellious against the authority which, during his boyhood, at least, the father had exercised in no uncertain manner. Any such rebellious impulses would have met with vigorous resistances on the part of the foreconscious, if directed at his so greatly loved father. They could, however, through displacement evade the repression and discharge themselves in some indifferent quarter as for instance against the railroad companies. In that connection he could act the way, which as far as his Unconscious was concerned, he would at times have liked to act towards his father, but from which he was withheld by resistances conditioned by love and respect.

Instances of this sort are very common. Some rule, prescription, specification or anything else giving the suggestion of authority is taken as an object to which to displace and discharge repressed impulses to rebellion and disobedience primarily referring to an authoritative parent—usually the parent of the same sex. I recall a young man who, if he saw a sign: "Don't walk on the grass," would go out of his way to walk on it. The legend: "No smoking" would cause him instantly to light a cigarette even though perhaps he had just finished smoking. The direction: "Slow down to ten miles an hour" would invariably impel him to speed up his car. The mania for doing things forbidden which so generally attacks boys or young men when they first go away from home to school or college is really a breaking through of the impulses of rebellion against the father which hitherto had been better repressed but now begin to find outlet by displacing themselves to almost anything that is prohibited. Often the thing done represents in a symbolic way some specific act forbidden or condemned by the father (usually a sexual one) and thus two sorts of impulses find a common outlet. According to Stekel and others, kleptomania has this origin. The thing stolen is usually symbolic of some sexual thing unconsciously wished for, and which in childhood the authority of one of the parents stood in the way of attaining. The stealing thus simultaneously expresses through displacement the desire for the thing or experience in question and the rebellion against the parent whose influence or authority originally interfered with its fulfillment. I have had one such case.

I live on Long Island and have my office in an office building in New York. One of my patients, a writer by occupation, with whom I was just beginning an analysis, opened the conversation at the third visit with the question: "How do you like having your office away from your house?" Upon my replying that I liked it very well, he continued: "Well, it's the only way to live. I've got to do something of the kind. I can't properly get down to work at home. There's something always interfering, and my writing suffers from it. I shall have to rent a room somewhere in an office building away from my house, where there will be no one to bother or interfere with me and then I can get down to real work and accomplish something, instead of puttering around as I do now."

He expressed himself with so much feeling

about the home interfering with his work that my attention was arrested at once, and I wondered if we were not dealing with a displacement. Cautious questioning confirmed my suspicions for it became quite apparent that whenever he showed a disposition to write, his wife religiously left him to himself, and took great pains that neither she nor the children ever disturbed him unless it was absolutely necessary. It further developed that he had not felt it any great handicap to have to work at home until perhaps seven or eight months before he came to me.

In view of these facts I at length said to him; "Perhaps work is not the only thing you want to do that the home interferes with." He seemed quite confused and startled for a moment and at last said with an embarrassed laugh: "I guess you hit it right that time," whereupon he went on to tell me that for two or three years he and his wife had been gradually getting out of touch with one another, and the state of sympathy and harmony which had marked the early part of their marriage had been slowly replaced by one of relative indifference. This had not disturbed him greatly at first for he had felt it to be a part of the natural course of things that married people should eventually become more or less tired of one another and thought that what he was experiencing was no exception to the general rule. Also he had vaguely felt that, as his devotion to his wife became less, that to his work became greater, a state of affairs with which he was quite well satisfied. But then, perhaps about a

year before he began treatment with me, he made
the acquaintance of a young woman, who as time
went on made it quite apparent that she admired
him exceedingly and would not regard any attentions from him as at all unwelcome.

Her obvious interest in him had at first merely
amused him and left him quite indifferent, but it
was not long before he found himself responding
to it with a warmth of feeling that surprised him,
and the next thing that happened was that when
one day they were left alone together for a few
moments, he threw his arms about her and kissed
her. After this he began to meet her occasionally
and indulge in some love-making, which however
did not go very far. He knew however that she
was a very sophisticated person and in his own
mind was perfectly satisfied that if he wanted
sexual relations with her, she would be completely
responsive. She was a very attractive and apparently passionate woman, and the knowledge of
what he might experience with her exerted on him
a powerful appeal, but nevertheless he hesitated
to go any further because he was married, and out
of regard for his wife. It was the state of conflict and uncertainty arising out of this situation
that was really the main reason for his not being
able to settle himself at his work. His feeling
that his home was interfering with his work was
really a displacement, though in a certain sense
there was an element of truth in this idea. It was
toward the possibility of a *liaison* with the young
woman that his home acted as an interference;
only secondarily and through this medium did

it interfere with his work. His desire to get a
room where he felt he could work more freely was
really a desire to get away from the inhibiting influence of his home upon his desires toward the
young woman, or (what is almost equivalent)
from the inhibition of his conscience.

There is a form of what might be called diffuse
displacement which results in a state in which
the person finds fault with nearly everything.
For instance, a woman when she goes out to dinner finds the food too hot or too cold, too salty or
not salty enough; the dress she buys is either too
tight or too loose, or else the wrong color. Always there is something wrong with her servants,
her house or her friends, in fact, everything she
comes in contact with. The explanation of this
continual dissatisfaction, apparently arising from
a multitude of minor things, is that it really had
origin in a dissatisfaction with her life with her
husband, but she had displaced it elsewhere.

In succeeding chapters we shall become acquainted with other clinical examples of simple
displacement, and no more need be given at this
point. We will consider instead some examples
of more complicated mechanisms, all of which
more or less involve displacement, but have their
special features and are known by different names.

(c) PROJECTION AND INTROJECTION

In early infancy the individual has no complete appreciation of where the self ends and the
external world begins. The small hand the baby
sees before him he does not recognize as a part

of his own person. The supply of milk that appears at such times as he is beset with hunger is not at first referred to the agency of another individual.

In the psychological sphere in adult life, particularly in abnormal cases, occur phenomena which parallel this early failure to distinguish between the ego and the non-ego. Thus on the one hand mental occurrences belonging to the ego are perceived by consciousness as of external origin, while, on the other, essentially external happenings are assimilated by the personality and made a part of the self. The former mechanism is known as projection, the latter as introjection.

The mechanism of projection is ordinarily one of defense. That which is perceived as of exopsychic origin represents trends or ideas which are painful to the conscious personality of the individual and out of harmony with the ruling impulses of the foreconscious. A completely successful repression such as he might desire would drive them entirely from the sphere of conscious perception; projection represents an effort at repression which is only partially successful. Failing to accomplish obliteration of the disagreeable presentations, the repression does succeed in more or less completely preventing the recognition of ownership. The presentations are then seen as of external origin, not as manifestations of tendencies of the individual himself.

A simple example of projection which borders on the pathological is the following. One of my patients, a widow of forty years of age suffered from a mild neurosis which came on shortly after her husband's death. At the time he died they had been living in a suburb of New York. She continued to live there for about a year after her bereavement and then moved to New York, feeling, as she explained to me later, that the atmosphere of this small town was largely responsible for the nervousness to which she was becoming subject. For, as she went on to say, in a place so small every one was interested in every one else's business and to live there meant being continually under the microscope. She knew, she said, that all the townspeople looked upon her as a "designing widow" anxious to entrap a second husband, and she could not speak a civil word to a man without the feeling that she was being watched and that everything she said or did was certain to excite malicious comment. This sort of thing made her extremely nervous and uncomfortable. It was to get away from it that she finally moved to New York.

Without denying that small town life does ordinarily give some objective basis for the notions of being watched and criticized from which this patient suffered, I early recognized that the external facts, whatever they were, did not represent the true cause of the patient's complaints. Her sense of being suspected really had origin in her own psyche. What appeared to her as thoughts of her neighbors was really her own ideas externalized through the mechanism of projection. For in a certain sense she *was* a designing widow and had reason to know it. Her married life, though not

positively unhappy, had not been entirely satisfactory, for her husband was a very matter of fact
person and failed to satisfy her sentimental longings.   In spite of her loyalty to him the reflection
had on more than one occasion crossed her mind
that his decease might mean the opening of the
doors to another relationship considerably more
romantic than what she had experienced.   Furthermore she found that the craving for physical
sexual gratification, which annoyed her little during her husband's lifetime, began after his death
to be a very insistent yearning with which she
found it very difficult to deal, and not unnaturally
she looked toward a second marriage as a means
of solving this problem.

But her conscience (foreconscious) was of such
a quality as to interpose resistances against these
various wishes.   She felt that loyalty to her husband's memory should prevent her from entertaining any dreams of a second and more satisfactory marriage, and that the longing for sexual intercourse, at least for a woman of her age, ought
not to be a troublesome factor, that she ought
easily to be able to suppress it.   Thus she refused frankly to admit to herself that she really
was a "designing widow" (in the sense that has
been indicated).   Consequently the idea that she
was, which she could not completely repress, was
then perceived by her consciousness as something
her neighbors thought, that is to say, as a projection.   Her moving to New York, which pur-
ported to be an attempt to get away from the suspicion and criticism of her neighbors, was really

an effort to escape from what she thought of herself and, naturally, was unsuccessful.

A second illustration of a very common form of
projection occurred in the case of a girl of eighteen who came to me suffering with attacks of intense pain in one side of her face. Her family
physician and one or two other doctors who had
seen her were not quite certain whether these
pains were of organic origin (tic douloureux) or
psychic, that is to say, hysterical; and she was sent
to me to have this question settled and, should the
condition prove to be one of hysteria, for analytic treatment. When, after the first examination,
I intimated to the girl and to her mother that the
malady was not organic, the young woman became very angry, and both to me and later to her
family expressed in no uncertain terms her very
great contempt for me in not being able to recognize an out and out organic disease when I saw
one. Nevertheless she eventually came to me for
treatment and I was finally able to establish that
her extreme emotional reaction against my view
as to the nature of her pain was essentially a
defense against the projected knowledge that I
was right.

For it appeared that these attacks of pain came
on when the young woman was indulging in erotic
day dreams, and then only; that she never had
them apart from these dreams; that they lasted
only as long as she kept on dreaming; and that
she could at any time stop them by stopping the
day dream. Thus she had every reason to know
that they were of psychic rather than of somatic

origin. She was a Catholic and she knew that
if she were to confess to the priest that she was
having such phantasies he would tell her they
were wrong and that she must stop them, a thing
she was unwilling to do. As a way of evading
this, her mind formed a compromise in the shape
of the pains, which served the purpose of a punishment and a penance for the phantasies she regarded as sinful, and thus in her opinion to a
certain degree absolved her from the obligation of
confessing them and from the sin of not doing
so.

What she attacked as a manifestation of my
stupidity was really a projection of her own unwilling knowledge that her pains were not organic.[1]

Another projection phenomenon displayed in
the same case is as follows. The analysis which,
once begun, proceeded for a time with fair promise of success, came to a standstill when the young
woman began to display toward me an attitude of
the most open hostility and antagonism. This
was shortly explained as having the following
origin. Her neurosis began at the time her parents interfered between her and a young man in
whom she had become interested and who pro-

[1] It is not rare to find neurotic patients who very much resent
being told that their trouble is psychic. In my experience this
always means that they not only have some reason for knowing
that the condition is psychic but that they connect it, usually
rightly, with something sexual of which they are ashamed. The
craving of the neurotic to find some physical cause for his trouble,
intestinal indigestion, eye strain, overwork, etc., is really an
effort to find some other explanation for the neurosis than the
sexual, which he vaguely senses to be its real cause.

fessed to want to marry her. Her hostility to
me, as she herself admitted, developed when she
came to the conclusion that the reason her parents sent her to me was that I might be able to
get so much influence over her as to make her
willing to give up the young man and conform to
her parents' wishes, a thing she had asserted
she never would do even if her life depended on
it. The more patient and sympathetic I was with
her and the more I professed to be quite indifferent as to what she did about the young man, the
more convinced she was that this was all a scheme
on my part to get her to like and trust me so that
eventually she would be willing to give him up
to please me, and consequently she became more
and more stubborn and antagonistic.

As a matter of fact she was quite correct in feeling that a strong influence was being brought to
bear upon her in the direction of making her give
in to her parents' wishes and renounce the young
man, but she was wrong in supposing it originated
with either them or me. In reality it came from
her own mind and consisted of her own impulses
and wishes to give up the young man in order
to please her parents and continue as a dutiful
daughter. Thus the force influencing her to give
up her lover, and which she perceived as emanat-
ing from me, was really her love for her parents
and her wish to do whatever was pleasing to them.
Her antagonism against me was really an antagonism to that part of her own self that interfered
with her romantic intentions.[1]

[1] It may be added that she had identified me with her father

It is to be noticed that in these and in all other examples of projection the reaction against the ideas projected is really a part of the resistances causing the projection and thus a part of the repressing forces. Were it not for these resistances (these objections) to the presentation in question, the ideas would be frankly admitted and there would be no projection. Thus, had not the girl just mentioned felt that there was a reproach contained in the assumption that her malady was of psychic origin, she would have been relieved rather than angered that such was my opinion of the case, or she would have honestly recognized it herself. The phenomenon of "the projection of a reproach" of which these cases are fair examples, is the basis for such common phrases as "A guilty conscience needs no accuser," "The wicked flee when no man pursueth," "It's only the truth that hurts" and the like.

The most elaborate examples of projection are furnished by paranoia or major psychoses of the paranoid type. Detailed studies of such cases are already to be found in the literature of psychoanalysis, the most noteworthy being Freud's analysis of the Schreber case, and shorter papers by Ferenczi, Brill and others. I will give some brief examples of cases approaching the paranoid type.

A young woman student had at various times a number of delusional attacks which invariably began with her becoming attracted by some one and transferred to me feelings that really belonged to him. Matters of this sort will be discussed shortly.

of her professors. She would for a time talk a great deal about him, of how able and attractive he was, but without intimating that she was falling in love with him. Then she would begin to think that he was falling in love with her. This would seem to please and amuse her at first, but soon she would get the notion that he was hypnotizing her, and her pleasure would be succeeded by anger. She would complain that through hypnotic influence he was putting into her mind all sorts of erotic phantasies about him, that against her will he compelled her to masturbate with him in mind, that by telepathic suggestion he gave her impulses to come to his apartment, to have sexual relations with him, etc., all of which would get her into a state of great rage and excitement and she would have to abandon her studies. Thereupon the attack would gradually subside, only to be repeated in connection with some other teacher when she resumed her work.

It is apparent that this patient's delusional ideas were nothing but a projection of her own erotic interests in her teachers. What she felt as an hypnotic or telepathic influence brought to bear upon her from without was simply an externalization of her own desires. Her anger against the teachers represented her pathological resistances against these desires. Presumably had she been able to regard her sexuality in a normal way, as something perfectly legitimate and wholesome, what appeared as delusional attacks would otherwise have been ordinary love affairs.

Some years ago I learned that the father of a girl I was treating in the clinic suffered from the delusion that his wife was untrue to him. He was madly jealous of the multitude of lovers he supposed she possessed and kept the house in a continual uproar with his threats and accusations. I thought little about his condition at the time, beyond sympathy for his family and some mild amusement at the idea of his wife (a somber, depressed and most unattractive Jewish woman well past the menopause) in the rôle of a Messalina, until there came to the clinic no less a person than the father himself, and the basis for his delusions was revealed to me. He had been impotent for ten years. This was the reason he thought his wife unfaithful to him. His own dissatisfaction at being impotent he had projected to her. She must, he believed, be dissatisfied with him. Then by elaborating this idea into the delusion that she consoled herself with other men he was able to reproach her in the same degree that he imagined she privately wished to reproach him.

Notions similar in content but somewhat different in origin are represented by a case of morbid jealousy in a woman. In this case the projected ideas did not quite reach the delusional stage. The woman was continually suspicious of her husband. If he displayed any ordinary civility to another woman, she thought he was trying to flirt. If he was late in coming home from his office, she was persuaded that a rendezvous with a chorus girl had caused his delay.

If he informed her he was called out of town on business, she would be convinced that this was merely a ruse to spend a week end with some one of his paramours. The chief argument on which she based her suspicions, which at the same time discloses their meaning, was that her husband rarely had intercourse with her more than once or twice a week. If he were not untrue to her, she felt, surely he would want intercourse more frequently than that. She knew men, she said, and no one could make her believe that anything short of having intercourse six or seven times a week would satisfy the creatures, and particularly such a man as her husband.

This woman's ideas of her husband's infidelity were really a projection of her own imperfect sexual satisfaction. For the facts were that to have intercourse only once or twice a week did not give her complete relief, but left her a prey to erotic longings in the intervals and inclined her to have day dreams of relations with men more passionate than her husband appeared to be. These, however, were facts that she could not face squarely. Her bringing up had led her to suppose that the woman should regard intercourse merely as a wifely duty to be submitted to with pious resignation out of consideration for the baser nature of the male. That a true gentlewoman could look upon it in any other way was almost unthinkable. Hence, when with intercourse once or twice a week she was incompletely satisfied, she was caught between the two horns of a dilemma. If she granted that this was enough to satisfy man's evil nature, and that her husband really was true to her, this involved the admission that she was more passionate and therefore more evil than even the man. But if she allowed that even a lady might need intercourse more than once or twice a week, it then followed that her husband, who, being a male and therefore infinitely more sensual than the female, must require it still oftener, which could only mean that he was satisfying himself elsewhere. She chose the latter alternative, for painful as it was to her to think her husband untrue to her, this was less painful than would have been the reflection that she was more erotic than he. Had her education, and consequently her foreconscious, been different, so that she could have recognized that passion in a woman is no disgrace, she could have perceived her imperfect sexual satisfaction directly instead of through the roundabout route of projection, and then perhaps, instead of pushing her husband further away from her through her unjust accusations, she might have rendered herself sufficiently attractive to him to bring about the satisfaction of her sexual needs.[1]

· · · · · · · ·

[1] These two cases are quite typical. Undue jealousy in a man usually means that he has, or thinks he has, some deficiency of sexual power. It means in a woman not, as many seem to think, that she is unusually in love with her husband but rather that she is not perfectly satisfied with him, and often, that she thinks if he really knew her, *he* would not be satisfied with *her*. In most patients suffering from morbid jealousy there is an overaccentuation of the homosexual component of the libido.

The mechanism known as Introjection, is as was said, a process almost the reverse of that of projection. Where in the latter case the individual narrows his ego to a degree that processes actually belonging to it are perceived as of external origin, in the former he broadens the self to include within it what really belongs to other persons or objects. Thus for example that which happens to some other person causes him to feel or behave as if it had happened to him instead. This involves something more than ordinary sympathy. There is a definite, though usually unconscious, sense of oneness or continuity with the other person. For this reason the phenomenon is commonly known under the term Identification.[1]

The phenomena of introjection or identification are very common and essentially normal. It is only when carried to extremes that identification becomes abnormal. It is for example a normal part of love. He who loves identifies himself with the love-object, and that person's pains or pleasures, successes or failures, honor or disgrace become in a measure his own. It expresses a sort of recognition of this love identification when we say of a married couple that the two have been made one.

[1] As we shall learn shortly, there are really two kinds of identification. The individual may identify himself with another person, which might be called subjective or introjective identification, or he may identify one person with another previously known person, and experience feelings toward, or see qualities in, the former that really belong to the latter. This is one of the many forms of displacement and might be called objective identification, but is usually spoken of as Transference.

We identify ourselves not only with loved persons, our friends and the members of our families, but also with things essentially impersonal or inanimate, our possessions, our country, its emblems, customs, institutions, etc. Thus we have a sense of identity with our house, our dog or our automobile, and see in them virtues peculiar and different from those of the houses, dogs or automobiles belonging to other people and which, in all tangible respects, are equal or superior to our own.[1] The resident of New York or Chicago experiences a glow of personal pride on listening to some comment on the greatness of his city (to which in all probability he has not made the slightest contribution) or the dweller in the country may feel a flash of resentment on hearing some slur at country customs or country manners even though he is as thoroughly sophisticated and unprovincial as well could be.

We have also a great tendency to identify ourselves with people of importance who excite our admiration but whom we do not, in any ordinary sense, love. Such identifications usually correspond to a wish fulfillment. The inmate of an insane asylum who proudly informs us that he is Alexander the Great and conquered the world, or that he is Jesus Christ and saved it, is merely displaying an exaggerated form of the same kind

[1] A person who suffers from a feeling of inferiority may not show this normal overestimation of his own possessions, but on the contrary project to everything that belongs to him some of his own feelings of insufficiency, so that whatever he has never seems to him as good as the equivalent thing possessed by somebody else.

of identification which enables us to find pleasure in such a statement as that our handwriting closely resembles ex-president Roosevelt's, or that our new maid was formerly in the employ of John D. Rockefeller. Identifications of this sort which often lead to imitation have much to do with the rapid spread of fads or fashions when once adopted by the great or near-great.

We may now consider some examples of identification which are taken from the domain of the pathological, though not all of them are in themselves abnormal.

A young woman who came to me complaining of insomnia and a depression of two years standing, mentioned during the course of the second visit that the night before she had dreamed of Evelyn Nesbit Thaw. I asked her, very casually, what she thought of Mrs. Thaw, whereupon she at once launched upon a most vehement and passionate defense of that celebrated young woman. Since her emotion concerning Mrs. Thaw, whom she had never even seen, was obviously excessive, I concluded the patient must identify herself with her. Inasmuch as her defense had to do entirely with the question of sexual temptations to which that lady had been alleged to have succumbed, I also decided that she too must have yielded to some temptations of that character, and that such was the basis of the identification. And this proved actually to have been the case. The patient had been seduced two years before and this experience was one of the chief determinants of her state of depression. Her defense of Mrs.

Thaw was then in essence a defense of herself.

Several years ago I was standing on the platform of an elevated railway station waiting for a train when a doctor with whom I am acquainted came up and spoke to me. We entered the train together and while we were talking he noticed in the headlines of the paper I had been reading the statement that the Philadelphia physician, Dr. Crippen, had just been executed in England for the murder of his wife. My companion at once dropped the subject which had previously engaged us, and began to talk about the case of this unfortunate doctor and the impression it had made upon him. Ordinarily, he said, he had taken no interest in murder trials and had been completely indifferent to the fate of the murderer, but this case had affected him profoundly. Almost against his will he had followed it in the papers, continually hoping that either the doctor would be acquitted or at least get off with life imprisonment. For, as he explained, it had seemed to him that for a doctor to have to suffer the death penalty, a man of education and culture and devoted by profession to the prolonging of life, was something unspeakably horrible and unjust. If such a man did commit murder there must surely have been, he felt, many extenuating circumstances. ''Who knows,'' he cried, rather excitedly, ''just what sort of woman that man's wife was? May be he married her with the best intentions in the world, only to find that instead of a friend and companion he had on his hands a regular she-devil who continually pestered him in all those sleek and fiendish ways of which only a woman is capable! Who knows? Perhaps if all the facts came out, the world which now blames him would in true justice feel that his wife, who broke no law, really deserved death more than he!"

At this point something in my expression must have betrayed that I involuntarily saw more meaning in his remarks than he had expected to convey, for he interrupted himself to say, with a laugh: "Oh, you analyst! I suppose you know all my secrets now! Well, go ahead and tell me what you have discovered."

I protested with well intended mendacity that I had discovered nothing and, as by that time the train had reached my station, we parted. A couple of weeks later I happened to meet the doctor again, whereupon he said: "I know that the other day you suspected that everything is not well with me, so I may as well tell you the truth, for I really want your advice." He then went on to say that his wife had turned out to be anything but the sweet and amiable companion he had expected when he married her, but that she was selfish and ill tempered and apparently bent on doing everything in her power to make him miserable and unhappy. He was profoundly distressed, for he was very much in love with her at the time they married, and even though that love had considerably waned, he still could not resign himself to seeing her as apparently she actually was, a thoroughly selfish, unscrupulous and malicious woman. He had tried to be patient and to please her in every way, feeling all the time that

it was perhaps his fault that she behaved in such
a manner, and that if only he made more effort
or understood better how to please her, the happy
state he had imaged before their marriage might
really be brought about. On the other hand,
though he rarely complained to her, he was becoming increasingly subject to internal spasms
of rage and resentment against her and at such
times there would flash into his mind all sorts
of murderous thoughts, prayers that she might
die, images of himself choking her or smashing
her head against a wall and other phantasies of
a similar character, the like of which he had never
experienced before. It was bad enough, he felt,
to have had to make such unpleasant discoveries
concerning his wife's character without being
compelled to add to them equally unpleasant ones
concerning his own.

It requires no further discussion to render perfectly clear why this doctor felt as he did over
the case of Dr. Crippen. His compulsive sympathy for that unfortunate man was essentially
sympathy for himself. For on the basis of the
murderous thoughts which, in spite of himself,
his wife inspired in him, he identified himself
with the murderer. He felt as if he too were on
trial, and his wish for the acquittal of the accused and his sense of injustice at the execution
were conditioned not by any actual facts of that
man's case but by features of his own.

It may be remarked incidentally that this case
of what appeared to be exaggerated sympathy is
quite typical of manifestations of that kind. The

person sympathized with is very frequently, as in this case, some one with whom the sympathizer unconsciously identifies himself and his great concern is thus not so entirely altruistic as it might at first glance seem.

Another and slightly different example of identification is as follows. I was treating a young man for homosexuality and during the course of one of the early visits he recalled that shortly after puberty there was a time when his feelings toward girls had been quite normal, but that his mother had so vigorously opposed all his interests in the opposite sex that after a year or more of struggle with her he finally gave in, and thereafter had only homosexual attachments. After having lived over again during this visit the bitter conflict he had had with his mother, which until he spoke of it on this occasion had for the most part faded from his mind, he remarked that he felt this discussion meant a great step toward recovery. He added that before he began the treatment he had had a feeling that we would suddenly come upon some discovery, whereupon he would all at once be well, and he now felt that the recollection of this warfare with his mother was that which he had been expecting. Upon my asking him what gave rise to this expectation, he replied that probably it was some case that he had read about but could not at the time recall. Shortly we discovered that the case was one mentioned by Dr. A. A. Brill, of a young man who suffered from an obsessive idea that he was only killing time, and took all sorts of precautions in order never to waste a minute. From the analysis of a dream Dr. Brill discovered that the figure of the old man representing Father Time was in this patient's case a symbol for the father and that his fear that he was killing time really represented a repressed wish to kill his father, which explanation the patient accepted and the obsession at once disappeared. My patient, from reading this case, developed the expectation that he too would get well in this sudden way. This meant that he unconsciously identified himself with Brill's patient. The basis for this identification was the wish that his mother would die. Such a wish was altogether foreign to his conscious thoughts, but existed as an unconscious one. So when he read Brill's case the idea of its similarity to his own instead of being presented to his consciousness directly and in some such form as: "I am like that man *because I wished my mother dead,*" appeared as an identification phenomenon in the shape of the expectation: "In the analysis I too will get well through a sudden discovery." He felt that the discussion of the conflict with his mother was a matter of great import, because it tended to bring to his mind that it was in this relation that the wish that his mother might die mainly arose. The identification contains the thought: "If my mother were out of the way I would be sexually normal," and this idea we can accept as pretty nearly correct, if for the word "mother" we substitute "mother's influence."

(d) RATIONALIZATION

It may have struck some of my readers that the patients who furnished the various examples of psychopathological reactions which have been described must have been singularly blind about themselves not to recognize at least in some cases, that these reactions were determined by their complexes and not to realize what the reactions meant. One might even go so far as to feel that neurotics, if these cases represent any fair sample of them, must be a rather stupid lot. As a matter of fact, neurotics, as a class, are rather above the average in intelligence (compulsion neurotics especially), and their failure to understand themselves is neither a function of a lack of intelligence nor of the neurosis as such, but results rather from the resistances, numerous parallels of which are to be found in the mental lives of even the most normal. The most well balanced people have many peculiarities and shortcomings which are all too apparent to their friends and acquaintances but to which they themselves are serenely blind. In fact it may be said with a fair degree of accuracy that neurotics are less blind to the workings of their own minds than are normal people, in the sense that the neurosis represents an *unsuccessful* effort to become oblivious to the same things that normal people succeed in ignoring completely. The normal man, who feels that his every action springs from reason rather than from his complexes, is deceiving himself more than does any neurotic.

This may seem a rather unreasonable and un-
justifiable assertion and therefore demands explanation. Ask of any normal man: ''Why did
you do that? Why do you like this? Why do
you dislike the other?'' and he is pretty certain
to give you an explanation that seems plausible
and to his mind completely satisfactory. He will
not reply: ''That action or feeling came from
some of my complexes or was, I suppose, the result of something in my Unconscious and I don't
understand it myself.'' Never, practically, will
one hear such an admission, or anything that is
the equivalent of it. Our actions and feelings,
even when most illogical and wholly determined
by unconscious factors, rather than by reason and
judgment, seem to us either perfectly logical and
reasonable and determined on such a basis, or
else accidental and requiring no explanation at
all. This, as was mentioned in the second chapter, is accounted for by the fact that those reactions which are determined by our complexes and
our Unconscious are almost invariably *rationalized;* that is to say, furnished with an apparently
reasonable and plausible explanation, often manu-
factured *ex post facto,* and which is more acceptable and agreeable to us than would be a correct understanding of the real motive forces. In
the case of intelligent neurotics these rationalizations are often so extremely plausible that the
analyst has to be constantly on his guard lest he
himself be deceived by them and overlook the unconscious factors really at work.

One of my patients confessed to me that it had

always been his intention to marry a rich girl, though as a matter of fact the girl he had married had no money at all. Before he became engaged he had taken advantage of every opportunity to meet, and be in the society of, rich girls, hoping to find one that would be attractive and at the same time willing to marry him. I felt somewhat surprised that his devotion and industry in this direction had met with so meager a result, and so expressed myself, whereupon he explained that all the rich girls he had ever met were so spoiled by their money and so utterly selfish that no matter how rich they were he would not marry any one of them. All of them, he said, put clothes and dances and yachts and cars, and all the other things that money could buy, ahead of love and sympathy and companionship, which, he assured me, were to his mind the vital features of marriage. But though I did not feel in a position absolutely to deny that great wealth may have a prejudicial influence upon character, the fact remained that this man had known a great many girls with money, and it did seem rather unlikely that every single one of them had exactly the same group of faults which he seemed to discover in them. His failure to carry out his intention to marry a rich girl (a thing he had many opportunities of doing) was, it appeared to me, due in all probability not so much to the alleged defects in the character of the young ladies, as to certain peculiarities of his own, while the explanation he offered was not the true one but a rationalization. The real determining factor, as at length appeared, was his own money complex. He felt that rich girls would be more interested in money than in companionship because to a certain extent he was that way himself. Since he doubted if he could care for a girl who was not rich, he was compelled also to doubt whether, since he was not rich, any such girl would care for him. He could feel sure of the love only of a girl who had no money at all, for such a one would appreciate, he felt, the moderate amount of money he did have.

One of my patients was engaged before he came to me to a rich girl and expected to be married in about a year. He then received the news that the parents of his intended lost all their money and that contrary to his expectation his bride would be penniless. He then insisted that they be married right away. The reason that he gave for this was the extremely convincing one that since the girl's parents could now support her only with difficulty, he felt that it was only right that he should step in, even though at some inconvenience, and care for her himself. The real reason was as follows. He had known the girl only slightly when he became engaged to her, and it was the fact that her parents had plenty of money that had been one of her attractions. An important reason he married her earlier than he had expected was that he was afraid that some one might think that now her parents had lost their money he would want to back out of the engagement, *which, as a matter of fact, was the very thing he did want to do,* though he would not admit it even to himself.[1]

Another patient gave me a very lengthy and rather logical explanation of why he was in favor of woman suffrage. The further course of the analysis revealed, however, that the basic reason for his position was his racial complex. He is a Jew and had felt very keenly the effects of the anti-Semitic prejudice that prevails in New York. He sympathized with women because he, like them, belonged to a group often regarded inferior and which is denied some of the rights and privileges that certain others may enjoy. His interest in equality of the sexes was really a manifestation of his more intimate and personal interest in equality of races.[2] The reasons given for his position were simply a rationalization.

At the time of the presidential campaign of 1916 another patient gave me a very logically formed set of reasons why in his opinion every one should vote for Mr. Wilson's reëlection, the principal ones being variations of the theme: "He kept us out of war." The real reason that this patient on all occasions took Mr. Wilson's part and defended him and his, at that time, unwarlike policies, was that the patient felt himself to be a coward and afraid to fight. He really thought Mr. Wilson belonged in the same category and

[1] This reaction is obviously an over-compensation. Fortunately the marriage turned out very well in spite of this unpromising beginning.

[2] In cases such as this the castration complex is sometimes an important factor.

secretly despised him as he despised himself,
meanwhile defending and making excuses for him
as he himself wished to be defended and excused.
The perfectly plausible reasons he gave for his
approval of Mr. Wilson really had practically
nothing to do with his position in the matter but
were simply rationalizations of the attitude determined by his complexes.

In the case of another patient who with the
greatest bitterness attacked the President in his
efforts to avoid war, meanwhile giving a most
plausible and reasonable explanation of why he
did this, was also displaying a purely complex-
determined reaction.   This young man had quar-
reled with his family, thinking that rather than
avoid an open break with him they would give in
and do a certain thing he wanted.   He sadly mis-
judged them for not only did they fail to be disturbed by the prospect of a rupture, but appeared
to be totally indifferent as to his fate, after it occurred, so that he not only failed to gain what he
wanted but lost many things he had previously
enjoyed.   Thus not only had he reason to feel that
he had made a great tactical mistake, but at the
same time he suffered from a certain sense of
guilt for the attitude he had taken.   But he was
unwilling to admit to himself or to anybody else
that he had been wrong in quarreling with his
family or that there was any reason he should feel
guilty over it.   Hence he was compelled to hate
Mr. Wilson or any one else who championed peace
or condemned war, for it was as if that person
were telling him in general terms what his con-

science was insisting in particular ones, namely that peace was right and his quarreling wrong.[1]

I noticed that a married woman, a patient of mine whom I had seen only four or five times, was invariably dressed in black. I supposed she was in mourning, though she had said nothing about a death having occurred in the family, and at last I asked her about it. She replied that she was not in mourning and that the reason she wore black was that she thought such material was more durable. This explanation seemed to me rather unsatisfactory, for in the first place the woman was sufficiently well off not to have to be concerned about the durability of her clothing, and in the second it was summer time, when black clothing is particularly uncomfortable and nobody wears it unless there is some reason for so doing. It later developed that her habit of dressing in black had a symbolic significance and that her ex-

[1] As familiar as I am with the frequency with which people's opinions on all sorts of objective matters are determined by their complexes rather than the actual merits of the case, it has been a never failing source of surprise to me to see the extent this has been true in regard to the present war and Mr. Wilson's policies. In the case of every one of my patients, and for that matter of all other persons with whom I am well enough acquainted to be able to judge of their complexes, the individual's opinion, whether pro-German or pro-Ally, pro-Wilson or anti-Wilson, was largely and in most instances wholly determined not by the facts known to him with regard to any one of the questions, but rather by his own intimate complexes. The reasons given for his opinion, though in many cases most plausible and convincing, proved on close examination to be little more than rationalizations. I doubt if any one unfamiliar with actual psychoanalytic work can realize or believe how entirely these statements are true, not only of neurotics, but of normal persons as well.

planation that such clothing is more durable was simply a rationalization of that action. She was dissatisfied with her husband who was a rather prosaic individual and paid little attention to her; though as a girl she had been very popular and liked pretty clothes and masculine admiration. Her humdrum husband had failed to satisfy her craving to be admired while her conscience forbade her seeking to gratify it elsewhere. Her dressing in black was a symbolic expression on the one hand of her wish to be a widow and receive attention as of old, and on the other of penitential impulses for her guilty feeling that it was her inordinate fondness for clothes and admiration that made her unhappy with her husband, who in many respects was a very considerate and worthy man.

(e) VARIOUS DEFENSE AND DISTORTION MECHANISMS

There are a great many symptoms or symptom-like formations which serve as defenses against a sense of guilt. One of these consists in displacing the guilt affects, which repression has failed to prevent, to the idea of some other and lesser male-faction than that from which they really have origin. Thus a patient of mine who had volun-teered to help one of her neighbors in caring for a very sick old woman, fell asleep while watching at the sufferer's bedside and was in consequence half an hour late in administering a dose of medicine that the doctor had ordered. When a few days later the old woman died, my patient began to reproach herself as being guilty of her death, feel-

ing that if she had given the medicine on time
it might not have occurred. This was despite the
fact that the old woman had an incurable illness
from which recovery was impossible, and that the
death occurred at just the time it had been pre-
dicted by the doctor. The guilty sense of having
caused the old woman's death really came from
another quarter. My patient was approaching
the forties without having married, a circumstance largely attributable to her mother's interference and tyranny, for she had rarely permitted
her daughter to have any suitors and had soon
interfered in the case of the few that did present
themselves.

The daughter had wished (even at times consciously) that her mother, who was not in the
best of health, would die before it would be so
late as to place marriage out of the question.
When her mother did die, a few months before
the old woman just mentioned, my patient had a
vague sense that her evil wishes had killed her.
The guilty feelings arising in this way she was
able to keep down until, at about the time of the
death of the old woman neighbor, they were augmented by the effect of a certain sexual temptation to which she was unexpectedly subjected.
Then, no longer able to suppress her sense of
guilt entirely, she partially escaped from it by
means of the displacement just described.

Another method of defense against guilt complexes consists of various sorts of penitential
measures or ceremonies. The action of the
woman who wore black in the summer time was

in part conditioned in this wise.   Another example
is that of a salesman whose business it was to
secure advertising for a certain magazine.
Though for a time very successful at this work,
his sales at length began to fall off very considerably, to such a degree, in fact, that he eventually lost his position.   The reason for this
change was that he had become, as he expressed
it, "over conscientious."   Instead of enthusiast-
ically explaining to the prospective advertisers
the great advantages to be expected to result from
buying space in the magazine, as at first he had
done, he would ask himself: "Now really would
this man's business profit by the kind of advertising I am supposed to sell him?" a question that
he often felt had to be answered in the negative.
On such occasions he would be impelled to advise
the prospective purchaser, against buying and
naturally made no sale.   He expressed the situation to me by saying: "I've gotten so that I
can't stand it to feel that my clients are not going to get full value received."

The origin of this compulsion, for such it was
(in many instances he advised against the pur-
chases of advertising where it really would have
been of advantage to the buyer), was from quite
another matter in his life, in which he had a much
more logical reason to feel that he was not giving
value received.   He had made the acquaintance
of, and eventually seduced, a somewhat innocent-
minded and unsophisticated young girl, who,
though he had never said so in so many words, had
all along had the impression that he intended to

marry her. He had not disabused her of this notion, for on the one hand he wished to continue his sexual relations with her, and on the other dreaded the storm of tears and reproaches which he knew would be forthcoming as soon as she knew how she had been duped. Meanwhile he tried to excuse himself by believing that the girl was not really as innocent as she appeared to be and that if she was foolish enough to expect him to marry her when he had never in so many words promised that he would, there was nobody to blame but herself. Failing then to give value received in this quarter he tried to make up for it in another, and through the falling off in his commissions and the eventual loss of his position, suffered an essentially self-inflicted punishment for the sin he really believed he was committing in spite of all his efforts to persuade himself otherwise.

A patient of mine who lived on the seashore where there was an excellent bathing beach of which nearly every one took advantage, had a marked aversion to going into the water, in spite of the fact that he was well able to swim. It was not through any idea of danger, and he had almost as much dislike of taking a cold bath in the tub in his house. Hot water he did not mind. He could remember a time in his childhood when he had no such aversion, but enjoyed going in swimming with the rest of the boys.

The explanation of this antipathy is to be found in what is known as the "Small Penis Complex." Little boys, of say four or five years of age, when passing through the period of sexual investigation, are often profoundly impressed with the difference in size between their own organs and those of grown men, the older brother or the father. From these comparisons arises a feeling of envy and jealousy and also a sense of inferiority, and this forms a nucleus for a complex which grows and persists long after the impressions with which it started have faded from conscious memory.

It is a common experience for a person who as an adult revisits for the first time some place in which he lived when a small child, to be much astonished to see how much smaller are the rooms and buildings and how much shorter are the distances, than he had remembered them. This is paralleled in the formation of the small penis complex. The memory impressions of the adult organs with which the little boy first compared his own keep in the Unconscious the original ratio of bigness, so that despite later comparisons in adolescence or adult life, which logically should serve to dispel the original sense of genital inferiority, it nevertheless persists. It is as if these old memory impressions, which became progressively magnified through the period of growth and so preserved their original ratio, remained as the final criteria of comparison. Naturally the person may be conscious only of the *feeling* of inferiority and through various defenses more or less escape awareness of the *idea* that this has a genital basis. Thus the person who unconsciously projects to the female his own high estimation of the significance of the size of the penis is apt to be backward with women, and to feel that he has little sexual desire, the real reason being that he fears revealing to the woman the (often purely imaginary) smallness of his genitals.

This patient's aversion to swimming had somewhat this origin. Some of his early painful comparisons were made at the country swimming hole where he and the rest of the youths of the community were wont to bathe in a state of nature. It did happen that he matured rather slowly, and most of the boys of his age developed genital hair and the other signs of sexual maturity before he did. He was painfully conscious that their organs were larger than his; and particularly so when he had been in the water, the coldness of which caused his penis to shrink into almost complete obscurity. As may easily be seen, swimming or cold bathing tended in later life to stimulate the small-penis complex through reviving these old memories, and thus threatened to bring into his consciousness, despite his defenses, ideas and affects that were very painful to him. As a defense his aversion or resistance to the complex was then transferred to appear as an aversion to bathing (i. e. to a stimulus of that complex) a mechanism much the same as that, by which as we shall see later, some of the symptoms of anxiety hysteria are formed.

Another and very familiar defense against a sense of guilt is exemplified by the common washing compulsions or ceremonials. A sense of moral impurity or uncleanness of whatever origin is replaced by the notion of physical uncleanness or defilement, which the patient then seeks to get rid of by continual washing and scrubbing.

Even more common, though less often recognized, is a certain feverish devotion to religion or to church or charitable work. In women particularly this is a very common defense against a sense of guilt arising from the masturbation conflict. Feeling herself to be ''bad'' the patient devotes herself to those activities which because of their nature tend to give her a feeling that she is ''good,'' which then serves as an antidote for her inculpatory affects.

Still another very common defense phenomenon is that of finding fault with others for shortcomings of which one is possessed oneself, though unwilling to admit it. It is as if one were making an effort to bring those about him down to the same level where he feels himself to be. A number of the examples which have been given to illustrate other points are at the same time instances of this mechanism. For instance the woman who was continually accusing her husband of infidelity was really at the same time defending herself against the guilty sense of having been unfaithful to him in her thoughts. The man who felt that rich girls put the things that money could buy before considerations of love and sentiment was only accusing them of what he vaguely felt himself also to be guilty. In the case described in Chapter VII we shall find some excellent examples of this form of defense. I may also mention one from my own personal experience. I found at one time that I was becoming very impatient at what I was pleased in my own mind to call the stupidity displayed by a woman I had been analyzing for some time with very meager success. If, for instance, I explained something to her, and, as often was the case, she did not grasp my meaning, or asked me to explain the thing over again, I would feel exasperated at her dullness in failing to comprehend what seemed to me very simple. On one or two occasions when she had made some feeble complaint to the effect that she was not improving very much, I had felt an unreasonable impulse to tell her that a person with no brains need not expect to get well rapidly by a method that required understanding.

It is true that this patient was not remarkably intelligent, yet, as it at length occurred to me, I was at the same time analyzing another young woman who was no more intelligent than she, but toward whom I never felt irritable, and if she asked me to repeat or clarify an explanation I did it with complete patience and good nature. The first patient was not, as I had sometimes told myself, too stupid to be analyzed, for as I knew, once I stopped to think of it, I had had good success with other patients no more intelligent than she, and in some instances her mental inferiors. Finally I realized that the reason I felt irritated with her, and in my own mind called her a fool, was that the circumstances were such that she was making me feel that I was one.

The reasons for this were as follows. She was referred to me by a certain doctor who had never

sent me any cases before and who I knew from conversations I had had with him was rather skep-
tical as to the value of psychoanalysis. He had
been rather interested in the case of this patient
and had for a long time tried to cure her himself
by various physical means. I suspected that one
reason he sent her to me was that he had at last
gotten tired of her continued complainings, more
than that he had any deep faith in my being able
to do her any good. When I saw the patient for
the first time I thought the case would not be a
very difficult one, and I was malicious enough to
take pleasure in the thought that when I did cure
her, I would wind up the thoroughly good-natured
arguments I had had with him about psychoanalysis by the triumphant statement that it had
succeeded when his methods, carried out for even
a longer time, had met with absolute failure.   I
knew also that if I did succeed with this case, the
doctor in question, who has an excellent practice
among well to do people, would send me other patients, a consideration to which at that time at
least I was anything but indifferent.   For these
reasons I accepted the woman for analysis even
though, as I knew, I would have to treat her for
a smaller fee than I was in the habit of charging.
But after the analysis was begun I found that the
case was really a much more difficult one than I
had expected, and that there was a certain amount
of danger that instead of my being able to report
triumphantly to my friend that I had succeeded
where he had failed and to enjoy the rewards of
this success in the shape of other patients referred

by him, he would be able to crow over me and to say that the method I had so stoutly defended was no better in results than his own. In addition to this I would have to reflect that instead of my acquaintance with this patient reacting to my profit, in the form of new cases referred by him, I would have nothing to compensate me for the time I had spent on her but a fee so small as to constitute no reward at all. Thus though all these facts were not ever continuously before my mind, nevertheless I had some basis for feeling that I was a fool or had made a fool of myself, and I could not see the patient without being, so to speak, unconsciously reminded of them. The irritation I experienced was really not so much a product of thoughts about *her* stupidity as about my own. With the other patients who were equally or even more slow of comprehension I had felt no irritation, for there was nothing in the situation to injure my self-esteem. I may add that once I had faced these facts which I was involuntarily trying to escape from, I was able to dispel my sense of irritation with the woman and to make of the analysis a fairly complete success.

A mechanism of disguise or defense which is most commonly observed in the compulsion neurosis is that by generalization. Feelings which in the patient's consciousness are attached to a class or group really refer in the unconscious to a special one of its members. This is exemplified by the case of the young woman who had an antipathy to *all* blond, blue-eyed men, which was really founded on repressed wishes concerning one particular man of that type. The woman who was converted to Christian Science and "hated" *all* doctors concealed within this generalization mixed feelings of love and resentment toward one particular member of the profession. Brill reports the case of a Hebrew who suffered from the obsessive idea that the Gentiles were going to kill all the Jews.[1] This obsession had origin in a death wish against one particular Jew, namely, the patient's father.

(f) TRANSFERENCE

Among the phenomena occurring under the head of Displacement we became acquainted with a form of identification which I suggested might be called subjective or introjective identification. This was to distinguish it from the other and even more important variety which we might designate as objective identification, but which we shall consider under the more commonly used term of *Transference.*

In subjective identification, as was said, the ego is broadened to include within it other persons or objects that are really external. In objective identification, or transference, the individual, instead of identifying external objects or persons with himself, identifies them with each other, and behaves or feels toward one in a way that is appropriate to, and conditioned by, experiences and impressions which really refer to the other.   The subject is usually not conscious of the existence

[1] "Psychoanalysis"—Chapter on the Compulsion Neurosis.

of the identification nor as a rule does he remember at all completely the experiences from which the transferred feelings really arise.

To make clear what is meant by transference I will give an instance of it from my own life. I was at one time confronted with a very difficult problem in my personal affairs which I soon felt was too much for me to solve alone and would necessitate my seeking some help and advice. There were among my friends three men with whom I was very intimate, to any one of whom I might have gone in this emergency with every assurance of receiving full coöperation and most valuable advice. Instead of doing this, I went to a fourth man about whom, though I had some pleasant acquaintance with him, I really knew very little, and whom I could hardly regard as a friend. I had in fact no logical grounds for believing that this man, whom we may call X. was really qualified to give me the help I needed, or that I could safely trust him with full knowledge of the situation. I now know that I could not have chosen a better person, yet for all the information at my command then, he might very well have been the worst.

When I went to him I had no realization that I was doing a very illogical and possibly unsafe thing. Such a possibility had not occurred to me nor did I think there was anything peculiar in my choosing him in place of some one of the three other men who, under the circumstances, were the logical persons for me to go to, until my wife expressed her surprise at what I had done.   Then all at once I realized how strange my choice had been.

As soon as I asked myself the reason, it came to my mind that during the night preceding the day I went to see X. I had had a dream in which appeared certain perplexities, which, I could readily see, represented the problem then confronting me, and I called to my assistance a certain man named T., who had been a member of the household during my childhood.   It then at once became clear to me why in my difficulty I had so unhesitatingly gone for help to X.   For, as I now realized for the first time, X. and T., though of very different ages, *look* a great deal alike.   On the basis of this similarity in appearance I had unconsciously identified X. with T.   Consequently I felt toward X. the sense of trust and confidence that, on the basis of childhood experiences, I really had reason to feel toward T.   In short, I felt and acted as if I were dealing not with the relative stranger X. but with T., a person whom I could logically regard as a tried and true friend.   Incidentally it may be remarked that X. and T., though alike in appearance and, as I can now say, in being equally dependable friends to me, are, in most respects, about as unlike as two persons well could be.

My failure to go with my problem to any one of the three intimate friends I have mentioned also appears to be, in part at least, the result of a transference involving them.   When as a little boy I got into difficulties and needed some help,

I always went by preference to T. rather than to
my father or grandfather (in whose home I spent
a large part of my boyhood) not only because I
had the greatest confidence in T.'s ability to help
me but because I was sure that he would be tolerant and sympathetic, as at times the others were
not. If, as was usually the case, the trouble I
got into was a result of some deviltry or mistake
of mine, T. would be just as good-natured about
helping me out of it as if I had been perfectly
blameless. With my father or grandfather, however, I ran a certain danger of being scolded and
told that if through my own fault I got into
trouble, it was only what I deserved. The difficulties which led me to consult X. would not have
arisen had I not made certain mistakes of a character not calculated to enhance my self-esteem.
My three friends, who were the logical persons
of whom to seek advice, as my father and grandfather had been in my childhood, were, it so happened, the sort of persons who, whatever mistakes they might make, would surely have avoided
the kind which at that time was the cause of my
perplexities. In this respect I could identify them
with my father and grandfather who were entirely
superior to the deviltries responsible for most
of my childhood worries. For this reason I expected (very unjustly, I think) that my friends
would blame me for the mistakes I had made as,
without being quite ready to admit it, I was then
blaming myself. I projected to them my own self-
criticism, which was originally parental criticism.
My behavior and feelings throughout are thus

seen to be a repetition of reactions carried out many times in childhood and were conditioned almost entirely by experiences of the past and only partly by the actual facts of the present. That I was so fortunate as to find in X. an equally dependable ally as in my boyhood T. had been was simply a stroke of great good luck.

The point in this example to which I wish especially to call attention is that the practically complete transference and identification had such a really insignificant basis, a not even striking similarity in appearance between the two men. But there is nothing unique about this. Psychoanalysis furnishes multitudes of examples of transference of even the profoundest of feeling, where the features common to the two persons identified are of the most trivial character—the manner of holding a cigar, the color of the hair, some little mannerism or trick of speech, etc.

That such insignificant stimuli should have at times the power to produce such profound and apparently disproportionate reactions seems at first thought hardly credible, or at least without parallel with anything else within the sphere of our observation. Nevertheless there is a parallel to be found (perhaps it is really the same thing) in certain phenomena that have been observed particularly by students of animal behavior. Pawlow, Watson, Lashley and others,[1] have shown

[1] Pawlow—"Investigation of the Higher Nervous Functions."
Watson—"The Place of the Conditioned Reflex in Psychology" —*Psychological Review*, Vol. XXIII, No. 2.
Lashley—"Human Salivary Reflex and its Use in Psychology" —*Psychological Review*, Vol. VII, No. 6.

that when the primary stimulus of a motor or secretory reflex is associated a number of times with an indifferent stimulus, then this indifferent stimulus alone may have the power of exciting the whole efferent part of the reaction. Let us consider an example. The sight of food is a stimulus which normally excites the flow of gastric juice in the dog. Now suppose that for a period a bell is rung in a dog's hearing each time just before food is shown him and he is fed. When at length he has sufficiently associated this really indifferent stimulus with the appearing of the food, then the ringing of the bell alone will be sufficient to activate the efferent paths constituting the "motor pattern" and produce a pouring out of gastric juice. This is known as a "conditioned reflex." The principle holds good not only for secretory reflexes but also for affective and apparently for motile responses as well.

These observations that a small and indifferent part of the stimuli corresponding to an original "sensory pattern" gain through temporal association the power of exciting the whole motor pattern and efferent discharge are perfectly paralleled by and, to my mind, identical with what in human beings we call transference. In the example of transference I have cited, my feelings and behavior toward X. really represented a sort of "conditioned reflex." My action and my affective state were really produced by the excitation of an old efferent pattern marked out in my childhood by contact with T. That which excited this pattern was the relatively unimportant visual stimuli corresponding to those features in the appearance of X. which, though I was not conscious of it, were reminiscent of T. They were thus a small and indifferent portion of what corresponded to the original sensory pattern. The fact then that even trivial similarities may serve to produce apparently disproportionate affective transference is not a phenomenon really unique and without parallel but rather a manifestation of something fundamental in animal reaction.

We may now ask how and when those motor patterns are formed which, when excited by stimuli from new objects, produce the reactions called transference. What is the source of that which is transferred? We may answer that the most important of these patterns are formed in childhood, usually before the end of the sixth year, and that the first source of the affects transferred is to be found in the relations of the child to his parents and to the other persons constituting his early environment. This brings us to a matter to which brief reference was made in the first chapter but which we must now take up in considerable detail, namely the formation of those important constellations known as the Œdipus and the Electra complexes, as well as those usually less significant ones which refer to the brother or sister.

To this end I can do no better than to quote directly from Freud.[1] As he has boldly stated, a sexual preference becomes active at a very early

[1] The paragraphs here quoted are from Freud's "Interpretation of Dreams," Chapter V. I have made some changes in their original order.

period. "The boy regards the father as a rival in love; the girl takes the same attitude toward the mother, a rival by getting rid of whom she cannot but profit."

"Before rejecting this idea as monstrous, let the reader consider the actual relations between parents and children. What the requirements of culture and piety demand of this relation must be distinguished from what daily observation shows us to be the fact. More than one cause for hostile feeling is concealed within the relations between parents and children; the conditions necessary for the actuation of wishes which cannot exist in the presence of the censor are most abundantly provided. Let us dwell at first upon the relation between father and son. I believe that the sanctity which we have ascribed to the injunction of the decalogue dulls our perception of reality. Perhaps we hardly dare to notice that the greater part of humanity neglects to obey the fifth commandment. In the lowest as well as in the highest strata of human society, piety towards parents is in the habit of receding before other interests. The obscure reports which have come to us in mythology and legend from the primeval ages of human society give us an unpleasant idea of the power of the father and the ruthlessness with which it was used. Kronos devours his children as the wild boar devours the brood of the sow; Zeus emasculates his father and takes his place as a ruler. The more despotically the father ruled in the ancient family, the more must the son have taken the position of an enemy, and the greater must have been his impatience, as designated successor, to obtain the mastery himself after his father's death.   Even in our own middle-class family the father is accustomed to aid the development of the germ of hatred which naturally belongs to the paternal relation by refusing the son the disposal of his own destiny, or the means necessary for this.   A physician often has occasion to notice that the son's grief at the loss of his father cannot suppress his satisfaction at the liberty which he has at last obtained.   Every father frantically holds on to whatever of the sadly antiquated *potestas patris* still remains in the society of to-day, and every poet who, like Ibsen, puts the ancient strife between the father and son in the foreground of his fiction is sure of his effect.   The causes of conflict between mother and daughter arise when the daughter grows up and finds a guardian in her mother, while she desires sexual freedom, and when, on the other hand, the mother has been warned by the budding beauty of her daughter that the time has come for her to renounce sexual claims.   All these conditions are notorious and open to every one's inspection."[1]

[1] H. G. Wells in "Ann Veronica" has given expression to the father complex in the following words of his character Capes: "I don't believe there is any strong natural affection between parents and growing up children. There was not, I know, between myself and my father—I bored him. I hated him. I suppose that shocks one's ideas. It is true. There are sentimental and traditional deferences and reverences, I know, between father and son, but that is just exactly what prevents the developing of an easy friendship. Father-worshiping sons are abnormal—and they are no good. . . ."

"It is found that the sexual wishes of the child (in so far as they deserve this designation in their embryonic state) awaken at a very early period, and that the first inclinations of the girl are directed towards the father, and the first childish cravings of the boy towards the mother. The father thus becomes an annoying competitor for the boy, as the mother does for the girl, and we have already shown in the case of brothers and sisters how little it takes for this feeling to lead the child to the death-wish. Sexual selection, as a rule, early becomes evident in the parents; it is a natural tendency for the father to indulge the little daughter, and for the mother to take the part of the sons, while both work earnestly for the education of the little ones when the magic of sex does not prejudice their judgment. The child is very well aware of any partiality, and resists that member of the parental couple who discourages it. To find love in a grown up person is for the child not only the satisfaction of a particular craving, but also means that the child's will is to be yielded to in other respects. Thus the child obeys its own sexual impulse, and at the same time reënforces the feeling which proceeds from the parents, if it makes a selection among the parents that corresponds to theirs.

"Most of the signs of these infantile inclinations are usually overlooked; some of them may be observed even after the first years of childhood. An eight-year-old girl of my acquaintance, when her mother is called from the table, takes advantage of the opportunity to proclaim herself her successor. 'Now I shall be Mamma; Charles, do you want some more vegetables? Have some, I beg you,' etc. A particularly gifted and vivacious girl not yet four years old, with whom this bit of child psychology is unusually transparent, says outright: 'Now mother can go away; then father must marry me and I shall be his wife.' Nor does this wish by any means exclude from child life the possibility that the child may love her mother affectionately. If the little boy is allowed to sleep at his mother's side whenever his father goes on a journey, and if after his father's return he must go back to the nursery to a person whom he likes far less, the wish may be easily actuated that his father may always be absent, in order that he may keep his place next to his dear, beautiful mamma; and the father's death is obviously a means for the attainment of this wish; for the child's experience has taught him that 'dead' folks, like grandpa, for example, are always absent; they never return.

"Being dead means for the child, which has been spared the scenes of suffering previous to dying, the same as 'being gone,' not disturbing the survivors any more. The child does not distinguish the manner and means by which this absence is brought about, whether by traveling, estrangement or death."

Feelings of hostility and death-wishes are inspired not only by the parent of the opposite sex but in the relation of children to their brothers and sisters. Freud goes on to say: "I do not know why we presuppose that it (the relation of brothers and sisters), must be a loving one, since examples of brotherly and sisterly enmity among adults force themselves upon every one's experience, and since we so often know that his estrangement originated even during childhood or has always existed. But many grown up people, who to-day are tenderly attached to their brothers and sisters and stand by them, have lived with them during childhood in almost uninterrupted hostility. The older child has ill-treated the younger, slandered it and deprived it of its toys; the younger has been consumed by helpless fury against the elder, has envied it and feared it, or its first impulse towards liberty and first feelings of injustice have been directed against the oppressor. The parents say that the children do not agree, and cannot find the reason for it. It is not difficult to see that the character even of a well-behaved child is not what we wish to find in a grown up person. The child is absolutely egotistical; it feels its wants acutely and strives remorselessly to satisfy them, especially with its competitors, other children, and in the first instance with its brothers and sisters. For doing this we do not call the child wicked, we call it naughty; it is not responsible for its evil deeds either in our judgment or in the eyes of the penal law. And this is justifiably so; for we may expect that within this very period of life which we call childhood, altruistic impulses and morality will come to life in the little egotist, and that, in the words of Meynert, a secondary ego will overlay and restrain the primary one. It is true that morality does not develop simultaneously in all departments, and furthermore, the duration of the unmoral period of childhood is of different length in different individuals. In cases where the development of this morality fails to appear, we are pleased to talk about degeneration; they are obviously cases of arrested development.

"Many persons, then, who love their brothers and sisters, and who would feel bereaved by their decease, have evil wishes towards them from earlier times in their unconscious, which are capable of being realized in the dream. It is particularly interesting to observe little children up to three years old in their attitude towards their brothers and sisters. So far the child has been the only one; he is now informed that the stork has brought a new child. The younger surveys the arrival, and then expresses his opinion decidedly: 'The stork had better take it back again."

"I subscribe in all seriousness to the opinion that the child knows enough to calculate the disadvantage it has to expect on account of the newcomer. I know in the case of a lady of my acquaintance who agrees very well with a sister four years younger than herself, that she responded to the news of her younger sister's arrival with the following words; 'But I sha'n't give her my red cap anyway.' If the child comes to this realization only at a later time, its enmity will be aroused at that point. I know of a case where a girl, not yet three years old, tried to strangle a suckling in the cradle, because its continued presence, she suspected, boded her no good. Children are capable of envy at this time of life in all its intensity and distinctness. Again, perhaps, the little brother or sister has really soon disappeared; the child has again drawn the entire affection of the household to itself, and then a new child is sent by the stork; is it then unnatural for the favorite to wish that the new competitor may have the same fate as the earlier one, in order that he may be treated as well as he was before during the interval? Of course this attitude of the child toward the young infant is under normal circumstances a simple function of the difference of age. After a certain time the maternal instincts of the girl will be excited towards the helpless new-born child.

"Feelings of enmity towards brothers and sisters must occur more frequently during the age of chilhood than is noted by the dull observation of adults." [1]

[1] Before going any farther let us be perfectly clear about what Freud does *not* mean by the above quoted remarks. He does not mean that the Œdipus complex consists, as some seem to think, merely of a wish on the part of the four or five year old boy to have intercourse with his mother. As a rule, boys of that age do not know that intercourse exists and (except out of curiosity or a desire to experience everything the father experienced) probably would not greatly care for it if they did know. There are, however, cases of more or less marked sexual precocity which present exceptions to this rule, but a strong desire for intercourse for its own sake belongs not to the infantile but to the adult sexuality, and does not appear as a dominant impulse until the primacy of the genital zone is established and the sexual synthesis is fairly complete. The dreams or phantasies of intercourse with the mother (conscious day phantasies of this character are by no means uncommon about the time of puberty and in many instances for some time after) are not manifestations of the

In these ways, through repeated excitations and discharges, certain reaction patterns are formed corresponding to each one of the persons important in the child's environment. They are well defined and more or less permanently fixed by about the time of the beginning of the latency period and before the end of the sixth year. Their form or content depends not only on the nature of the impressions received from the persons constituting the infantile environment but also upon the child's constitutional make-up. These patterns the individual carries with him throughout life and in larger or smaller measure they serve to determine the form or quality of his reactions to all succeeding persons. He has a tendency to repeat in all later contacts the modes of reacting represented by the primary efferent patterns. His feeling or attitude to any new person is in part determined independently of the

Œdipus complex in the infantile form but with the addition of new contributions from the beginning adult sexuality.

In the second place Freud does not mean, as again many have seemed to think, that the little boy's feeling toward the father or the other children felt as rivals is *all* hostile. Such a state of affairs almost never exists. There is always (at least in my experience) love mixed with the hostility, no matter how great the latter may be, and in many instances the degree of love existing alongside the hate or jealousy is of no mean proportions. Furthermore, it should not be understood that a hostility existing toward a parent in childhood is never to be replaced by love in later years. In childhood the father and the father-imago are essentially one. In later life they may not coincide at all. The real father may thus be loved while the father-imago remains invested with the full measure of infantile hate. *Mutatis mutandis* the same may be said in regard to the mother-imago and mother love.

actual sum of peculiarities or total make-up of this person, but is also partly determined by that one of the original sensory patterns with which the stimuli proceeding from this person happen to coincide.

The extent to which the individual's later reactions follow the old patterns and the degree to which these patterns are modified or added to by new impressions and experiences varies a good deal with different individuals. It may be said, however, that those of neurotic predisposition and those who, after attaining adolescence are kept by objective or other conditions longest under the influence of the family, have the greatest tendency to repeat in their feelings and behavior the infantile modes of reacting and to retain the original efferent patterns in the least modified form.

To express some of this in more strictly psychoanalytic terms,[1] there is formed in childhood an "Imago" corresponding to each one of the persons of the family, and these *imagines,* which represent a precipitate of a large group of emotionally toned experiences, are permanently retained by the individual in the Unconscious. Upon each one is fixed a varying amount of the libido (hostile

[1] I hope I need not apologize for borrowing certain terms from the behaviorists to express strictly psychoanalytic ideas. It is to the behaviorists rather than to the "orthodox" psychologists, that psychoanalysis will, it seems to me, look for help and cooperation in the future, and I would like to see the terminology of the two schools interchangeable as far as possible. The most understanding and valuable contribution to psychoanalytic literature yet made by a member of another school is from a behaviorist, Prof. E. B. Holt. ("The Freudian Wish.")

or tender) which is not actually applied to reality, and this tends to become transferred (temporarily or permanently) to those persons of later life who can be fitted into the infantile imago, and in such connection to discharge itself in repetitions of the corresponding infantile reactions in so far as subjective inhibitions and external circumstances will permit.   Thus a man who as a child hated his father tends in later life to hate in like manner those persons, say his employers, who have some features in common with the unconscious father-imago, often when these features are of themselves indifferent ones, and neither they nor any others give logical grounds for hate.   In the same way he chooses his love-objects after the model of the mother.   The more closely a woman tends to coincide with the unconscious mother imago the more is she likely to be loved, while toward those who fail to recall the adored parent he tends to remain cold.

It should perhaps be said that the unconscious imago of father, mother, sister or brother is not necessarily an accurate picture of the person in question.   On the contrary it is usually a very untrue one, as might be expected.   The real mother is seldom as angelic or as beautiful as the boy of five thinks her, nor the father the cruel and powerful tyrant he can appear in his son's eyes. But the fact that in his later years the boy may clearly see that his mother is not an angel nor his father an enemy does not prevent him from retaining in the Unconscious the quite unaltered parental *imagines* formed in early years. Thus it is quite possible for a person to be displaying hostile reactions to surrogates for the father (persons unconsciously identified with the father imago) while with the real father he is the best of friends.[1] In the normal course of things the Œdipus (or Electra) attitude toward the real parents, which has experienced an amelioration or apparent disappearance during the latency period, is to some extent restored for a time with the onset of sexual maturity, but then, as the adolescent gradually transfers his libido to objects outside the family, it ceases to exist as such, even though in the most normal the influence of the parental *imagines* always continues to play an important rôle. In neurotics the infantile attitude may be kept up toward the real parents, even consciously, but in any event the amount of libido fixed upon the parental *imagines* in the Unconscious (as distinguished from that which is applied to real objects in the external world) is with them disproportionately very large. The fact that in the Unconscious the infantile attitude to the parents or their surrogates persists indefinitely is in line with

[1] Such statements as that a patient "hates his father" or "is in love with his mother" have been used rather carelessly by some psychoanalytic writers when it was not the real father or mother but the parental imago that was meant. Of course cases in which the patient in every sense of the word hates the real father or is in love with the real mother are not at all uncommon, but this does not justify us in failing to distinguish in our reports whether it is the real parent or the distorted subjective conception of the parent (the parental imago) which in any given case is hated or loved.

what was said in the first chapter in regard to the processes of the Unconscious being unoriented as to time and reality.

Imagines of later persons as well as those of the infantile environment may also be formed and retained in the Unconscious as the basis for still other identifications and transferences. For example, as described in Freud's "Bruchstücke einer Hysterie Analyse" (Sammlung kleiner Schriften zur Neurosenlehre, Bd. II) his patient Dora identified Freud with Herr K., the man she had loved, and applied to the former certain sentimental and revengeful impulses which really referred to the latter. In succeeding chapters of the present book we shall meet with similar examples, for instance in the case of Miss S. (Chapter IX) and in the case of Stella (Chapter VII). It may be said, however, that, as a general if not always demonstrable fact, these transferences from one to another person of adult life are really in the last analysis transferences from the infantile imagines. Thus, had the work been carried far enough, it might have been clearly revealed that Dora's love and revenge impulses for Herr K. which she transferred to Freud, had earlier been similar feelings for her father which she had transferred to Herr K.

In regard to the fidelity which our reactions bear to early impressions it might be said that we resemble certain primitive races such as the Bushmen of Australia, who have practically no abstract words or ideas. In place of such a word as *hard* the savage thinks *like a stone; long* is *like a river; blue* is *like the sky.* In the same way, to our unconscious thinking, Miss Jones is not *beautiful, amiable* or *sympathetic,* nor Mr. Smith *overbearing, quick tempered* or *in the way,* but *like Mother, like Father,* or *like brother* or *sister,* as the case may be. But in a certain sense neurotics, and to a less extent all of us, exceed the limits indicated by this feature of savage thought and language. The savage's idea of a path which is long may be *like a river* but he does not act toward the path as if it were a river, and, for instance, try to swim in it. Yet the qualities such as beauty in a woman or overbearingness in a man which to the Unconscious are *like Mother* or *like Father,* lead us, within certain limits, to feel, and even to act, as if the case were not one merely of *like* but, more or less completely, of *is.* For example, a wealthy young man became infatuated with a divorcée considerably older than himself, who, as was clearly apparent to every one but him, was a thoroughly unscrupulous adventuress. But in his eyes she was the purest, truest and best of all women. His friends who tried to save him from her clutches by bringing forth evidence from her past record or present behavior to show that she was absolutely mercenary, were to his mind but slanderers made malicious through envy of his love. He confided to her all his intimate affairs, allowed her to extract large sums of money from him on the flimsiest of pretexts, and put himself absolutely in her power with childlike trust in her being heart and soul devoted to him. The explanation is that

certain features of this woman, her being older,
having belonged to another, her treating him like
a small boy, these, together with some vague
similarities in appearance, caused an unconscious
identification with his mother (a sense not merely
of *is like* but of *is*), whereupon the whole motor
pattern corresponding to the mother-imago was
brought into play, and he experienced toward her
all the feelings of love, trust, and devotion which
had been felt toward the actual mother, but which,
as any one but himself could clearly see, were
pitifully inappropriate here.

Reactions from the father complex are exemplified in the case of a male patient, an able and
fairly successful professional man, of considerable wealth and social standing, who complained
of often being overawed by persons who, in many
cases his reason told him, were really beneath
him. If a loud voiced aggressive man made a
statement, the patient was impelled to agree with
him, even when he knew the other to be wrong.
When a street-car conductor would shout roughly:
"Move up forward!" he would feel constrained
instantly to obey, even while he realized that perhaps nobody else in the car was paying the slightest attention. Once when on going to a hotel he
found the room assigned to him was almost unin-
habitable, and he went to the clerk to protest, that
individual's somewhat cold and insolent glance so
overcame him that he instantly abandoned his
purpose and asked for some postage stamps. An
agent was able to sell him a rather large policy of
life insurance, which he had not the slightest de-

sire to purchase, because the man had such a commanding presence and authoritative manner that the patient lacked the courage to say No. These are only a few of a great many instances of a similar nature, which even went so far that on one occasion he caught himself saying "Yes, Sir" to a waiter whose severe countenance and forbidding mien had half consciously impressed him. With persons more logically deserving of respect he was equally, if less conspicuously, unassertive. Meanwhile he hated those persons who overawed him, and hated himself for being unable to prevent it.

The significance of these reactions is of course quite simple. Indications of authoritativeness, dictatorialness, sternness or severity in another man (especially an older man) produced an identification with the father and caused a transference-reaction in the shape of the mixed feelings of submissiveness, fear and obedience, and the less clearly perceived ones of hate, rebellion and antagonism, which were appropriate to the father alone. The rough order of the street-car conductor or the forbidding countenance of the waiter which should at most have only served as a *reminder* of the father (an *is like* reaction), instead activated the whole motor pattern corresponding to the father and resulted in a reaction of identity.

The feelings belonging to the father complex may be transferred not only to logical surrogates for the father (the teacher, employer or any other person in authority) but likewise are capable of being brought into play by essentially impersonal

things.   As in the life of the little boy restraint,
control and punishment are ordinarily represented by the father, thus whatever in later life
restrains, prohibits or threatens ill consequences
may be unconsciously identified with the father.
Thus what was primarily the rebellion of the boy
against his father's authority may in later years
be directed to religion, the law, convention, etc.,
and the person so becomes an active atheist, an-
archist or railer at conventional restraints.   Or if
over-compensations have developed, he may display the other extremes of religious fanaticism,
over-conscientious and scrupulous obedience to
every sort of code, standard or prohibition, or of
great devotion to the state or ruler.   One of my
patients who belonged in the category of compensatory over-conscientiousness well described himself by saying: "I have always been so afraid
of doing something wrong that I have never yet
done anything right." [1]

Other examples of objective identification and
transference are as follows.   A patient who suffered at times from psychic impotence and who as
a rule seemed to care little for women, was most

---

[1] The cases we have cited to illustrate other points contain
instances of transference. For example the girl suffering with
a pain in her face had identified me with her parents (really
with her father) and her antagonism to me (corresponding to
the notion that I was desirous of breaking up her love affair)
was a transference of the similar feeling she had had for her
father. Underneath her antagonism was the affectionate transference, originally the wish to do what he wished in order to
please him. The example of the man who would not submit to
the tyranny of time-tables shows a different transference from
the father.

attracted by comparatively ignorant servant girls or nurse maids older than himself, and as a rule only by those who were very thin and dark. His only serious love affairs were with such women, and in these relations he was completely potent. His preference for women of this type was especially striking, since he had always lived in most refined surroundings and was a man of unusual intelligence and culture—in short, one who would be expected to find congenial only women who possessed cultural and educational attainments comparable to his own. But such women, though he was perfectly capable of experiencing the greatest admiration, respect and liking for them, never aroused in him any sensual emotion or desire for physical contact and caresses. One peculiarity of his attachment to the women who did sensually attract him was that he was very jealous, not of grown men, but of the children under their care, and quite unreasonably suspected that some sort of sexual practices were going on.

The peculiarities of this patient's attitude toward women is readily explained on the basis of identification and transference. The patient was the oldest of several children. He had been the favorite of his mother, a woman of great force and brilliance, as well as exceptional culture and refinement, who had lavished upon him the wealth of affection she was unable to bestow upon her quarrelsome and alcoholic husband. The patient was attached to his mother most deeply, and regarded her as the most wonderful, pure and angelic of all the women that had ever lived. When he

was about five years old his mother was away for
some months, leaving her children in the charge
of a nurse who had for a long period been in the
employ of the family. This nurse began the practice of having one of the children sleep with her,
usually the patient, but sometimes one of the other
children. He awoke one morning before she did,
and finding that the bed covers were thrown back
so she was partially exposed, he began a cautious
investigation of her genitals, in the midst of
which she woke up and discovered him. Instead
of scolding him, as his mother had done when on
certain occasions he had displayed some sexual
curiosity, the nurse laughed and kissed him, and
then exposing herself still further encouraged him
to go on with his investigations. After this nearly
every morning she would play with his genitals,
often taking them in her mouth, and would encourage him to look at and handle hers. He took
no little pleasure in this, and in the affection and
petting he now received from her; and on those
occasions when she took one of the other children
to sleep with her, he was mad with jealousy, fearing that she might carry on with the others the
same practices he wished to be reserved for him.
The morning sexual play continued until after
his mother's return, when she somehow discovered it, and, in an extremity of rage and horror,
turned the nurse out of the house. Her vehement
expressions of disgust and the attitude of shrinking and aversion which she for some time displayed toward her small son, gave him the impression that what had taken place was unspeak-

ably evil, and that both he and the nurse were somehow contaminated for life. This very perceptible change in his mother's attitude toward him caused him the most acute and profound distress.

These events, the memory of which had in large measure faded from his mind, to be recalled or reconstructed as here given only in the course of the analysis, were mainly instrumental in determining the peculiarities of his adult love life. The nurse was a thin and very dark woman. Those nurses or servants with whom the patient fell in love and experienced full sexual attraction were persons whom he unconsciously identified with her on the basis of similarity of appearance and social level. These external similarities caused him unthinkingly to expect a total similarity, which included a willingness to participate in about the same sort of sexual experiences he had known from his childhood.[1]

But while he tended to identify nurses and servants with the "bad" nurse of his childhood and because of their real or fancied badness to feel comparatively free sexually with them, the superior type of woman, who showed signs of refinement and culture, he identified instead with his mother, who had been horrified at what took place with the nurse and whom he considered immaculate and far above such base interests as those of sex. To

[1] He was best satisfied when in his relations with these women the earlier practices were reproduced, perferring them to intercourse, though often feeling some hesitation in stating this preference.

think of sexuality in connection with such women was to his mind a sacrilege, while in addition there existed the unconscious expectation that they would be horrified and disgusted by any display of erotic tendencies on his part as, in his childhood, his mother had been. For this reason he could love them only the "pure" way he had loved his mother. His sensual longings were inhibited by anything in them reminiscent of her and he was impotent in consequence.

With these examples we may be prepared for the mention of another and most important aspect of the question of transference, which we have not yet considered, namely the transference to the physician which occurs in every analysis. Many have seemed to think that this transference consists in little more than the development in women of love wishes for the doctor. But the case is not so simple. Any conceivable sort of impulse or feeling that the patient has previously experienced may be transferred to the analyst, irrespective of his age, sex, personality or any other external factor. The patient may, in other words, unconsciously identify the analyst with any previously known person of either sex, and feel or act toward him accordingly. The transference is never love or hate alone, but always a mixture of both sorts of feeling, though one may predominate and for a time obscure the other. For this reason we distinguish the "positive" (affectionate) from the "negative" or hostile transference.

Because of the nature of the relationship the

doctor (if a man) is most commonly identified with the father and consequently the feelings transferred are in women predominantly love wishes and in men hostile ones, envy, jealousy, etc. But this is not invariably so. The doctor may be identified with brother, mother or sister (despite difference in sex) or with persons belonging to the patient's adolescent or adult life. He may at one time be identified with one person, and later with quite another.

The transference which occurs in the analysis is not created, but merely uncovered, by it. Patients carry on the same transferences with other physicians under different therapeutic régimes, and to just the same degree. The transference to the physician is simply one phase of the neurotic's "passion for transference" generally, and finds expression in every contact of life.[1]

There is no analysis in which transference does not occur and in which it is not of vital importance. Its proper handling is the most difficult but the most vital part of psychoanalysis. In the clinical chapters we shall deal with examples of such transference.

[1] See Ferenczi: Introjection and Transference, Chapter II of his "Contributions to Psychoanalysis."

CHAPTER V

A NEUROSIS, especially when it suddenly breaks out in a person previously in seeming good health, has the appearance of something bizarre, foreign and devoid of all continuity with the rest of the individual's mental life. No data within the reach of his consciousness serve satisfactorily to explain its advent or its meaning, or to connect it with the main trends of his ordinary thought. The malady appears not to be of endopsychic origin, but more as if the mind had been invaded by a strange something which, like an infectious disease or a demoniac possession, would have origin primarily from without.

The seeming discontinuity between the neurosis and the rest of the individual's personality and psychic life is not real but only apparent. It is conditioned by the fact that the malady has origin in trends which are unknown to the patient, rather than in those whose existence he realizes. As soon as these unconscious processes are known it is easy to see that there is a continuity between the neurotic symptoms and all other elements of the patient's mental life—a continuity which is everywhere complete. The neurosis is neither an invasion of the personality by something foreign, nor a neoplastic excrescence which develops on its surface, leaving the underlying strata unchanged, but rather a composite expression of its totality, an extract which contains something of all its vital constituents.

The necessary condition for the processes of the Unconscious to manifest themselves in this abnormal way (as neurotic symptoms) is a failure of repression. The efferent avenues to discharge as affectivity or action are normally under the control of the foreconscious and conscious systems. Only those trends come to expression which are in accord with their specifications and are passed by their censorship. When a neurosis comes into existence it means that the sway of these normally ruling forces has in some degree been broken through. The trends of the Unconscious which in this way come to the surface as symptoms are not necessarily greatly different from what a normal person would possess. The essential pathologic feature is the failure of the repression. Thus an outlet is gained by forces which in the normal would either be repressed completely or their energy diverted to paths of discharge which presented no conflict with the ruling trends residing in the foreconscious. The content of the Unconscious in both normal and neurotic is qualitatively about the same.

The failure of repression which allows the Unconscious to manifest itself in what we know as symptoms is, however, in the neurosis, never complete. The repressing forces are not overthrown *en masse* (as in certain forms of psychosis) nor do those of the Unconscious gain full license to express themselves. The failure of repression is only a partial one. To some degree the repressing forces give in to the repressed, and the repressed to the repressing. The result, the neurosis and its symptoms, is thus a sort of compromise brought about by mutual concessions on the part of forces which actually are at war.

While the repressing trends sacrifice something in allowing to the repressed any manifestation at all, they in their turn make a reciprocal sacrifice in the form of limitations as to the modes in which they are to be expressed. Though allowed some expression they are restricted to such varieties as *appear* to conform with the censorship and show no open disharmony with the individual's ethico-esthetic feelings and his ego-ideal. Trends really incompatible with the superior strata of the personality and which a perfect repression would exclude, now secure representation in consciousness under the condition that they be so disguised and distorted that their true meaning is not revealed. The neurotic symptoms, like the dream, are then manifestations of the Unconscious, accomplished by means indirect, mendacious, and equivocal. The qualities of the symptoms are neither wholly those of the Unconscious, nor wholly those of the higher systems, but in varying degree partake of the nature of both.

As we know, the Unconscious can only wish. It has no other energy than conative tensions; its active content is all desire. The forces which break through the repression and supply the mo-

tive power for the neurotic symptoms are wishes
of the Unconscious. The symptoms (again like
the dream), are an attempted realization of one or
more unconscious wishes. But we can say something about the nature of these wishes. ''According to a rule which I had always found substantiated,'' writes Freud, ''the symptom signifies
the representation (realization) of a phantasy
with a sexual content, and so a sexual situation. I
might better say, at least one of the meanings of
a symptom corresponds to the realization of a
sexual phantasy, while for the other meanings
there is no such limitation of content.''[1] The
wishes which the symptoms attempt to realize, in
other words, belong in the main to the holophilic
instinct.

Statements of this sort have excited a great deal
of opposition. Why, many have asked, must the
central factor of the neurosis be a sexual one?
Why cannot conflicts between non-sexual wishes
produce symptoms? Why may not cases occur
in which the sex factor plays no important part?

I do not know that these questions really have
to be answered. The essential matter at present
is not so much *why* the sexual factor is the central
one in the neurosis but that it *is*. Freud's statements are based on empirical observation, not on
theoretical speculation. I am well aware that certain individuals have published reports of cases
in which, they assert, the sexual factor was absent, and that all the symptoms were to be ex-

[1] "Bruchstück einer Hysterienanalyse," Samml. kl. Schr. z.
Neurosenl. II.

plained on other grounds. But there are no real exceptions to Freud's rule. I do not hesitate to assert that the sexual factor was present in these cases but that the observer failed to see it. This is evident ordinarily from the reports themselves. For on the one hand they show the sexual element present in some veiled form, and on the other that the observer was totally ignorant of the means (and often of the need) of overcoming the patient's resistances in order to allow this factor to come to clear expression.

No one would be so absurd as to assert that persons exist who have no sexual instinct at all. The most frigid woman has a sexual instinct, even granting (what is most unlikely) that she has not and never did have any conscious sexual feelings. And if she has a sexual instinct, it must play *some* part in her mental life, even supposing (another impossible state of affairs) that it is wholly confined to the Unconscious. In the face of the numberless observations which found the sexual factor present and dominant in the neurosis, the only sort of case report that should have any weight against Freud's statement would be one which not only connected the symptoms with exclusively non-sexual factors, but at the same time traced the sexual instinct through all its ramifications and showed what it *was* doing and how it *did* manifest itself. Nobody has ever done this or apparently ever attempted it. Those who assert that the symptoms in their cases were of non-sexual origin tell us nothing of how the sex impulses were disposed of in these patients. With a force so subtle, so pervasive and so wide in its radiations as the sex instinct no one should trust himself to say where it *isn't,* unless he knows in fullest detail where it *is.*

My own experience is that the sexual factor comes to expression in every analysis almost at once—usually within the first two or three visits. And I am sure that for this result no special technique or dexterities are required; about all that is necessary being to let the patient talk. On the other hand there is something required of the analyst. Neurotic patients are quick to sense what sort of impression they are making. And if the doctor is himself tied up with sexual resistances and repressions, so that he cannot look upon the content of the patient's "confession" without prejudice and without emotion, and simply as a matter of biological fact, the patient, in many instances, will divine this beforehand and the confession will consequently never be made. Nobody can thoroughly investigate the permeations of the sex impulses in another person without having first traced them in himself. And this he cannot do alone. It requires the help of another person to overcome the resistances (which all of us have) and until these are overcome and one is permitted to see himself clearly, he will be blind to whatever in his patients he also possesses but would not wish to see in himself. A person can not see through the disguises of sexuality in his patients when in himself the same or similar disguises exist unpenetrated.

When I say that the doctor's own blindness

rather than any real absence of the sexual factor
was responsible for the cases reported as exceptions to Freud's rule, I intended no reproach to
these men, for I believe that they are thoroughly
sincere. The reproach, if there is any, belongs
not to them but to our unnatural and hypocritical
cultural and conventional standards, in the face
of which, for those who accept them, self-deceit is
well nigh unavoidable and only ignorance is bliss.
As long as we are taught and believe that there
is something disgraceful about having a sex instinct, we have either to give up being honest with
ourselves or else to give up our self-respect.

To the question with which we began the discussion, Why is the sexual factor dominant in every
neurosis? I shall not attempt to make any detailed reply. The answer is perhaps to be sought
in the direction indicated by Meyer when he says:
"No experience or part of our life is as much
disfigured by convention as the sex feelings and
ambitions."[1] That is to say, if we had other impulses which throughout the whole life of the individual were so consistently and unremittingly
warped, cramped and deformed in every conceivable and unnatural manner, and they had the same
strength to rebel against such treatment as have
the sex impulses, *then* we might have neuroses in
which they and not the sex factor played the
dominant rôle.

The statement that the wishes which the neu-

[1] Adolf Meyer: *A Discussion of Some Fundamental Issues in
Freud's Psychoanalysis, State Hospitals Bulletin*, Vol. II, No.
4, 1910.

rotic symptoms attempt to realize are predominantly sexual requires some qualification. The word sexual must not here be interpreted in its popular sense. The wishes in question belong more to the infantile than to the adult sexuality. The basic ones are continuations and descendants of holophilic impulses normally present in infancy or childhood but which in a perfectly evolved sex life become subordinate to the genital primacy, give up their energy to sublimation formations or subside into a state of latency and perfect repression. But in the neurotic they either retain measures of energy that should have been employed elsewhere, or else, having been temporarily deprived of such activation, they regain it through a damming up of libido consequent upon failures to secure satisfaction through the external world. It is from that portion of the individual's sexuality which has failed to complete the normal ontogenetic evolution, rather than from the normally synthetized and adult portion, that the motive force of the neurotic symptoms is mainly derived.[1]

[1] Some years ago a prominent neurologist said to me: "Freud's theory that the neuroses depend upon unsatisfied sexual wishes is absurd on the face of it. Why at least fifty percent. of neurotic women haven't any desire for intercourse at all."

I quote this as a fair example of some of. the criticisms of Freud's views. It shows quite typically how ignorant many of his critics are on the one hand of the facts of the sex life, and on the other of the theories they are criticising.

It is not Freud's theory that a *conscious* desire for *intercourse* is responsible for the neurosis. In fact the presence of a well developed desire of that character instead of indicating that a woman was likely to develop a neurosis would more reasonably

But to say that the wishes which are expressed
in the neurosis have the character of infantile sexuality rather than that of adult life is the same
thing as saying they or their sources are essentially perverse. For we have learned that the
characteristic feature of the infantile sexuality
is that it is "polymorphous-perverse." Both
neurosis and perversion represent a disposition of
a portion of the libido to channels at one time
normal but from which, for an adult love-life, its
main currents should be withdrawn and employed
elsewhere. Those tendencies which, in the perversion, are continued on the surface and consciously, are in the neurosis maintained in the
Unconscious in subjection to varying degrees of
repression. The neurosis, as Freud expresses it,
is the *negative* of the perversion.[1] Both represent
a partial arrest of development. Meanwhile it
may be added that though every neurosis is an
attempted realization of infantile, sexual and perverse wishes, not every wish that the neurosis
attempts to realize is either infantile, sexual or

signify that she would *not*. It is the *unconscious* and *repressed*
sexual wishes of the patient which furnish the neurosis with its
motive power. The desire for intercourse is *only a small part of
sexuality*, not the whole of it, as this speaker seemed to think
and it is often the least among those sexual wishes which go
to form the neurotic symptom. "Frigid" women are no more
lacking in sexuality than are "passionate" ones but are more
likely to develop a neurosis. As a matter of fact, many of the
women who are anæsthetic during intercourse are continually
indulging in erotic day dreams, and in many cases are chronic
masturbators.

[1] Freud: "Selected Papers on Hysteria and Other Psychoneuroses," Chapter IX.

perverse. The neurotic symptom is almost invariably a condensation product, expressing *several* wishes, and is thus "overdetermined." Non-sexual, non-infantile and non-perverse wishes may furnish determinants, but they alone do not *cause* the neurosis.

What has been said about the libido remaining in channels of distribution corresponding to developmental phases that should have been left behind brings us to the important matter which is technically known as "fixation." James points out a phenomenon which he calls "the inhibition of instincts by habit." "When objects of a certain class elicit from an animal a certain sort of reaction," he writes, "it often happens that the animal becomes partial to the first specimen of the class on which it has reacted and will not afterwards react on any other specimen.

"The selection of a particular hole to live in, of a particular mate, of a particular feeding ground, a particular variety of diet, a particular anything, in short, out of a possible multitude, is a very widespread tendency among animals, even those low down in the scale. The limpet will return to the same sticking-place in its rock, and the lobster to its favorite nook on the sea-bottom. The rabbit will deposit its dung in the same corner; the bird makes its nest on the same bough. But each of these preferences carries with it an insensibility to *other* opportunities and occasions —an insensibility which can only be described physiologically as an inhibition of the new impulses by the habit of the old ones already formed.

. . . A habit, once grafted on an instinctive tendency, restricts the range of the tendency itself,
and keeps us from reacting on any but the habitual object, although other objects might just as
well have been chosen had they been the first-
comers.'' [1]

This establishing through use or habit of a
partiality for particular specimens of general
classes is apparently the same thing as that which,
when occurring in the human sexual sphere,
Freud calls fixation.   For the holophilic impulses,
when repeatedly gratified either singly or in conjunction by a given person (or object), tend to
become partial to that particular person and correspondingly insensitive to others of the same
class.   These impulses or their libido are then
said to be ''fixed'' on that person or the corresponding ''imago.''   Normal love constancy is an
example of an ''inhibition by habit'' or ''fixation''
which involves the main current of the libido and
practically the whole group of the synthetized
holophilic impulses.

But what James has said concerning the tendencies of an impulse to become fixed upon the
object which has gratified it also applies (at least
in the case of the human holophilic impulses) to
the *aim* as well, that is, to the type of action which
gratifies the impulse and gives the libido discharge.   A peculiarity of the holophilic impulses
is that they are not in the beginning specific with
regard to aim.   Each one may secure gratification in *many* ways, or through any one of a num-

[1] William James: ''Principles of Psychology,'' Vol. II, page 394.

ber of really quite different actions, in distinction
to the hunger impulse which can be satisfied in no
other way than by eating. Were it not for this
non-specificity of the holophilic tendencies, such a
thing as sublimation, where the libido belonging
to a holophilic impulse finds satisfaction in actions
that are not sexual at all, would be quite impossible. But, through repeated activity, part or all
of the libido of an impulse may become inhibited
by habit or fixed on the sort of action that produced the gratification, whereupon the claims of
the impulse to that extent become specific; its
libido is deprived of the original mobility, a preference is established for this particular sort of
action, with a corresponding indifference to others
which might also have represented possibilities of
satisfaction. In fact the tendency of the libido to
form fixations applies not only to aim and object
but in some degree to the whole *ensemble* of
repeated gratifying experiences, even including
incidental and essentially indifferent features of
external circumstance associated with the gratification.[1] The essential point in all this is that the
greater the portion of the individual's libido
which has undergone fixation, the more circum-
scribed is the range of its possibilities for application and the more the individual is limited to
loving certain particular objects and in certain
particular and definite ways.

I said in the first chapter that though autoerotism preponderates in the picture of the infan-

[1] Compare what has already been said concerning the conditioned reflex, in the section on Transference, page 197.

tile holophilic activities, nevertheless there is some object-love even in these early years, namely that which the child feels for the members of the family. A second object-selection occurs after puberty when the sexual synthesis has been completed and object-love is the main feature of the sexual life. It has also been indicated (in the section on Transference) that the first or infantile object-selection has a lasting influence, more profound in some persons than in others, throughout the individual's life. In other words, a varying portion of the individual's libido is fixed upon the unconscious *imagines* of the loved persons of early years and strives continually to repeat the early love experiences, either in phantasy (conscious or unconscious) or in the form of transferences to new persons who can be identified with and form acceptable substitutes for the old.[1] This unconscious portion of the libido has a directing

[1] We must not be confused by such cases as the one mentioned in the section on transference of the man who reacted to many persons, including street car conductors and a waiter, as if they were his father. At first glance such a case might not seem to be the inhibition by habit through which the individual "will not afterward react on any other specimen of a certain class." It seems rather the reverse of such inhibition and as if habit, instead of limiting the numbers of a class to which the individual would react, had abnormally increased them. The case is only an apparent contradiction to the rule. Psychologically the patient was not reacting to *different* members of a class, now a conductor, now a waiter, etc., but rather to the same person all the time, namely the father. The fidelity of the fixation was so great that it required only, as it were, a *part* of the father (loud voice, stern manner, etc.) to touch off the reaction. The possibilities of reacting to *a waiter, an hotel clerk* or *a conductor* were ignored.

influence in the second object-selection. For instance, the man is most drawn to those women who
give promise of satisfying these unconscious
strivings—those who present such qualities that
give rise to an unconscious identification with the
imago of mother, sister or some other loved
woman of the years of childhood. This influence
is perhaps most apparent in the first love affairs
of a young man which quite frequently are with
a woman considerably older than himself, in many
cases a married woman, while he tends to show
toward her more or less of the same respectful
adoration he felt for his own mother.[1]

But though the influence of the first object-
selection always makes itself felt in the second, it
cannot be said to dominate the picture in the case
of normal people. The normal person reaches
adult life with a wide range for object choice.
Thus a healthy man can fall in love almost equally
readily with any one of a large number of women,
and when, through the accident of propinquity or
some similar factor, he has done so with one of

[1] Does the woodpecker flit round the young *ferash?*
Does the grass clothe a new-built wall?
Is she under thirty the woman who holds a boy in her thrall?
RUDYARD KIPLING: *"Certain Maxims of Hafiz."*

I was a young un at Oogli,
Shy as a girl to begin;
Aggie de Castrer she made me,
And Aggie was clever as sin;
Older than me, but my first un—
More like a mother she were—
The Ladies.

Many of this writer's stories give good pictures of object-selection dominated by the mother complex.

them, he is satisfied with her, and relatively indifferent to others for an indefinite period. In other
words, his sexual ideal is quite inclusive and his
love specifications are not very strict.

But with the neurotic it is otherwise. His love
specifications are much more strict and numerous,
his sexual ideal is exclusive, his requirements for
loving are difficult to fulfill. Instead of his being
able to content himself with any one of a large
number of women, there are but few whom he
could fall in love with and find satisfying for long.
This results from the fact that a larger portion of
his libido is fixed upon the images and the aims
corresponding to the first object choice. His
tastes in love matters are already formed when
he is still a child, and, up to a certain point, their
demands are peremptory and inexorable.

Fixation means, ordinarily, that the greater
portion of that libido which is distributed to the
infantile channels and strives to repeat the early
love experiences, can only to a limited degree
be gratified by reality. For on the one hand,
there are lacking in reality the objects that would
gratify these earlier formed wishes, or external
obstacles would stand in the way of such gratification, even if the objects were available; and, on
the other, the situations necessary to gratify these
wishes cannot be realized because of internal
inhibitions. That is to say, the unconsciously
desired object is an incestuous one, or the desired
aim perverse; hence the constellation meets with
resistances on the part of the foreconscious which
not only prohibit real gratification of the wishes,

should real gratification be possible, but also prevents the individual from becoming aware of their
existence. The wishes in question have, in other
words, to remain unconscious and repressed instead of being directed to real and external
things; and in the main no gratification is possible
save when a breaking through the censorship allows their representation in consciousness in such
forms as neurotic symptoms and dreams.[1]

[1] It has seemed to me that somewhere in this problem of fixation is to be sought the answer to that very baffling question,
In what respect is the constitutional neurotic different from the
normal person, fundamentally? Jung has said: "In a certain
sensitiveness," which to my mind is about the same as saying:
"In possessing a greater tendency to form fixations." Neither
statement, it must be confessed, means very much. I am, however, of the opinion that "the greater tendency to form fixations"
is not something primary or inherent but secondary to a sexual
precocity. The neurotic is a person who has learned to love and
hate too soon. His holophilic feelings possess almost adult
intensity while, in years and in his modes of reaction, he is still
a child. The greater tendency to form fixations is, then, it seems
to me, simply a result of this holophilic prematurity. It is as if
the holophilic impulses tend to become fixed when they attain a
certain level of intensity or possess a certain measure of libido.
Thus if this intensity is reached prematurely, a premature fixation occurs. This is in accord with the observations that external factors such as repeated seductions or too much love and
petting from the parents, both of which tend to develop intense
love emotions in the child, have almost the same tendency to pre-
dispose to a neurosis as the constitutional factors.

I should perhaps emphasize that I mean not a qualitative but
a quantitative precocity. So far as I know there is no essential
difference *in kind* between the infantile holophilic impulses and
interests of a normal child and those of one who will later become
a neurotic. The basic difference is, it seems to me, that those
of the latter are *more intense,* and represent a greater measure of
libido. On the other hand, it is just as possible that it is not
so much the intensity as the frequency of the reactions which is

The practical element in the question of fixation is that the points at which fixation occurs (whether they be fixation in respect to object or in respect to aim) are *loci minoris resistentiæ* in the synthesis of the holophilic impulses. Whatever portion of the libido is subject to fixation diminishes the amount which is left free for distribution to aims and objects of the external world. And when that portion which has been directed and satisfied externally is, through meeting with some obstacle, loss or disappointment, cut off from that which had satisfied it, a damming up of the libido all too readily occurs and the tension has a tendency to expend itself in those directions which *formerly* afforded an outlet. In other words, the libido is apt to *regress* to earlier lines of discharge and thus augments that portion already fixed and imperfectly satisfied. The unconscious strivings for repetition of the infantile gratification experiences thus receive a powerful reënforcement, which menaces the previously serviceable repression and may be strong enough to break through it and form a neurosis. This regression doubtless follows the same familiar principle that the tensions corresponding to states of temporary excitement may overflow through earlier channels of discharge, and produce reactions which are entirely unoriented with and unadapted to the

the deciding factor for fixation. The same reaction patterns which exist in the normal child may be worn more deeply in the neurotic through being more often traversed. All this, again, does not mean very much.

realities of the immediate situation. For in- stance, a German living in this country who has habitually spoken and thought in English for years nevertheless will, if very angry or otherwise excited, relapse into his mother tongue, despite the fact that perhaps none of his hearers can un- derstand a word he says. Examples such as this are within the sphere of every one's experience.

When I was an interne in Bellevue I was struck by the fact which at that time I could not inter- pret, that oftentimes a man in sudden and intense pain (such for instance as might be caused by manipulating a fracture) would call for his mother. To hear wails of "Mama! Mama! Help me!" from some of those hardened old repro- bates of the alcoholic or prison wards whose grim, craglike faces gave as little suggestion of the lurking presence of soft memories of mother love as would the rock of Gibraltar, was indeed a thought-provoking experience, particularly if one happened to know that the mother in question had been in her grave for years, assisted thereto by unfeeling abuse received at the hands of the wailer. The essential futility of the reaction (calling for help to a person neither present nor living), its implicit lack of orientation as to time and reality, its infantilism and its utter discon- gruity with all that ordinarily held sway in the individual's character, might well have prepared me for the regressions I was later to see expressed in neurotic symptoms, whose only essential differ- ence is that they are not so short lived.

But the regressions of the dammed up libido to

the old paths left by earlier real or attempted discharge is not merely one from the present back to the past, but from the real and the external inward to the imaginary. The libido, or a portion of it, is withdrawn from reality, the individual losing some of his interest in the world and persons about him, and this energy is then applied to phantasy, and seeks gratification according to the old pain and pleasure principle which attempts to satisfy all wishes by the hallucinatory route. This process has been generally known as Introversion, according to the convenient term which Jung introduced. Introversion is an essential preliminary to the production of any neurosis.

The great increase in the amount of libido which normally attends the attainment of puberty usually results in a period of masturbation in which phantasy supplies the sexual object, chosen after the model of the infantile *imagines*, but which reality still withholds. Later the libido gradually becomes transferred from these phantasies and goes over into action which shall eventually win real satisfaction from real objects in the external world. Now, introversion reverses this process. The libido is withdrawn from those actions which might serve to win a sexual object and real satisfaction in the external world. Instead of to the real sexual objects and gratifications thus despaired of, it is directed to *phantasies* of gratification; first perhaps to conscious ones, but shortly it regresses still further to phantasies which are unconscious. The phantasies thus re-activated are either those which were once

conscious, in the form of some of the masturbatic
phantasies of puberty, which were later forgotten,
or those which had been formed in the Unconscious and were never known to the individual.
In them the external sexual object of adult life is
usually succeeded by an incestuous one corresponding to the infantile *imagines,* while perverse
aims take the place of those of normal sexuality.[1]
This return of the libido from reality to refill
the channels left by the infantile holophilic reactions and revivify the old unconscious phantasies
corresponding to the incestuous images and perverse aims is an invariable and necessary preliminary to the production of any neurosis. The
neurosis has origin from *the introverted portion*
of the libido which, partially overcoming the repression, seeks to realize unconscious phantasies
corresponding to an earlier developmental phase.

[1] Any given symptom is ordinarily a condensation product corresponding to the attempted realization of *several* unconscious
phantasies, not all of which are necessarily infantile nor for that
matter, even sexual, though the central ones are usually both.

When I say that the neurosis attempts to realize the now unconscious phantasies corresponding to the abandoned masturbation of puberty, I hope this may not be construed to mean that
masturbation either directly or indirectly *caused* the neurosis.
One could more truthfully say that it was not the masturbation
but the giving it up which caused the neurosis, inasmuch as it is
the damming up of the libido and not its gratification which
produces neurotic disease. Both the phantasies attending the
masturbation and the neurosis have a common "cause" for they
express the *same* trends. Masturbation is normal or abnormal
in youth according to whether it expresses normal or abnormal
wish constellations.

Cp. Freud: *Hysterical Fancies and Their Relation to Bisex-
uality in* "Selected Papers on Hysteria and Other Psychoneuroses,"
Chapter IX.

But the neurosis is not only an attempt to gratify, after the manner of the old hallucinatory method, wishes belonging to the Unconscious which are returning from repression. It may also serve to secure gratification for other and even conscious wishes and not through essentially phantastic but through real means. The first form of wish fulfillment Freud calls the primary function of the neurosis, the latter its secondary function. For, at least in any cases of long standing, the neurotic *uses* his illness as a means or instrument to various ends. Though when the neurosis first breaks out, it is regarded by the patient as wholly a calamity, he begins at length to make capital out of it, after the manner, as Freud expresses it, of a workman who, having lost his legs in an accident, becomes a street beggar, thereby converting what was at first wholly a loss into an important business asset. The neurotic takes advantage of his illness to gain attention, sympathy and love, to avoid things disagreeable, to revenge himself on others, or to punish himself and do penance for what he conceives to be his sins. And just as a legless mendicant with a well established begging business, who has become adjusted to a life of that sort and forgotten the trade by which he originally earned his bread, might hesitate to take advantage of the opportunity, should he find his legs could miraculously be restored; so the neurotic is loath to give up what the neurosis gains for him, and the more it wins him through its secondary function the greater will be his resistance against the analysis or any other procedure which seeks to bring about a cure.

In pointing out that the neurosis is a wish realization from the side of the unconscious part of the personality, we must not lose sight of its other aspect, namely that, considered from the point of view of the upper strata, consciousness and the foreconscious, it is a defense. It signifies a withdrawal from and a denial of facts that are disagreeable, a purposive blindness to what the patient does not want to see. For, whatever an individual's conscience, standards or ideals may be (and in this respect persons differ enormously) the trends from the Unconscious which are seeking expression are of the very sort which, according to *his* lights, are the most undesirable to have, and the most painful and mortifying to acknowledge. The neurosis is thus an effort to maintain the individual's narcissistic satisfaction or self esteem; a sort of self-deception which attempts to treat as if non-existent whatever trends in his make-up are uncongenial and would lower·him in his own eyes. It tries to prevent the displeasure which results from the perception of a disparity between the real self and the ideal set for the self by denying that there is any disparity. These resistances, at the same time, are an expression of the ethical part of the personality, and reflect a moral struggle and an effort on the part of the individual to be what he thinks he ought to be, a yearning to live up fully to his own ideals. Some who read reports of analyzed cases get the impression that the neurotics are by nature exceptionally immoral or even unmoral people. But this is because the analysis is particularly devoted to the study of the unmoral (instinctive) tendencies. The truth is that neurotics are very moral people (too moral, perhaps) despite the fact that their behavior would not in every instance appear to confirm such a statement. Compared with the average normal people their moral impulses are unusually strong and compelling. For whatever they do that is not moral, they have to pay in remorse and self-reproaches to a degree which, in spite of all their displacements and defensive mechanisms, exceeds that which the ordinary person suffers for any equivalent misconduct.

If it now be asked what is the immediate cause for the regression of the libido and introversion which is manifested by the breaking out of a neurosis, no better way of reply can be found than by quoting at length from Freud's illuminating paper on this subject.[1]

"The cause of neurotic illness easiest to find and understand is that external factor which may be described as *deprivation*. The individual is healthy as long as his need of love is satisfied by a real object in the external world; he becomes neurotic as soon as this object is taken away from him, without his finding a substitute for it. Fortune and health, misfortune and neurosis here coincide. A cure is brought about more easily by fate, which

[1] Freud: *Ueber die neurotischen Erkrankungstypen*, Zentralblatt f. Psychoan. Bd. II., 1912, pages 297–302.

may send a substitute for the lost possibility of satisfaction, than by the physician.

"In this type, which includes the majority of people, the possibility of disease therefore begins only with abstinence, a fact from which one may estimate how significant the cultural limitations upon accessible satisfaction may be in the etiology of the neurosis. Deprivation acts pathologically because of the fact that it dams up the libido and so puts the individual to the test of how long he can endure this increased psychic tension and what course he will pursue to free himself from it. There are only two possibilities of remaining healthy in a long continued actual deprivation of satisfaction, first that of transforming the psychical tension into kinetic energy which continues to be directed towards the external world and finally forces from it a real satisfaction of the libido; second, that of renouncing the love satisfaction and sublimating the dammed up libido by turning it to attainable aims which are no longer erotic. That both possibilities are actually found in the fate of mankind shows us that misfortune is not absolutely coincident with neurosis and that deprivation is not the only deciding factor for the health or illness of the individual. The result of deprivation is primarily that it brings into action the previously latent dispositional factors.

"Where these are sufficiently strong, there is a danger that the libido will become *introverted.* It turns away from reality, which on account of its obstinate denial has lost interest for the individual, turns to the life of phantasies, where it creates new wish formations and revivifies the traces of earlier, forgotten ones. As a result of the intimate interdependence of the phantasy activity and the repressed and unconscious infantile material existing in every individual, and by virtue of the fact that phantasy activity is exempted from having to conform to reality,[1] the libido can revert further, find infantile channels by way of *regression* and strive toward the aims corresponding with them. When these strivings, which are incompatible with the actual circumstances of the individual, have gained enough intensity, there must occur a conflict between them and the other part of the personality, which has retained its true relations to reality. This conflict is compromised by symptom formations and comes out as a manifest illness. That the whole process comes from the actual deprivation is shown by the fact that the symptoms, with which the level of reality is again attained, are substitute satisfactions.

"The second type of the exciting cause for the illness is not at all as obvious as the first, and as a matter of fact may be discovered only by penetrating study in conjunction with the 'doctrine of complexes' of the Zurich[2] school. Here the individual becomes ill not as a result of a change in the external world, which has put deprivation in

[1] *Formulierungen über die zwei Prinzipien des psychischen Geschehens*, Jahrb. f. Psychoanalyse, Bd. III.

[2] Jung: *Die Bedeutung des Vaters für das Schicksal des Einzelnen*, Jahrb. f. Psychoanalyse, I, 1909.

the place of satisfaction, but as the result of a fruitless effort to get the satisfaction which is accessible in the world of reality. He becomes ill in the attempt to adapt himself to reality, and to fulfill the *demands of reality,* an attempt in which he meets with insurmountable internal difficulties.

"It is desirable to distinguish the two types of illness sharply from each other, more sharply than observation generally permits. In the first type a change in the external world is the prominent feature, in the second, the emphasis falls on the internal change. According to the first type one falls ill of an experience, according to the second, of a developmental process. In the first case there is set the task of doing without a satisfaction, and the individual falls ill of his inability to endure the privation; in the second case the task is to exchange one kind of satisfaction for another, and the person is wrecked by its difficulty. In the second case, the conflict between the effort to remain as one is and the effort to change oneself according to new designs and new requirements of reality exists from the beginning; in the first case it arises only after the dammed up libido has chosen new and at the same time unacceptable modes of satisfaction. The rôles of the conflict and the early fixations of the libido are incomparably more striking in the second type than in the first, where such impracticable fixations arise only as the result of the external deprivation.

"A young man who has previously satisfied his libido by phantasies terminating in masturbation, and now wants to exchange this régime, so near

to autoerotism, for real object love; a girl who has
given her father or her brother her entire affection
and now in her relations with her lover ought to admit into consciousness the previously unconscious,
incestuous libido wishes; a married woman who
desires to give up her polygamous tendencies and
prostitution phantasies, in order to be a true wife
to her husband and a blameless mother to her children—all these fall ill of the most praiseworthy
efforts, if the earlier fixations of their libido are
strong enough to resist a displacement, a matter
in which disposition, constitutional make-up and
infantile experience are the deciding factors. In
a way they all suffer the fate of the little tree in
Grimm's fairy tale, that wanted to have other
leaves. From the hygienic standpoint, which to
be sure is here not the only one, one could but wish
that they still had remained as undeveloped, as
inferior and as irresponsible as they were before
their becoming ill. The change which the patients
strive for, but produce only incompletely or not at
all, has regularly the value of progress in the sense
of the real life. It is another matter if one
measures them with an ethical standard. One
sees that people quite as often fall ill if they wish
to give up an ideal as if they wish to attain it.

"Despite the very significant differences between the two types of becoming ill, they yet coincide essentially and are easily reduced to a unity.
Falling ill from deprivation also comes under the
heading of a failure to adapt to reality, in the case,
for example, where reality refuses satisfaction of
the libido. Falling ill under the conditions of the

second type reduces to a special case of deprivation. In it not every form of satisfaction by
reality is withheld, but merely the one which the
individual insists is the only one for him, and the
deprivation comes not directly from the external
world, but primarily from certain strivings of
the ego. The deprivation remains the common
element. As a result of the conflict which immediately takes place in the second type, both kinds
of satisfaction, the accustomed and the newly
striven for, are inhibited. This amounts to a
damming up of the libido with the same results
which follow it in the first case. The psychic
processes on the path to symptom formation in
the second type are rather clearer than in the first,
as the pathogenic fixations of the libido had not
first to be established here but had been in force
during the period of apparent health. A certain
degree of introversion of the libido already existed; a part of the regression to the infantile is
dispensed with by the fact that the development
did not have to travel back over the entire way.

"The next type which I will describe as a becoming sick through an arrest of development,
appears as an exaggeration of the second type,
the falling ill through the demands of reality.
There is no theoretical requirement for differentiating them, but there is a practical one, since it is
a question of persons who fall ill as soon as they
leave the irresponsible age of childhood and therefore have never reached a phase of health, i. e. of
a wholly unlimited efficiency and well being. The
essentials of the disposing process are quite clear

in these cases. The libido has never abandoned
the infantile fixations, the demands of reality do
not suddenly burst upon the partly or wholly
mature individual, but arise from the fact of becoming older, for quite obviously they continuously change with the age of the individual. The
factor of conflict here recedes before that of defect, and yet, according to all our other views we
must assume an effort to overcome the fixations of
childhood, otherwise the issue of the process could
not be a neurosis but only a stationary infantilism.

"As the third type has shown us the dispositional factor almost isolated, the fourth, which
now follows, calls our attention to another which
plays a rôle in all cases, and, for that very reason,
might be overlooked in a theoretical discussion.
Thus we see individuals falling ill who were well
previously, but to whom no new experience has
occurred, and whose relation to the external world
has suffered no change, so that their falling ill
must impress us as being spontaneous. Closer examination of such cases shows us that a change has
taken place in them nevertheless, and one which
we must consider of the greatest significance in
the causing of illness. As a result of attaining a
certain period of life and in connection with regular biological processes, the *quantity* of libido in
their spiritual economy has had an increase which
of itself is enough to upset the balance of health
and produce the conditions for a neurosis. Such
rather sudden increases of libido are familiar and
are regularly connected with puberty and menopause, and the attainment of a certain age in

women. In many men they may be manifested
also in still unknown periodicities. The damming up of the libido is the prime factor here; it
becomes pathogenic as a result of the *relative*
deprivation on the part of the external world,
which would still permit the satisfaction of more
limited demands of the libido. The unsatisfied
and dammed up libido can open the path to regression and kindle the same conflicts which we have
posited for the absolute external denial. We are
thus reminded that we should not lose sight of the
quantitative factor in any consideration of the
etiology of the illness. All other factors (deprivation, fixation, arrest of development), remain
without effect if they do not relate to a definite
measure of libido and cause a damming up to a
definite height. This quantity of libido which
seems to us requisite for a pathogenic effect, is of
course not measurable. We can postulate it only
after the illness has taken place. In only one direction can we estimate it more closely; we may
assume that we are not dealing with an absolute
quantity but with the relation of the actual amount
of libido to that quantity of libido which the individual ego can control, i. e. maintain in tension,
sublimate or directly apply. Therefore a relative
increase of libido quantity may have the same
effect as an absolute one. A weakening of the
ego by organic disease or by a special requisition
upon its energy is able to cause neuroses which
otherwise would have remained latent in spite
of any disposition.

"The significance in the causation of the illness

which we must grant to the quantity of the libido agrees very well with the two main principles of the doctrine of the neuroses which have been gained from psychoanalysis. First with the principle that the neuroses arise out of the conflict between the ego and the libido, second with the view that there is no qualitative difference between the conditions of health and neurosis, that the healthy have to struggle much more vigorously with the task of controlling the libido, but that they succeed better.

"It still remains to say a few words about the relation of these types to experience. When I think over the patients whom I am just now analyzing, I must say that none of them is a pure example of any one of the four types of falling ill. I rather find in each one of them a bit of deprivation operative alongside of a partial inability to adapt to the demands of reality. The concept of arrest of development, which coincides indeed with the rigidity of the fixations, comes into view in all, and we can never neglect the significance of the quantity of the libido, as before mentioned. Indeed I learn that in several of these patients the illness has appeared in installments, between which were intervals of health, and that each one of these installments may be reduced to a different type of causation. The putting forward of these four types has therefore no great theoretical value; they are merely different ways of establishing a certain pathogenic constellation in the spiritual domestic economy, namely the damming

up of the libido, against which the ego, with the
means it has, cannot protect itself without injury.
The situation is in itself pathogenic only by virtue of the quantitative factor; it is not a novelty
introduced into the mental life by the intrusion of
a so-called 'cause of disease.'

''A certain practical significance we gladly con-
cede to these types of falling ill. In individual
cases they may be observed in their pure state.
We should not have noticed the third and fourth
type, if they had not contained the only causes
for the illness of many individuals. The first
presents to us the extraordinarily powerful influence of the external world; the second, the no
less significant rôle of the make-up of the individual which resists this influence. Pathology cannot give the correct solution to the problem of
the cause of the disease as long as it concerns
itself merely with the distinction of whether these
affections are of *endogenous* or *exogenous* nature.
Against all experiences which point to the significance of abstinence (in the broadest sense) as the
cause it must always raise the objection that other
persons suffer the same fate without falling ill.
But if pathology emphasizes the idiosyncracy of
the individual as the essential for illness and
health, then it neglects the fact that persons with
such peculiarity may remain healthy for a very
long time, as long as they are permitted to retain
it. Psychoanalysis has suggested our giving up
the fruitless antithesis of external and internal
factors, environment and constitution, and has

taught us regularly to find the cause of the neurotic disturbance in a definite psychic situation
which may be produced in various ways."

. . . .

While we still have in mind the question of the
damming up of the libido, it may be well to enter
into some general considerations concerning a
common result of this damming up, namely morbid fear or "anxiety," a symptom which, as Jones
remarks, is undoubtedly the most frequent one in
the whole realm of psychopathology.[1]

First let us ask what is the difference between a
fear that is morbid and a normal fear. In the
quality of the emotions themselves there is nothing which would invariably distinguish them.
Though in morbid fears there is often a prepon-
derance of the physical manifestations, this is by
no means invariably the case. Nor is the intensity of the emotion a definite index. Morbid fears
are usually more intense than any fears that a
normal person suffers under ordinary circumstances, but situations of great danger can produce perfectly normal fears which are quite as
intense as any morbid ones. What really distinguishes the two sorts of fears is the fact that,
as Jones points out, a morbid fear is a *relatively
excessive* one.[2] It occurs on occasions where a
normal person would either feel no fear at all or

---

[1] The word anxiety, as used in psychoanalytic writing, has
about the same significance as the German word *Angst*, i.e., an
intense fear. The words fear and anxiety are, however, often used
interchangeably.

[2] Jones: "Pathology of Morbid Anxiety" in his *Papers on Psychoanalysis*.

else a less intense one. An additional fact is that normal fears are usually short in duration, while morbid ones may be very persistent. None of these criteria is, however, absolute. The basic difference between a morbid and a normal fear is one of origin, and this is not revealed to superficial observation. A normal fear is a reaction to an external, material situation or condition of which the individual is clearly aware. A morbid fear, on the other hand, has its real source in an internal and psychic situation, of which the individual is unconscious. The external stimulus which *evokes* an attack of morbid fear is not, as the patient may think, the *cause* of the emotion, but merely serves as a cue to set off a reaction which has its real source elsewhere.

The essential cause of morbid anxiety or fear is a damming up of the libido. The fear is an overflow phenomenon, the result of the pent up energy forcing a way of escape despite opposition or repression. The dammed up wish-energy which the repression withheld from action now breaks out as feeling. The effect of the repression has been to transform this energy into fear. Morbid fear, in other words, is really desire—in the broad sense, sexual desire—which various inhibitions have diverted from more natural channels of expression.

That morbid anxiety really results from desire seems, at first thought, hardly credible. A wish and a fear are so utterly unlike in their qualities that it seems impossible that ever under any circumstances the one could be the cause of the other.   Nevertheless, the more we become acquainted with the facts relating to the situation, the less improbable all this seems.

Let us ask what an emotion is, and see if this does not throw some light on the question.   An emotion, one might say, is an undischarged action, a deed yet retained within the organism.   Thus anger is an unfought combat; fear an unfled flight. Perhaps it would be more accurate to say that an emotion is *a state of preparedness* for action, which however in many ways is almost the action itself.   The involuntary nervous system is excited in the same way as in action.   The same changes take place in the blood.   A state of tonus is produced in the same voluntary muscles that would be innervated to produce the action itself.   Thus Crile writes: "There is (in emotion) a specific stimulation or inhibition of every organ and tissue in the body, in accordance with the rôle each is to play in the intended adaptive muscular response. Blood is transferred from the parts non-essential to muscular action (the stomach, intestines and genital system) and concentrated upon the machinery necessary to muscular action (the heart, lungs, central nervous system and skeletal muscles).   The circulation is accelerated, metabolism is increased, the production of waste products is at its maximum, the breath comes faster, the heart beats quickly, the skin is moist from excessive perspiration, the limbs tremble, the extremities tingle, every detail of the intended muscular action is simulated."[1]   The organism

[1] Crile: "Man, an Adaptive Mechanism."

is like a car which, with throttle open, spark advanced and engine racing, throbs and trembles with liberated energy, while the clutch which shall connect this power with the locomotor machinery is not yet thrown in. The identity of emotion and action goes so far that, as Crile points out, strong feeling results in the same fatigue phenomena (subjective and objective signs of exhaustion, histologic changes in various organs) that would result from the exertion itself. In short, emotion is the same as action in practically every respect, save that of massive movement.

But what is of particular interest is the fact that, as shown by Cannon, by Crile and by others, there take place, in strong emotion, characteristic changes in the blood content which anticipate and prepare for great exertion, such as that of combat or flight. Iodized protein, Crile thinks, is thrown out in abnormal amounts from the thyroid in strong emotion and has the effect of sensitizing the organism by facilitating the passage of electrical currents through semi-permeable membranes, and so lowering the threshold to all stimuli, and increasing the energy transformation. As Cannon showed, there is an increased amount of sugar furnished to the blood, which increases the capacity of the muscles for work and thus prepares for struggle or flight. Similarly as he demonstrated there is an increased output of adrenin, which not only aids in bringing out sugar from the liver's store of glycogen, but has the property of restoring to fatigued muscles the same readiness for response which they had when fresh.

It has the further effect of constricting vessels in such parts of the body that are not active in exertion and thus driving the blood to those regions where in strong effort it is most needed. It also relaxes the muscle fibers in the bronchioles and favors respiration as in preparation for great effort. The clotting time of the blood is at the same time decreased as if to prepare for the possible wounds that might come in the course of combat.

The emotion, from the point of view of physiology, *is* these various preparatory changes in the content of the blood, in the innervation of the various muscles, endocrine glands and other viscera. The emotion, from the point of view of psychology, is the afferent, sensory report of these changes. Thus, as James epigrammatically expressed it, we are afraid because we tremble, not that we tremble because we are afraid.[1]

One is accustomed to think of sexual emotion, or excitement, as being something essentially very different from all other emotion, say anger or fear, and so it is from the subjective side. On the other hand, from the physiological point of view, it is not so different as one might expect. In fact it can be shown that these states of sexual tension and of fear are so closely related that it need not be considered surprising that one merges into the other—i. e. that a condition of tension or prepared-

[1] William James: "Principles of Psychology," Vol. I, page 450.
The state of tension or tonus, which, according to the channels along which it is expressed, is either emotion or action, is the physiological equivalent of what in Freudian psychology is spoken of as the unconscious wish.

ness which is primarily sexual can give the subjective report of fear. But to show this is as far as one can go at present. Our knowledge is insufficient to explain *why,* under some circumstances, a damming up of libido *must* be felt as fear and what are the exact details of the process. We have to be content with knowing that this relationship, which clinical observation demonstrates certainly to exist, is, on physiological grounds, well within the bounds of the eventually explicable.

Popular opinion would regard sexual emotion or excitement as conditioned mainly by an accumulation of semen in the testicles. This notion is obviously incorrect, for sexual excitement occurs in children long before there is any seminal secretion, in males castrated after puberty and in women, who have no specific external sexual secretion. About the same sort of objection applies to the theory that sexual excitement is wholly dependent on accumulations of internal secretions from the specifically sexual glands. In short, the sexual secretions, either internal or external, probably are not the chief immediate basis for sexual excitement, but at most supply only its specific factors.

Cannon, Crile and others seem to think that there occur in sexual emotion the same blood changes anticipatory of exertion that take place for other emotions, namely an increase of thyroid products, of adrenalin, of sugar, etc. It is perhaps, then, not unreasonable to think that sexual excitement has both specific and non-specific components. The specific factors would very likely include the accumulations of internal secretions of the sexual glands, and the stimuli represented by the pressure of seminal secretion upon the walls of its receptacles. Most, if not all of them, would come into play only in adult sexuality. The non-specific elements would be changes in the blood content and in the sympathetic-autonomic balance, much the same as those that prepare for any sort of vigorous action or exertion such as attack or flight.

Sexual emotion, tension or preparedness is less dependent on external stimulation than are other normal emotions. We do not feel continuous normal anger or fear unless we are continuously subject to an external menace. But sexual tension or preparedness may arise in the absence of any external stimulation and tends to persist until relieved by some suitable action, of which coitus, in the adult, is normally the most satisfactory one. Thus, in the absence of actions adequate in quality or in frequency to discharge the libido, there may come about a state of organic sexual preparedness which is chronic.[1] In other words a lack of adequate sexual outlet (and by this is not meant simply abstinence from intercourse) may result in an accumulation in the blood of abnormal quantities of thyroid bodies and perhaps of sugar, adrenin and other substances which constitute an important part of the state of preparedness for *non-sexual* exertion such as attack or flight, and this very likely is accompanied by corresponding

[1] This does not mean that the individual need be continuously *conscious* of sexual desire.

changes in the sympathetic-autonomic balance. It is not then difficult to imagine that this accumulation and these changes in the involuntary nervous system which have so much in common with the states of preparedness from which come the afferent reports known as anger and fear, could reach such a point as either to create abnormally low threshold and exaggerated reaction to slight occasions for normal anxiety or fear (e. g., an excessive anxiety over what would normally be a matter for slight worry) or even give the afferent report of fear (or anger) in the absence of any special external stimulus.[1]

Certainly the clinical facts are in accord with this hypothesis. In 1895 Freud wrote a paper describing a condition which had formerly been classed as one of the varieties of "Neurasthenia" which he named *Anxiety Neurosis*.[2] The symptoms were (1) general irritability and hyperes-

[1] It cannot be advanced as an objection to this hypothesis that if a damming up of the libido can cause fear it also ought to cause anger, for the reason that, in certain cases, it *does* cause anger (or at least an over intense reaction to what in normal persons would cause but slight irritation). The constant state of irritability, exasperation or ill temper (in short, of chronic anger) which is manifest in some nervous people is so familiar as hardly to require comment. Why a damming up of the libido should more frequently cause fear than anger is a question that cannot yet be answered more than to say that conditions of inhibition or repression which are usually in part responsible for the damming up are surely closely allied to fear; while anger more nearly coincides with the freer or self-assertive state of mind that leads to or goes with an adequate sexual outlet.

[2] *Ueber die Berechtigung von der Neurasthenie einen bestimmten Symptomen-komplex als "Angstneurose" abzutrennen.* Brill's translation appears in "Selected Papers on Hysteria and Other Psychoneuroses.

thesia, (hyperacusis, insomnia, etc.), (2) anxious expectation, fearfulness, worry, with perhaps occasional severe attacks or seizures of intense anxiety, and (3) somatic symptoms such as disturbances of heart action, attacks of dyspnœa, of sweating, trembling, vertigo or diarrhœa.

This condition Freud considered an "Actual Neurosis" (as distinguished from a psycho-neurosis, an essentially psychic disease) which arose under such conditions as lead to "an accumulation of somatic sexual excitement" which had not been allowed to become elaborated into psychic excitement or to obtain adequate discharge. Conditions such as those of voluntary sexual abstinence, the practice of coitus interruptus or reservatus, or the failure of gratification in the woman which results from premature ejaculation on the part of the man, he found to be typical for its causation. The establishment of a better régime (for instance, the substitution of coitus condomatus for coitus interruptus) which made full sexual gratification possible, had in many cases the effect of removing all symptoms.

These symptoms which Freud describes indicate very clearly the presence of the endocrine factors and correlated disturbances of the sympathetic nervous system.[1] The condition of general irritability (i. e. of lowered threshold and too

---

[1] Freud has pointed out the resemblance of the physical accompaniments of the anxiety attacks to those of sexual excitement—rapid heart action, hurried breathing, perspiration, dryness of the mouth, involuntary muscular contractions, etc. They also resemble those of angry excitement.

ready response to all sorts of stimuli) is what we expect from an abnormal amount of thyroid secretion in the blood. It is altogether like that which occurs with Graves's disease (a condition, by the way, in which morbid anxiety is often a prominent symptom) or can be produced by the administration of thyroid. The palpitation, diarrhœal attacks and other symptoms are apparently the same as those occurring with hyperthyroidism of other origin. The vaso-motor symptoms and others referable to the sympathetic nervous system might indicate the presence of an excessive secretion of adrenalin or might be the effect of thyroid bodies themselves. (Elliott [1] asserts that adrenalin can produce every result of stimulation of the sympathetic nervous system except an increase in the secretion of adrenalin.)

Anger, hate and the impulses to overcome or attack blend with the sexual sadistic, aggressive and self-assertive reactions, while fear and the impulses to submission or flight are likewise shaded into the masochistic reactions. The sadistic impulses and the combative or destructive impulses were doubtless identical early in phylogenetic history, if not indeed in the ontogenetic. We know how readily, either in animals or in man, a state of anger or the act of attacking may be converted by relatively slight changes in the incoming stimuli into fear or flight, and *vice versa.* It is not so very strange, then, if we find the energy corresponding, in the broad sense, to sexual excitations or tensions shifting from pro-

[1] Quoted by Cannon.

gressive or aggressive manifestations and becoming fear in much the same manner as rage or anger may readily become fear.   Coitus, as many have said, is, in a way, an overcoming, a struggle, a combat, and this might prepare us for the fact that the impulses thereto, and particularly those that have their somatic fulcrum in the voluntary muscular system, undergo the same shifts and transformations as do those of anger and combat which are designed for self-preservation.

At any rate, and however we explain it, there is abundant and incontrovertible evidence that dammed up forces corresponding to inhibited, or ungratified, or undischarged impulses that, in the broad sense, we must call sexual, do certainly result in fear.   Perhaps for all practical purposes we have sufficient explanation in the following principles suggested (in a somewhat different connection) by Spencer.   "It is an unquestionable truth that, at any moment, the existing quantity of liberated nerve force, which in an inscrutable way produces in us the state we call feeling, *must* expend itself in some direction—must generate an equivalent manifestation of force somewhere."   "Overflow of nerve force, undirected by any motive, will manifestly take the most habitual routes; and, if these do not suffice, will next overflow into the less habitual ones."[1]   In short, the holophilic energy (and by this is meant not simply the desire for coitus), if denied an adequate natural outlet, sublimated or otherwise, will force

[1] H. Spencer: "Essays, Scientific, Political," etc., quoted by Darwin in his "Expression of the Emotions."

for itself an unnatural one. It *"must* expend
itself somewhere."[1]

So much for the physiological aspects of the
question. Let us now look at it from the psychological point of view. The biological function or
purpose of fear is protective or preservative.
Every one of us alive to-day owes his existence to
the fact that his human and prehuman ancestors
were afraid. It has often been stated that the
human skin, with its acute sensitiveness to pain,
is a better protective medium than the enormously
thick and tough hide of the rhinoceros, or the bony
casing of the armadillo. In the same sense it may
be said that a readiness to fear is as valuable a
protection as the poison fangs of the serpent or
the strength of the elephant.[2] That is to say, fear
constitutes an insurance for the preservation of
the animal or species by compelling withdrawal
from situations that threaten injury or death, or
by prohibiting approach to such situations.

It hardly seems probable that in morbid fear
the emotion has lost this biological significance.
At most we should expect that there could be only
a miscarriage of it. Normal fear, however, is
provoked only by external conditions or objects.

[1] We cannot even attempt to explain on a physiological basis
why morbid fear attaches itself to certain special objects and not
to others.

[2] As Crile points out, animals like the rabbit, antelope, horse,
monkey and man, which depend for self-preservation on a swift
locomotor reaction, exhibit fear and an irrepressible impulse to
flee from danger. The skunk, however, whose chief means of
protection is its odor; the porcupine, defended by its quills; the
turtle, protected by its shell; the lion and the elephant, secure
in their superior strength, show little if any fear.

Morbid fear has origin from conditions that are internal. This seems to us something entirely novel. Nevertheless it is not. We have seen that in infancy there is no accurate distinction made between the ego and the non-ego. A similar state of affairs may also exist in adult life. Objects or persons really external are felt as a part of the self (identification) while processes really belonging to the individual's own psyche are perceived as influences arising from without (projection). This really is the expression of a general principle. That is to say, the ego has a tendency to treat all sources of pleasure, whether they be internal or external, as a part of the self (for instance, the identification that comes with love); while to all sources of pain or displeasure, whether they are inner or outer, it tends to react as if they were hostile and a part of the external world.[1] That the ego can react to really endopsychic processes or conditions as if they were external and hostile is really then no absolute novelty to us.

Morbid fear seems to occur according to the principle just stated. Though it is justifiable to speak of morbid fear clinically as being converted libido, this may not be entirely accurate, as Jones points out.[2] The morbid fear is perhaps not the libido itself, converted, but rather a *fear reaction against the libido*. That is, the repressed libido, striving for forms of wish-fulfillment, which from the point of view of the individual's conscious and

[1] Compare Freud's "Triebe und Triebschicksale," Int. Zeitschr. f. ärzt. Psychoanalyse, Vol. III, 1915.
[2] L. c.

foreconscious trends, are repugnant and would cause *displeasure,* is treated like other sources of displeasure, as something external and hostile, and so provokes the protective reaction of fear.

The prayer: "Lead us not into temptation" in a certain sense implies that the individual is afraid of his own desires. We often hear it said that a certain man is his own worst enemy, which means that his welfare is menaced, as through a hostile influence, by wishes that are really his own. In morbid fear it is as if such a statement were taken literally, and the individual reacts to what is really a part of himself as if to an enemy. When a woman, finding herself in danger of being forced to have intercourse with a strange man, reacts with fear, we call the emotion normal. If, however, the impulse that threatens to force her into sexual relations with a stranger is her own dammed up libido, and the danger is thus one that arises primarily from within, we call the fear abnormal, though in each case the impending experience which she dreads is exactly the same.

Morbid fear is then an excitation of the normal fear instinct provoked, however, by the individual's own sexual impulses, which, breaking through the control of the higher psychic systems, threatens to become a menace. Naturally the more powerful the unruly impulses and the greater the failure of repression, the more intense will be the morbid fear. In one sense morbid fear is not morbid at all. It is rather a *normal reaction* to the danger arising from an *abnormal condition*—the damming up of the libido to a point where it breaks through foreconscious control.

As I have pointed out elsewhere, the existence of a causal relationship between desire and fear has not everywhere been unsuspected, even before Freud. Certain writers such as Krafft-Ebing, Nyström, Rohleder, Kisch, Leyden [1] have noticed that sexual abstinence resulted in states of anxiety and nervousness. There has also been some popular recognition of this fact. I have used the following story to bring out the latter point.

The traditional Miss Antique came to the boarding house table one night in a state of great excitement. "Oh," she cried, "I've had *such* an experience! Just now as I was coming home through a dark and lonely street I saw a Man! And, My Goodness, how I did run!"

"You don't say so!" returned one of the boarders, looking up with an expression of sympathetic interest, "and did you catch him, Miss Antique?"

To illustrate the point in question this story does not have to be true. Women of the sort it describes unquestionably do exist. And their exaggerated fear of men has, in other instances than that of the cynical boarder, been correctly interpreted as an over compensation for unsatisfied desire.[2]

We have offered two explanations of the origin of neurotic fear from dammed up desire, a physio-

[1] See H. Ellis: "Sex and Society."
[2] Fielding and Dickens, among other writers, show a keen insight into defensive reactions of about this sort.

logical and a psychological one. The latter seems to me the more satisfactory and perhaps the best substantiated. As a matter of fact it is probable that both are correct. In one case what we would call the strictly physiological factors may predominate, and the psychic ones in the next, while both are, in varying degrees, involved in all.

This may be paralleled with the fact that morbid fear cases may have two types of origin. In one the damming up of the libido results primarily from physical factors, in the other mainly from psychic ones. Where the essentially physical factors form the starting point (as for instance where coitus interruptus, or premature ejaculation on the part of the husband, leaves the woman ungratified) the symptoms may be done away with by establishing a better régime (coitus condomatus in place of coitus interruptus) which allows the woman's gratification to be completed. A damming up which arises as the result of psychic factors (repressions, resistances and conflicts) is not noticeably affected by any alteration of the physical factors in the sex life.

Pure cases of the anxiety neurosis, which correspond to the first type of origin, and which, when Freud first described the condition, he regarded as an ''actual'' neurosis (a non-psychogenic malady), probably do not exist. It now seems quite certain that even in those cases where the physical factors interfering with discharge of the libido are the primary and significant ones, psychic conflicts come into play secondarily and have a rôle in the formation of the symptoms—conflicts which,

---

however, may subside as soon as the physical primary factors are properly attended to. But the anxiety neurosis nevertheless remains as a valuable concept, and represents a real condition, even though it cannot be observed clinically in a pure state. The anxiety neurosis is now included within the term anxiety hysteria, which at one time was reserved for those cases where primarily physical factors played no important rôle. It may be added, however, that even in the cases which are most truly "psychical," the physiological element of endogenous intoxication by retention of secretions is without doubt always present and has a definite rôle.[1]

In the hope of correcting certain false impressions that may have arisen in the course of this discussion, let us again warn against taking the word sexual in a too narrow sense, and regarding genital sexuality as the whole of sex. When we say that for health any individual requires an adequate sexual outlet, it must be understood that this outlet may be secured in a great number of different ways. A person may be having regular and frequent sexual intercourse (excessive intercourse, in fact) without this affording him an adequate outlet or preventing his libido from becoming dammed up. On the other hand, another person may not be having intercourse at all, and yet his sexual outlet be entirely adequate, for he can work off most of his libido through sublimations

---

[1] Cf. Jones: "The Relation Between the Anxiety Neurosis and Anxiety Hysteria," *Journal of Abnormal Psychology*, Vol. VIII, 1913.

and in aims that of themselves are not erotic. If all that is required for an adequate sexual outlet were frequently repeated orgasms, then masturbation would cure every neurosis.

CHAPTER VI

NOT very long ago practically all neurotic disturbances which on the one hand were not manifest cases of hysteria nor on the other of major psychoses, were as a rule grouped indiscriminately under the one designation of Neurasthenia. Though this easy if slipshod diagnostic practice is not yet entirely done away with, even among neurologists, nevertheless most neurologists and psychiatrists now clearly recognize that what was formerly called neurasthenia really comprises several distinct disease entities differing from one another in clinical characteristics and pathological structure, and that, as applied to most, if not all of them, the term neurasthenia is a decided misnomer. For most of these conditions are not, strictly speaking, *nervous* disorders at all. They are states of *mind*, psychological disturbances; and the nerves, as such, are not immediately involved in their pathology. The term "nerve weakness," whether in English or Greek, is therefore a poor name to apply to them.

A group of cases most obviously purely psychological and among the first to be recognized as such are those which Janet rescued from the diagnostic waste basket and designated by the name psychasthenia. They comprise the variously called obsessions, fixed ideas, morbid fears (phobias) doubts, compulsions and impulsions. Later observations, particularly those by Freud, resulted in the division into two groups of these cases which Janet included under the one term psychasthenia. One contains certain fear states or "phobias" of which agoraphobia is a type, and is designated by Freud as anxiety hysteria. The other is now usually known as the compulsion (or obsessional) neurosis. We shall begin with a consideration of the latter condition.

Let us study some examples. A man killed a fly which annoyed him by buzzing about the room. Hardly had he done so when there came to him the thought, accompanied by an intense feeling of horror and fear: "My God, what if I should kill a *person* like that!" He was not conscious of ever having had a desire to kill any one; he was not really in fear that he ever would kill any one, but nevertheless the thought "But wouldn't it be awful if I did?" stuck in his mind for months at a time and he was utterly unable to banish it.

A young married woman, who happened to be watching another woman who was seated at a window across the street, suddenly discovered that she could not get the thought of this other woman out of her mind. She *had* to think of her, she did not know why nor to what end, but she could not stop it. These thoughts, accompanied by a sense of apprehension and depression, persisted for the greater part of the time for four or more years. These two cases are examples of what are known variously as compulsive ideas, fixed ideas or obsessions.

An intelligent young Jewish girl, who was herself not at all superstitious, was induced by a relative to consult a fortune teller in reference to a love affair. Shortly afterwards she was suddenly seized with a terrific fear that the fortune teller was exerting some sort of magical spell over her and that as a result she would go insane. She knew this was perfect nonsense, yet the fear continued to force itself upon her with remarkable intensity and she was absolutely powerless to drive it from her mind. (Obsessive or compulsive fear.)

A young woman, whenever she uses the word "I" is tormented by the question "Who is *I?* What is it?" To use or to hear the word "My" has a similar effect. "Who is *My?*" she has to ask herself. "*My* is not my body or I wouldn't say '*my* hands.' It's not my mind or I wouldn't say '*my* mind.' Who or what then is it?" She felt continually impelled to ask other people these questions, and many had tried to answer them or convince her that they were unanswerable, but to no avail. "I've *got* to know!" she would say. "I *must* find out. I never can rest until I do." All the time she suffered from a tense, anxious feeling which, it seemed to her, could be relieved only by her finding the answers she sought. (Compulsive thinking, *Grubelsucht.*)

A boy in high school was supplied with some second hand books. He began to doubt the accuracy of them, for, as they were not new, he thought they might be out of date, and what he read might not be the truth. Before long he would not read a book unless he could satisfy himself that it was new and the writer of it an authority. Even then he was assailed with doubts. For he felt uncertain as to whether he understood what he read. If for example he came across a word of which he was not sure of the exact meaning, he could not go on until he had looked up the word in a dictionary. But as likely as not in the definition of the word there would be some other word with which he was not entirely familiar and he would have to look *that* up, so that at times half an hour or more would be taken up in reading a single page, and even then he would feel doubtful as to whether he had gotten the exact truth. (Compulsive doubt.)

A young woman was impelled at frequent intervals to rip up her clothes and make them over again, feeling that she could improve their fit. Another was forced to eat bread in enormous quantities. Still another had to count ten before every contemplated action and then while carrying out the action she would have to tell herself what it was she was doing. Thus if she were going out she would have to say: "Now I am putting on my hat; now I am opening the door; now I am going down the steps; now I am turning the corner, etc." Before beginning each of these actions she would have to count ten. These are cases of compulsive or obsessive actions. In each case the patient *had to* obey the impulse in question. An effort to resist it invariably resulted in an unbearable sense of tension and anxiety which was relieved only when the act was carried out.

Now what feature have these cases in common to be classed as compulsions? In what does a compulsion consist?

From the point of view of the patient the term compulsion is accurately descriptive of his own feeling with regard to his symptoms. The compulsive idea, fear or impulse, as the case may be, appears in his consciousness as something foreign which is forced upon him as if from without. There is to him a sense of *must*-ness which invests the compulsive activities. He is *compelled* to think, to fear or to act in a certain definite way, although his reason and his inclinations are opposed to his so doing.

From the point of view of the observer the essential fact of a compulsive symptom would appear to consist in a *mesalliance* between affect and idea-content. This *mesalliance* is most commonly quantitative. The emotion or impulse appears altogether excessive for its ideational accompaniment. The fear of the young woman that the fortune teller was driving her insane by means of magic might not have seemed excessive, *had she really believed that he had that power,* but as a matter of fact she did not believe it, and was quite convinced that he was merely an ignorant charlatan. Thus the amount of her fear was entirely disproportionate to her ideas of the thing feared. In the same way it was quite reasonable for the high school boy to wish to assure himself that the books he studied were reliable and that he under-

stood what he read, but his feeling in the matter
was altogether excessive in proportion to the likelihood of his receiving any serious misimpression
either through inaccuracy of his books or a failure
to understand all the words he read.

There may also be a qualitative disharmony in
addition to a purely quantitative incongruity between the affective and idea content of a compulsive symptom. Such was the case in the example
of the patient who could not stop thinking about
the woman across the street. There was a quantitative incongruity inasmuch as the woman across
the street was a perfect stranger and there was no
apparent reason why the patient should have any
emotion about her at all. But the *kind* of feeling
which accompanied her thoughts was also *qualitatively* unsuitable, for there seemed to be nothing
in the woman's appearance or the patient's conscious knowledge of her to account for the fact
that thinking of her gave rise to apprehension and
gloom.

It would seem, on approaching the matter as
we have done, that the chief problem presented
by compulsive phenomena is that of explaining
the lack of accord between affect and idea. If
the considerations represented by the idea-content of a compulsive symptom are obviously inadequate to account for its emotional content, we
feel then that we must account for the emotional
content in some other way. It would seem, in
short, that the affects must have some other
source than that represented by the ideas to which
they are attached. But if in pursuance of this

hypothesis we ask of a patient: "Is there anything in your life that troubles you, or that could
give rise to the strong emotions of which you
complain?" he replies: "No, nothing at all. If
I could only get this terrible fear out of my mind,
I'd have nothing else to bother me, and I'd be
perfectly happy and well." In the face of such
an answer, unless we are willing to abandon our
hypothesis entirely, we are forced to conclude
either that the patient is lying or that he does
not know.

But with these last words *he does not know* we
have hit upon the truth of the matter. If we were
acquainted with every detail of the patient's mental life, it would at once be plain that there are
most adequate reasons for the strong affects in
question, but that he was not fully aware of them,
that they were partly unconscious. Or we might
find that though he was conscious of the causes
of the strong affects, he was not conscious of them
as causes of these affects, that, in other words,
he did not recognize the connection between the
affect and its cause. The apparent dispropor-
tion between affective and ideational content in
the compulsion would then be seen to be due to
the fact that the affects had been attached to
the wrong ideas. Of the right group of ideas
(those in full accord with the affects) he had
been at best only dimly conscious while the connection of these ideas with the "morbid" impulse
and emotion he had not recognized at all.[1] In
other words, to seek to explain the phenomena

[1] This fact alone goes a long way toward explaining why logic

of the compulsion on the basis only of what the patient is aware of is really to seek the impossible. Their true significance does not appear until we bring the symptoms into relation with certain motives, wishes and considerations of which the patient has not complete comprehension and consciousness.

Such a word as "Unconscious" or "Subconscious" as applied to mental processes for most people smacks of the transcendental and the unreal. It seems to them hard to believe that ideas or impulses which are more or less unconscious can at the same time be significant and exert a potent influence in the individual's conscious life and conduct. And it often appears particularly hard to believe that unconscious or unrecognized thoughts produce *symptoms*, that is to say painful effects, sickness and suffering. "If there is anything in a person's life bad enough to make him sick, surely he'd know all about it" I once heard a prominent physician say, and this remark expresses a quite general feeling in regard to the matter.

But, as a matter of fact, all of us, even those who have been most vehement in denying the reality or significance of unconscious mental processes, do in a way recognize both their existence and their potence in determining human conduct, and we frequently interpret the behavior of our acquaintances upon such a basis. How often, for instance, do we hear some such statement as this:

and reason are powerless to dispel obsessions. Such attempts cannot be directed to the real (unconscious) cause.

"Stokes *thinks* he is in love with Miss Rhodes, but I'm sure he isn't. It's really her money he's marrying her for, but he doesn't know it." And what does such a statement imply, if not that Stokes is swayed by a powerful motive of which he is not vividly conscious? Who has not made remarks containing similar implications?

Even the physician quoted above, who does not "believe in" the Unconscious, gave evidence of a keen appreciation of the potence of the non-conscious factors in determining behavior. Commenting upon a woman who had suddenly displayed a fanatical and obviously neurotic enthusiasm and activity in the cause of woman suffrage, he said: "It isn't a *vote* that she wants." His meaning, obviously enough, was that what she did want was a man, and that her feverish activity in behalf of "the Cause" was really the product of repressed longings the reality and nature of which she was unwilling to recognize and admit —longings which were, in part at least, unconscious.

It is hardly to be denied then that an impulse or an idea does not have to be a clearly comprehended and conscious one in order to be of significance in the life of the individual. Consequently the statement that the real causes of the apparently exaggerated affects in the compulsion neuroses are for the most part unrecognized or unconscious is not really so much at variance with every day experience as perhaps it first appeared.

It is now to be asked what the reason is that the

forces causing the compulsive symptoms are not
apprehended by the patients. What is it that
prevents them from being aware of the factors
that are really at work? We had a hint of the
answer to such questions from the two examples
of unconscious influence that have been given.
For in both cases it will be noted that the unrecognized trend was of a nature which the individual would have been rather reluctant to admit of
possessing or giving in to. And if one searches
his memory for similar cases, as furnished by the
behavior of his acquaintances, he is quite certain to find this feature common to all. Such is
the explanation of why the neurotic patient does
not know the nature of the forces producing his
compulsions. For in the main these impulses
(and their representing ideas) are of such a kind
as to be repugnant to his conscious personality
and contrary to, or out of accord with, the trends
of his ethical self. The lack of knowledge is a
result of the automatic censorship exercised by
consciousness and the foreconscious,—an effect
of repression.

But, as has been many times indicated, the
fact that a wish is out of consciousness does not
mean that it has ceased to exist. Repression is
not annihilation. A wish which is repressed may
persist in the Unconscious entirely unchanged in
quality or intensity and in no way differing from
a conscious wish save in the one particular that the
individual has ceased to have awareness of it.

A neurosis is then a *partial failure* of repression. The repressed elements in such a case are

neither completely excluded from consciousness
nor have they wholly free entrance into it.   What
happens is that the repressed forces again manifest themselves in consciousness, not, however in
their original, but in a disguised and distorted
form which conceals their true meaning.   The
disguise corresponds to what is left of the repression, and in general the more extensive its failure, the less complete the disguise.

Depending to some extent on the degree of
failure of repression, we have three types of
neurosis: (1) hysteria proper, or conversion hysteria, (2) anxiety hysteria and (3) the compulsion
neurosis.   The mechanism or structure of the
symptoms differs with each type.   That which
returns from repression (the active element at
least) consists of instinctive and infantile wishes
and strivings which, as was said, are out of accord with the individual's adult and ethical self.
Now, in what we may call a wish-presentation
there may be distinguished two parts: a purely
energic element called by Freud the "affect-
sum" (Affektbetrag) which I have already mentioned as activation energy, and an ideational element.   Thus when, in the middle of the day I find
myself desirous of eating, I am able to divide
this presentation into its energic content (the
more or less undifferentiated urge or tension) and
its ideational content (thoughts of lunch instead
of thoughts of dinner, ideas of some particular
kinds of food, certain anticipatory images of eating, thoughts about where the meal is to be obtained, etc.)

In conversion hysteria the ideational elements remain repressed (unconscious) while the energic element (the libido) is employed in somatic innervation, sensory or motor, excitor or inhibitory, producing a purely bodily symptom (a pain, anæsthesia, spasm, paralysis or the like). The locus, thus over-innervated, is found, on analysis of the case, to bear a definite relation [1] to the nature and content of the wishes thus side-tracked and in some way represents an attempted fulfillment of them. In cases where the conversion is complete, the patient shows toward the symptoms the typical "belle indifference" of hysteria. Some of the activation energy may, however, escape somatic conversion and lead to the development of affects (anxiety, depression, etc.) in a varying degree. In the one case a woman tells us, for instance, that she has a perfectly excruciating pain in her abdomen, yet at the same time she is perfectly serene and smiling and seems totally indifferent to her "agony." But in the other, the patient is worried. She asks anxiously if the pain may be due to a cancer, she expresses a fear that her case is incurable, and she begs for some medicine to bring her relief. Since in cases of complete conversion no affects are developed, the repression or defense may be said to be fairly successful inasmuch as it is the purpose of repression to spare the individual the development of painful affects.

In anxiety hysteria and the compulsion neurosis, on the other hand, the repression is essentially un-

[1] Freud: "Sammlung Kleiner Schreften," Vol. II, Chapter I.

successful. The idea-content of the repressed presentation is withheld from consciousness and remains repressed. But the activation energy (the libido) goes fully over into affect development. In the former neurosis it is converted without loss into an equivalent amount of fear. In the latter there is again no loss, affects are developed proportionate to the amount of libido, which may take the form of fear or almost any other, usually unpleasant, feeling or impulse. The repressed idea is replaced in the individual's consciousness in each case by a substitute idea. In other words all that is accomplished by the repression is an avoidance of the ideas. By means of the mechanism of displacement the energies themselves break through the repression and fully manifest themselves in consciousness.

The energy displayed in the compulsive symptom (wish, fear, imperative impulse, prohibition, inhibition or what not) is *displaced* or *misplaced energy,* in other words a force designed for some other activities than that in which we find it expressing itself. The symptoms are thus *substitute activities* and take the place of some other form of action which has been inhibited. This will perhaps become clearer when we have considered the examples which follow.

I shall first take up some cases in which the energic element of the wish-presentations returning from repression entered into consciousness unchanged, that is, still in the form of a wish. The "compulsion" in these cases depends upon the fact that this wish-energy is attached in con-

sciousness to some new idea-content, is, in other
words, directed to a substitute, rather than to
what is actually wished for. With such a compulsion we are already acquainted, namely that
of the young woman who had a morbid impulse
to take drugs. A similar case is that of the
woman who suffered from an imperative craving
to eat bread. When a little girl, she, like many
other children, gained the impression that the
fertilizing substance entered the body by way of
the mouth, that pregnancy was brought about by
the mother's swallowing something—a seed or
some medicine. Bread is very familiarly the
"Staff of Life" and hence could be a symbol of
the penis. Her compulsion came on when, after a
not very happy wedded life, her husband died,
leaving her childless. The unhappiness of her
married life had caused the patient to resolve not
to make a second venture. But her natural cravings for sex satisfaction and for motherhood, thus
denied their natural outlet, were displaced, to find
expression in a substitute action. The symbolism
of the substitute action was, as is easily seen, com-
pounded partly from infantile and partly from
adult conceptions of the initial act of reproduction.

In these cases it is to be seen that practically
the sole effect of repression was to push the wish-
energy or libido away from its natural ideational
accompaniment over to a new one, thus producing
a compulsive wish and a compulsive action. In
another type of compulsion, repression not only
separates the wish from its original ideational ac-

companiment but also produces a transformation of the wish energy into anxiety. We have then a *compulsive fear*. Indeed it is not difficult to imagine such a thing occurring in the case first mentioned, that, instead of a *desire* for drugs and an impulse to take them, there had appeared a *fear* of drugs, or, as is usually the case, a fear of being poisoned. Such fears are not uncommon and, ordinarily, have precisely the same sexual significance as in the case we have mentioned. I have in mind a very similar case in which the patient, a young unmarried woman, suffered from a fear of dust, particularly a fear that she might swallow some accidentally. Thus, as soon as her food was cooked, she covered it with a carefully shaken napkin, which remained in place until she was ready to eat. Before she could bring herself to eat, she would carefully brush her clothes, dust the table cloth, and repeatedly wash and rinse her dishes, all for fear that some particle of dust would get upon her food and she would unknowingly ingest it. She was very conscious of the absurdity of her fear and often argued with herself saying: "Why should I be afraid? Dust couldn't hurt me, even if I ate a lot of it. It's perfectly harmless; in fact, according to the Bible it's what we are made of. So how could it do me any harm?"

But these thoughts, though not interpreted by the patient, disclose the meaning of the compulsion. Dust being "what we are all made of" is a symbol for the fertilizing substance, semen, and thus, to an unmarried woman, at least, is not in every sense harmless. Her fear of eating dust is similar in its symbolism to the other cases that have been mentioned and depends upon the same infantile theory of oral impregnation.

As I was careful to emphasize in the second chapter, the rôle of the foreconscious is not a purely passive one, or limited to the screening out of elements that would be objectionable to consciousness. It represents rather an active, positive force. A wish remains repressed only through the continuous activity of a counter-wish. That this is true the cases thus far cited do not sufficiently emphasize.

By virtue of the fact that repression is active and positive we often, and in fact almost invariably, find that the energy or driving force displayed in a compulsion is not derived from the repressed force alone but that *some of it is contributed by the repressing forces.* This is true to an even greater extent in the compulsion neuroses than in hysteria or anxiety hysteria.

This fact is indicated in the first case analyzed, as I may now mention, for the young woman had herself often felt that the desire to make herself sick was to some extent an impulse to self-punishment, an abortive suicidal attempt, so to speak, which was designed to expiate what she regarded as sinful in her thoughts and actions. This is very typical. A compulsion as a rule is a resultant of two sorts of forces, the one represented by the repressed wishes which are breaking through repression, the other (of a character directly opposite to the repressed) has its origin in the ethico-esthetic part of the self and corresponds to the repressing forces. The following is a good example.

A young professional man, unmarried, began to suffer from compulsive self-reproaches which came on rather suddenly after a disappointment in love. The reproaches concerned themselves with most trivial matters, as a rule, sometimes one thing, sometimes another, yet he was reproaching himself about something practically all the time, and in a seemingly exaggerated manner. Thus one day he went into a store to buy a straw hat. He selected one that suited his fancy, put it on and left the store. Hardly was he outside the door when the thought came upon him: "You ought not to have bought that hat." Absurd as it may seem, the sense of having done wrong which he experienced was of very great intensity. He continued on his way, arguing with himself to the effect that his feeling was absurd, that he had done nothing wrong, yet all the while the sense of self-reproach remained. Finally his distress was so great that he turned and began to retrace his steps toward the store, intending to exchange the hat for another one. On the way back he was assailed with new doubts, for he kept thinking: "Maybe it would be better if I kept this hat. Maybe I am making a mistake if I take it back." By the time he had reached the store, he had decided that it would be better to keep the hat, so he started for home again with his purchase still on his head. Before he had gone very far, the first sense of guilt again assailed him and finally he did return to the store and, when exchanging the hat for another one, felt considerably, if not entirely, relieved. He went through a similar performance on another occasion when he had gone to his bank to get a new check book. No sooner had he received the book than he felt he ought not to have it, that he must take it back, that he was doing a great wrong in delaying an instant. On still another occasion, a friend suggested to him that he ought to join a certain regiment. Without thinking of the matter at all seriously, he replied: "Well, perhaps I will join before long." Soon after leaving his friend the idea suddenly seized him: "You ought never to have said that. You shouldn't join the regiment," and he could not rest until he had gotten into communication with his friend and taken back his words. Having done so, however, he still felt dissatisfied, and kept thinking: "Maybe it would be better if I did join. Maybe I should not have said I wouldn't, etc." A day or two later, having berated himself continually in the meantime, he called up his friend and told him he had decided to join after all, and then immediately the first set of reproaches returned, so that still later he had to retract this decision, etc.

This patient, let it be understood, was a man of education and of unusual intelligence. Yet against these absurd doubts and fears he was absolutely powerless. And though continually beset with an overwhelming sense of doing wrong, he could not in any instance point out what there

was wrong in the things he had done, or explain
why he felt guilty and reproached himself. I
should add that there was apparently nothing in
his life that should give occasion for such feelings
of guilt, for he was a man of quite exceptional
morality, and commanded the liking and respect
of every one.

His peculiar symptoms are, however, by no
means inexplicable, if we take into account certain elements of his mental life that were not
clearly before his consciousness. He had, as was
said, been disappointed in love. The situation
and circumstances of the disappointment were
such as to give rise to a considerable degree of
resentment on his part toward not only the young
lady herself, but towards his family, his father
in particular. His hostility to his father was,
however, really a revival of earlier hostilities
dating from his childhood, which related to interference and punishment but which, for the most
part, were quite fully repressed and withheld
from his consciousness.

A knowledge of the existence of this hostile or
sadistic trend is sufficient to enable us to explain
the symptoms that have been mentioned without
taking up its origin in further detail. The explanation of his compulsion is really absurdly
simple. The straw hat which he selected in the
store had, at the back of the sweat-band inside the
crown, a tiny bow of red ribbon. This fact he
perceived as he examined the hat, without its
really arresting his conscious attention. But the
important thing was that the tiny red bow looked,

as he glanced at it, not unlike a small splotch of blood. Thus, for him to wear that hat was, in a way, *to have blood upon his head.* This was the reason he reproached himself. For if he had put into action the hostile impulses he was repressing, he would in fact have had blood upon his head; he would have murdered some one.

The incident of the check book depends upon a similar association of ideas. The one he first received at the bank had a bright red cover, thus suggesting blood, and to keep it suggested having "blood upon his hands." When he had taken it back and exchanged it for a yellow one, he felt considerably relieved.

In the same way the idea of joining the regiment had become connected with the repressed murderous trend, for there had passed through his mind the thought: "Suppose I join the regiment and there is a strike or a riot, for which the militia are called out.[1] *Then I might kill some one.*"

His compulsive vacillation is thus seen to have had its origin in two opposed and displaced trends. The one which led him to reproach himself for having purchased the hat, received the check book and promised to join the regiment was derived from his conscious, ethical, social and affectionate self. The other consisted of primitive, savage, asocial impulses, inhibited very naturally from direct expression, but nevertheless not kept entirely subdued by repression. It was the non-satisfaction of this trend which led him to criticize

[1] This was before the beginning of the European War.

his desire to take back the hat and the check book, etc. and was responsible for his lack of complete satisfaction when he had done so.

⌐ It is to be seen that in this case, if anything, more energy is contributed to symptom formation by the repressing forces than by the repressed. His compulsion for the most part was an *overcompensation* on the part of his conscious personality for his unconscious sadism. It was as if, vaguely perceiving his subliminal murderous tendencies, he could not be content merely with avoiding actual murder but must avoid also *everything even remotely suggesting it*.

We may now take advantage of this case to introduce a consideration of some typical features of the history and characteristics of compulsion neurotics. This young man was, as I have said, quite exceptionally moral in his ordinary behavior. He was a most dutiful son, devoted to his parents in a very marked degree. He was to all appearances good tempered, conscientious to a fault, and inclined more to gentleness and submissiveness than to aggression and pugnacity. But these traits, be it remembered, were expressions of his *conscious* personality.[1] The history of his early childhood presents quite a different picture. For as a very small boy he was very unruly, jealous and subject to most violent fits of anger and rage. He had also shown at times a certain tendency to be cruel to other children and

---

[1] The words "conscious personality" as used in this book mean the combined tendencies of the foreconscious and conscious systems.

to animals. His brother, of whom he was jealous at times, he had often wished dead, and on one occasion in a fit of anger nearly killed him.

Now this early history, or the equivalent of it, is typical of the compulsion neurosis. Careful study invariably shows that the so-called sadistic impulse (the tendency to aggression, anger, violence and cruelty, a trace of which is found in every person) is manifested very early in the lives of these patients and in a very vigorous form. But, and partly, no doubt, because of its premature display, the impulse early gets into disrepute, for, coming into conflict with the corrective discipline on the part of the parents, often not very gently administered, it succumbs to a premature and all too fundamental repression. This repression is often very complete by the fifth or sixth year of the child's life, and thereafter, instead of showing the sadistic tendencies which earlier manifested themselves, he is more apt to be distinguished by an exaggerated over-conscientiousness and even submissiveness, particularly to parental authority. What happens is as follows. The repression of the sadistic impulse produces not its annihilation but merely its transfer from consciousness to the Unconscious. And there, withheld from the neutralizing influence of conscious reasoning, this impulse and the phantasies derived from it are not only preserved without deterioration but may even grow in vigor and intensity. Thus, despite the fact that in many instances the individual's conscious life is apparently singularly irreproachable, nevertheless this life is lived coincidently with an undercurrent of impulses of anger, hate, hostility, and revenge and their corresponding phantasies. To compensate for this substratum of hostile trends the conscious qualities of love, sympathy, considerateness and scrupulousness are developed often to an unusual extent and participate in the task of maintaining the repression.

The period of apparent normality, but really of successful repression, which succeeds upon the earlier phase of more or less free sadistic activity is terminated with the outbreak of the neurosis when, the repression in part failing, the hostile tendencies are allowed a certain limited access to consciousness, subject, however, to disguise and distortion, particularly in the form of displacement. The symptoms produced by the return from repression are in part then derived from impulses, in the shape of hate, hostility, etc., coming from the Unconscious and in part from the highly developed conscious and foreconscious impulses of love and conscientiousness which serve as reaction against them.

The fact that the hostile responses (or rather the impulses so to respond) are for the most part confined to the Unconscious produces a very singular condition, namely, that the individual is able to have toward the same persons simultaneous impulses of both love and hate, both possessing a high degree of intensity. The love, no matter how great, fails to neutralize the hate, which is withheld from it in the Unconscious and merely accomplishes its repression.

The first effect of this strange constellation of the love-life is a sort of "weakness of will," an inability to make decisions in matters which pertain to love. For the unconscious hostility produces an inhibition or resistance in carrying out all those actions for which love would be the impelling motive. Thus important and decisive actions are put off, while those of minor importance are carried uncertainly, irresolutely and without any subjective sense of full satisfaction and finality. Evading major love decisions, the patient very typically concentrates his energies on matters preparatory to deciding, but here too the irresolution and lack of decisiveness displays itself and the patient is unable to achieve anything final, even in these minor matters. The aboulia, the inability to decide, thus does not long remain limited to the original love problems but gradually diffuses itself over all departments of the patient's life.

The further the spread of irresolution and doubt is carried, the greater is the tendency for thinking to take the place of action. "The native hue of resolution is sicklied o'er with the pale cast of thought"; doing is replaced by doubting, performance gives way to pondering.

The compulsions themselves represent an effort to compensate for the doubt and conflict in the love-life. The energy dammed up through the mutual inhibition of the opposed impulses of love and of hate is continuously seeking an outlet. Unable to discharge into the actions appropriate to its qualities, it forces for itself new avenues of outlet, somewhat in the manner that the current of blood, after ligation of an artery, tends to swell the smaller branches and establish a collateral circulation. Thus we find large amounts of energy discharging, or attempting to discharge, through channels represented by mental or motor activities of so little intrinsic dignity and importance as to be entirely out of accord with such great expenditures. These collaterals, tapping the store of energy corresponding to the impulses of love and hate denied expression elsewhere, are those strange phenomena which clinically we know as compulsions. Sometimes they give expression to a hostile impulse, sometimes to a tender one, but the rule is that the activity which becomes compulsive is one of a sort to give to the hostile and tender impulses a more or less simultaneous discharge, and thus represents a sort of compromise between them.

The compulsions are then, as was said earlier, *substitute activities* and come about through displacement. But the energy which is displaced is that derived from impulses of love and hate which have reciprocally inhibited one another. Depending on the extent to which thinking has replaced action, we have compulsive thinking or "ideas" (obsessions) instead of compulsive actions in the narrow sense. Whether the compulsive activities take the form of imperative wishes, impulses, doubts, etc., or that of *fears* depends on whether the original energic content retains more or less its true form or is transformed by the repression into anxiety or some similar emotion.

In the majority of cases there develop the so-called "measures of secondary defense." They are activities which occur after there has been a failure of repression, and have the appearance of being directed against the symptoms themselves.

For instance a person with a compulsive fear often has some formula or prayer which he repeats, or some gesture or rite which he performs in order to prevent the feared occurrence from taking place. But the measures of secondary defense are not sharply marked off, either clinically or psychologically, from the primary symptoms. For the secondary defensive action is usually found upon analysis to have received some of its motivation from the very impulses causing the primary symptom and against which it is intended to defend. For example a young man who suffered from an obsession that he was noticeably effeminate in appearance conceived the idea that by injecting himself with testicular extract he might gain a more virile and masculine aspect. This obsession, apart from the hostile elements in its motivation, was mainly dependent upon a repressed homosexual trend. Thus the measure which was intended to do away with the appearance of effeminacy (which was a projection, a substitution of an *outer* for the repressed *inner* perception of homosexual tendencies) was one symbolic of a coitus, in which the patient, in the feminine rôle, received the semen of the male.

A typical occurrence in the compulsion neurosis is that of "two-sided compulsive acts," where a hostile movement alternates with a tender one. They are a manifestation of the state of ambivalence, the coexistence of opposite trends of love and hate toward the same individual. Freud gives the following example.[1] His patient, a young officer, while walking along a street struck his foot against a stone lying in the roadway. The young man's fiancée was going away that day, and the thought came to him that on her way to the station her carriage might pass along this street and be wrecked on this stone, and she come to injury. In consequence he was compelled to pick up the stone and carry it to one side of the street. But a few minutes later it occurred to him that what he had done was very foolish and absurd, whereupon he had to return and replace the stone in its original position in the middle of the roadway.

Cases such as this one of Freud's or my case of the young man who had such a conflict about his straw hat show a type of symptom formation that is usually not to be found in conversion hysteria or anxiety hysteria. In those maladies the rule is that compromises are formed which satisfy opposite trends in a single presentation; here, however, the opposite impulses are discharged separately, first one and then the other, of course not without some attempt to rationalize into some semblance of harmony the contradiction between them. The patient's removal of the stone from the street is an expression of the overdeveloped

[1] "Bemerkungen über einen Fall Zwangsneurose," Jahrbuch f. psychoan. u. psychopath. Forsch. Bd. I., Hft. 2, 1909.

love impulses; but his action in returning it to its original position did not come from a purely objective judgment of his morbid act nor signify a healthy erasing of it, as the patient might have thought. It was in itself a compulsion, a part of the morbid action, and motivated by an opposite trend from that of the first part. The first part expresses the thought: ''I hope no injury befalls my beloved''; but the second does not mean, as the patient probably believed, ''I must not be so foolishly anxious about her'' but rather ''I hope something *does* happen to her.''

The state of ambivalence which distinguishes the compulsion neurotics seems to arise through a constitutional accentuation of the sadistic component of the holophilic instinct. The undercurrent of hostility which in these patients exists in all relationships is a continuation of the strong sadistic trends which in early childhood had succumbed to a premature and perhaps too extensive repression. The neurosis itself coincides with a fixation in, or a regression to, a certain stage in the evolution of the holophilic impulses which precedes the final genital organization. The holophilic impulses, as I said in the first chapter, are more or less independent of one another before puberty. Their complete synthesis into an harmoniously operating hierarchy under the primacy of the genital zone does not occur until the beginning of sexual maturity. Nevertheless, preceding this final synthesis, there are states of incomplete organization or synthesis, and the compulsion neurosis results from a regression to one of these, namely the so-called sadistic-anal-erotic organization. This is a stage in which the individual is past the predominantly autoerotic phase, and object-love has already been well established; but the primacy of the genital zone has not yet come about. A division of the holophilic impulses into antithetical groups which rule as "masculine" and "feminine" in the normal adult sexual life, has taken place, but the groups at this stage cannot be so distinguished, and are rather to be called "active" and "passive."[1] The active or sadistic group coincides with the instincts for acquisition and mastery and its main organic complement is the voluntary muscular and kinesthetic systems (as the genital system is the prime organic complement in the adult organization) while for the passive group the anal zone is the chief somatic focus. Each group has its sexual objects which are not necessarily alike or identical. A regression of the libido (after a period of more normal distribution) to the old channels marked out by the pregenital organization is the underlying essential factor in the outbreak of a compulsion neurosis.

A somewhat similar return, Freud points out, is at times to be observed in women when, having passed the menopause, the genital function is given up. They become on the one hand ill tempered, quarrelsome, tyrannical and malicious (sadistic traits), and on the other envious and ob-

[1] The antithesis "masculine-feminine" as distinguished from "active-passive" does not exist until the genital zones become the prime foci of sexual reference.

stinate (anal-erotic traits) though during the period of sexual functioning they had shown no such characteristics.[1] Thus, as he says, such characteristics, corresponding to a sadistic-anal-erotic organization of the impulses may not only be a precursor to the genital phase of the sexual life but likewise its aftermath. But whereas the post-climacteric regression meets with no particular opposition on the part of the individual, it is resisted in the case of compulsion neurosis, is confined chiefly to the Unconscious, and causes conflicts, reaction formations, compromises, compensations, etc. The character of the compulsion neurotic might be described as that of an ill tempered, willful sadistic child or of a querulous hateful old woman, upon which has been superimposed a corrective stratum of such qualities as sentimentality, over-conscientiousness and over-morality—which the tumultuous undercurrents continually threaten to break through. The compulsion neurosis is the negative of the sadistic perversion.

The curiosity impulse which, like the sadistic, has one of its roots in the acquisitive and dominative impulses is unusually highly developed in compulsion neurotics and may contribute a good deal to the clinical picture. These patients as a class are above the average of intelligence and are great thinkers, though their intellectual activi-

[1] Freud: "Die Disposition zur Zwangsneurose," Int. Zeitschr. f. Aerztliche Psychoanalyse, Vol. I, No. 6, 1913. Cp. Freud: "Charakter und Anal-Erotik," Sammlung kleiner Schriften zur Neurosenlehre, Bd. II or Brill: Anal-Eroticism and Character in his book on "Psychoanalysis."

ties, at least after the outbreak of the neurosis, are by no means regularly productive of any tangible or valuable results. But a good deal of the libido that in less inhibited persons would go over into action is in these cases taken over by channels derived from the curiosity impulse and expends itself in thought. "Where the curiosity impulse preponderates in the constitution of the compulsion patient, morbid pondering will be the chief symptom of the neurosis. The reasoning process itself becomes sexualized, while the sexual pleasure, which was already connected with the content of thought, now becomes diverted to the act of thinking, and the satisfaction of accomplishing an intellectual operation becomes felt as sexual satisfaction. This relation of the curiosity impulse to the reasoning process makes it particularly able, in the different forms of compulsion neurosis in which it plays a part, to tempt toward reasoning, where there is offered the possibility of pleasure gratification, the energy which labored in vain to express itself in action."[1] Freud is of the opinion that there occur cases of compulsion neurosis which have as their basis not the sadistic impulse but the curiosity impulse alone.

Compulsion neurotics have a certain typical peculiarity with regard to superstition and the possibility of the death of other persons. Though a great proportion are very materialistic and not religious, nevertheless they are almost invariably superstitious. Their superstitious ideas

[1] Freud: "Bemerkungen über einen Fall Zwangsneurose," Jahrbuch für psychoan. u. psychopath. Forschungen, Vol. I, 1909.

exist along side, and in spite of their materialistic convictions. As Freud expresses it, they are superstitious and at the same time not superstitious, having, as it were, *two* convictions on the matter, rather than the uncertainty of an unformed opinion. In many cases their superstitions are not of the sort current among the uneducated, but rather private ones which have a common origin with their neurosis.

The thoughts of the compulsion neurotics are continually occupied with the possibility of the death of others. "At first their superstitious tendencies had no other content, and in general perhaps no other origin. Above all things they need the possibility of death in the solution of their yet unsolved conflicts. Their essential characteristic is that they are incapable of decision, particularly in love matters. They endeavor to postpone each decision and, in doubt as to what person should be decided for or against, or as to what rule should be employed in making the decision, they follow the model of the old German courts, the processes of which were commonly ended by the death of one of the contesting parties before any judgment was handed down. So in each conflict they lie in wait for the death of some one significant to them, usually a loved person, whether it be one of the parents, or a rival or one of the love-objects between whom their inclination wavers."[1]

The superstition of these patients is related to and based largely on a belief (unformulated and

[1] l. c.

in the main unconscious) in the omnipotence of
their wishes, particularly their evil wishes against
others,—the so-called Omnipotence of Thought.
This is something, however, that is to be observed
more or less in persons with other types of
neuroses and in many normal persons. How such
a belief arises has been ably discussed by
Ferenczi and need not be considered here.[1] It
is sufficient for our purposes merely that we know
it exists.

Inasmuch as in the preceding chapters we have
heard so much about the highly important rôle
of the Unconscious in the neurosis, while in the
next chapter we are to consider a case in which
we shall find that a leading part was played by
factors which were not unconscious, it may be
well for me to say that in the compulsion neurosis
the rule is that the recent factors in the patient's
falling sick are not reduced to amnesia by the
repression, as is so often the case in hysteria, but
are dealt with by a different defensive technique.
In the compulsive cases the "infantile precursors
of the neurosis may sink into an (often incomplete) amnesia. On the other hand the recent
cause of the illness is retained in memory. The
repression has here employed a different and
really more simple mechanism. Instead of causing the trauma to be forgotten, it has withdrawn
the affect belonging to it, so that there is left in
consciousness an idea-content which is deemed
indifferent and non-essential. The difference re-

[1] Ferenczi: "Contributions to Psychoanalysis," Chapter VIII,
tr. by Ernest Jones.

sides in the psychic process which we must infer as being back of the phenomena. The result is about the same as in hysteria, for the indifferent ideas only seldom become reproduced and play no rôle in the thought activities of the patient. In differentiating the two forms of repression we can utilize the assurance of the patient that the content of the ideas recovered in the analysis was in the one case always known, and in the other had been forgotten for a long while.''

"It is therefore no rare occurrence that the compulsion patients who suffer from self reproaches and have connected these affects with false causes, make the correct confession to the doctor without perceiving that it is from what they have confessed that their reproaches are derived.''[1] And when it is explained to them what the relation is, they still fail to see it, saying: "Oh, *that* doesn't bother me. I never worried about it.''

I recall a striking example of this which, though I did not analyze the patient, is sufficiently convincing. One day as I was entering the rooms belonging to the neurological department at Cornell Dispensary, an intelligent looking young woman got up from the benches belonging to the skin department, which is next door, and stopped me.

"Doctor,'' she said, "is there any one in your department who knows how to hypnotize?''

"Yes,'' I replied, "why do you ask?''

"Because I want to stop smoking cigarettes,

[1] L. c.

and I can't. I thought maybe if I could be hypnotized it would help me. I've got to stop. The things are killing me."

"All right," I said, "come in and we'll see what can be done," and, sitting down, I began to take the usual routine history.

"Your age?"

"Twenty-five."

"Occupation?"

"I am a prostitute."

"What diseases have you had?"

"I've had gonorrhea and syphilis. I'm being treated for syphilis now in the skin department."

"Do you drink?"

"Yes, I drink quite a lot. I smoke dope and snuff cocaine a little too, but I don't think I have a real habit for them."

"How long have you smoked cigarettes?"

"Five years."

"How many a day?" (I expected her to say forty or fifty.)

"Oh, seven or eight."

"But that isn't very many," I said. "I don't believe seven or eight cigarettes a day would hurt you at all, to say nothing of their 'killing' you."

"But they *are* killing me. I know. I feel so nervous and worried and blue, and all the time I am always thinking I am going to die. It's the cigarettes that's doing it. I'll be dead or dippy, if I can't stop them soon." She spoke most earnestly and seriously.

"But maybe it is something else—for instance, the kind of life you lead, or having syphilis—that

really makes you feel blue and worried, and you
only think it's the cigarettes that are doing it.''

"No," she said, "it's the cigarettes. They're
what's killing me. I know, because I never felt
this way until I began to smoke them.''

"How long ago did you begin the sort of life
you are now leading?''

"Five years ago. I was a perfectly straight
girl up to then.''

"But that's just the time you began to smoke
cigarettes, isn't it?''

"Yes, that's right," she admitted.

"But," I asked, "since you began to smoke
cigarettes and to do these other things at just the
same time, how do you know which it is that makes
you feel badly? Being a prostitute and having
gonorrhea and syphilis might much more easily
cause a girl to feel blue and worried than smoking a few cigarettes. Don't you think it possible that some of these other things and not the
smoking are the real reasons why you do not feel
well?''

"No," she said, "I see what you mean, but I
don't agree with you. Somebody else might
worry about such things, but I never do. Old
R. E. Morse never bothers me. If I could stop
the cigarettes, I'd feel fine. They're what's killing me and nothing else.'' It was very apparent
that she really believed this, and that no ordinary
argument could shake her out of her conviction
—and this despite the fact that the girl was by
no means unintelligent.

The case clearly enough was one in which the

patient had made the "correct confession"[1] without realizing that what she had confessed was the real source of the affects that were troubling her. Naturally she could not become amnesic to the fact that she was a prostitute and a sufferer from venereal disease. She was, in other words, unable to defend herself against these sources of painful affects by completely forgetting them. The next best defense to denying their existence (amnesia) was that of denying their importance. "Somebody else might worry about these things, but I never do." This the repression could accomplish, whereupon the painful affects, which as depression, nervousness, etc., continued practically unaltered, she explained to herself as the result of something relatively innocent, namely the cigarette habit.

This defensive mechanism, of which we shall have further illustration in the next chapter, reminds one of the following familiar story. A sporty young man who was not feeling "fit," consulted a physician. "My boy," said the doctor, when he had made his examination, "you have been going too fast a pace. There lies your trouble. Wine, women and song are killing you."

"All right, Doc," replied the young man cheerfully; "I'll cut out singing."

This story serves to bring out an important point in connection with defensive displacement.

---

[1] Without doubt the "confession" was incomplete. I imagine that oral perversities or tendencies thereto constituted one of the sources of the displaced affects, and that this was one of the reasons why the cigarette habit was selected as a substitute idea, for it too had to do with the mouth.

If the young man confined his reformative efforts to the non-essential, singing, he would spare himself the renunciation of those other activities, which, being more pleasurable, would be harder to give up. Likewise the young woman, by making, as it were, a scapegoat of her cigarette smoking, dodged the problem of so reforming the rest of her life that there would be no cause for the development of guilt affects. She had thus, in the shape of whatever sexual satisfaction or pecuniary gain she derived from the sort of life she was leading, a certain "reward of illness," corresponding to the "secondary function of the neurosis."[1] This she would have to forego, if (her instincts and economic situation permitting) she abandoned such a life in favor of one more in accord with the demands of her conscience.

[1] Freud: "Allgemeines über den hysterischen Anfälle"; Sammlung kleiner Schriften zur Neurosenlehre, Bd. II.

CHAPTER VII

A COMPLETE report of an analysis would sometimes be as long as the stenographic report of a hard fought legal battle. An absolutely full analysis is impracticable as it would include an inventory of every thought and impulse the patient had ever had since birth.

The fact that up to the year 1917 there were not more than half a dozen comparatively complete reports of analyses published in any language, (one of Freud's was an unsuccessful case and the other a full analysis but incompletely communicated) has led me to give the following case in as great detail as the limits of this book allow. The ordinary objections against publishing such material are less weighty in the present case because the subject is a clinic patient whose friends are not likely to read it, and the circumstances of her neurosis were known only to her husband, who is now dead, to herself and to me.

The case is unsatisfactory because the work was interrupted and so the analysis is not a full one, but it is illuminating because of the documentary corroboration of the facts disclosed by the analysis and because of the clearness with which

308

it shows that the confessions of the patient were not "suggested" by the psychoanalyst. It confirms the correctness of some of Freud's conclusions as to the mechanism of neurotic disturbances, particularly the displacement of affects.

The case is also valuable in the light it throws on some points in psychoanalytic technique, showing as it does (1) the gross sexual element emerging first, (2) a non-sexual but exceedingly important factor disclosed later but with great resistance, (3) the insignificance from a therapeutical point of view of an apparent willingness to get well on the part of the patient, (4) the refutation of the charge that psychoanalysts read sex into everything and (5) the confirmation of the emphasis which psychoanalytic theory lays on sexual factors. The last point does not diminish the value of the present analysis as an illustration of the fact that other elements are not overlooked.

PART I. HISTORICAL

(a) Data of the First Visit

In May, 1911, there came to my office a small, plump, young woman who bore upon her round, good-natured-looking countenance an expression of distinct anxiety.

"Doctor," she said hurriedly, "I am afraid I am going insane. I once went to a fortune teller and I imagine he·is bewitching me; do you think it is all right for me to get married?"

This obsession had appeared in July, 1910, ten months earlier, when she was madly infatuated with a young man, and upon the advice of her cousin, a very superstitious girl, had sought the services of a fortune-telling magician. She had the idea that through his influence the young man would be stimulated to ask her hand in marriage.

Two days after this visit she was suddenly seized with a terrific fear that the fortune teller was exerting some spell over her as a result of which she would die. This fear of death was succeeded after a time by a fear of insanity. She soon sought treatment, and in November the obsession, which had continued with great intensity up to that time, almost completely subsided, only to appear again the following March (1911) in all its original intensity.

I was surprised to learn that the young man, Max by name, her infatuation for whom appeared to be the cause for her getting into all this trouble, was not the one she had in mind when she asked me about marriage. For in the early months of her illness, Max, serenely unaffected by the alleged powers of the man of magic, had passed out of the young lady's life. Another young man, whom we shall call Barney, had then presented himself and, swayed by no other form of sorcery than that which she herself exerted, had proposed to her and had finally been accepted.

The immediate cause of her great anxiety at the time she came to me seemed to be that the day set for her marriage to Barney was only three weeks off. She feared the fortune teller was making her insane and that she was thus destined to bring nothing but trouble and unhappiness upon her husband. She could not make up her mind what to do, for despite the fact that the various physicians she had consulted had without hesitation assured her that there was not the least likelihood of her ever losing her mind, she was not satisfied and could not banish the fear that in marrying she would do a great wrong to an innocent man.

I finally said that although I, too, was convinced that she was in no danger of becoming insane, I felt, nevertheless, that it would be well for her to postpone her marriage for some months in the hope that meanwhile she could get over her fears and thus take without any undue handicap the important step she contemplated.[1] But this, she

[1] Physicians are often consulted by neurotic patients contemplating matrimony who express some more or less vague fear that they may be impotent, or have syphilis, or suffer from some other ill which would render marriage inadvisable. They wish to be examined and assured that their fears are groundless, and as the physician usually does not find any evidence of the condition which the patient seems to fear, the assurance desired is as a rule promptly given. Now, as this case shows, one should, as a matter of fact, be extremely careful in such cases. The patient's fear that some condition exists which would prove an obstacle to marriage usually means either a *wish* that such were the case (showing that the individual in question is really of two minds in regard to the object of his affections and that to a certain degree he would welcome some excuse for not marrying) or that there actually is some reason why he ought not to marry, although *not* the one he fears. Both these things were true in the case of this young woman. But although in some cases it would be a serious mistake to advise the patient to go ahead and marry in spite of his fears, yet on the other hand there are cases in which to advise against marriage would be almost equally serious. In short, in most cases of this sort the physician has no way of knowing with any certainty what he should advise, unless he analyzes the patient, which unfortunately is in most instances imprac-

replied, was impossible. All the arrangements for her wedding had been made, the invitations had been sent out, and, finally, neither her own nor her fiancé's parents would listen to any proposal of delay. To follow my advice was out of the question.

After some further discussion relating to the treatment of obsessions and to the probability of her recovery, she told that she was very poor and asked if it would not be possible for me to treat her in a clinic. On this account I referred her to Cornell Dispensary.

(b) Results of the First Period of Treatment and Detailed History Obtained During that Time

At Cornell the young woman was treated for nearly a year with the ordinary medical remedies employed for such cases, and, in addition, with hypnotic suggestion administered once or twice a week by Dr. Stechmann or myself. Suggestion occasionally gave her relief which lasted for a few hours. Bromides and other drugs seemed to have no effect. Cold tonic baths received at another institution often gave her temporary relief. On the whole, however, she had not made the slightest permanent improvement at the end of this period of treatment. Her fear was just as intense and just as compelling as when I first saw her. Her marriage, which took place at the appointed time, seemed to have no particular effect upon her symp-

ticable. Cf. Jones, "Der Stellungsnahme des Aerztes zur den Aktual Konflikten," *Internationale Zeitschrift für Aerztliche Psychoanalyse*, Vol. III, 1915.

toms other than to cause temporary exacerbation of her fears just before it.

During this first period of the young woman's attendance at the clinic, although I made no real attempt at analysis, I talked with her from time to time and endeavored to obtain an accurate and detailed history of her neurosis and the events which attended its development. When, then, late in the spring of 1912 I decided to begin an analysis, I had at my command the following items of history. The patient, whom we may call Stella, was then twenty-three years old. Her family history was decidedly psychopathic. Her mother, two brothers, and her sister had at different times suffered from various forms of psychoneurosis.

The clinical past history which she gave contained nothing of particular interest. She had had the usual diseases of childhood, and had been inclined to be nervous as long as she could remember. Her menstruation had often been irregular and scanty. Sometimes weeks elapsed between her periods, and on a few occasions the interval had been as long as several months.

When thirteen and a half years old she had suffered, she stated, from some sort of nervous illness which lasted about two years. It was brought on, she believed, by the sudden death of an aunt about four years older of whom she had been extremely fond. The symptoms of this nervous illness she could not describe definitely, but she remembered that she lost weight, was very much depressed, and dreamed of her aunt nearly every night. One of the doctors who attended her made the statement that she was ''very poor in blood.'' She could not remember what her aunt died of, but thought ''it was from worrying about something.''

Physical examination was practically negative. The patient was well nourished, rather fat in fact; examination of the heart and lungs and nervous system failed to reveal anything significant. She had a moderate anæmia; the urine was negative.

Stella was born in a small village in Russia. Her parents were Hebrews, religious to the point of fanaticism and full of all sorts of Old-World fables and superstitious beliefs.

Stella's father, a Talmudic school teacher in his old home, had come to this country when she was five years old, but his family, which already included two boys both younger than Stella, did not join him until four years later.

In the New World little prosperity awaited them. The father, a man whose reputation for piety, honesty, and religious scholarship gave him no little standing in synagogic circles, did not shine in the world of business; and, although he managed to keep his family from falling into actual want, he was never able to provide any other home for them than a cheap flat in a lower East Side tenement.

When Stella was sixteen the family, by that time augmented by the arrival at different intervals of three more boys and one girl, threatened to become an economic problem so far beyond her father's power of solving that she sought employment in order to lighten his burdens. She soon obtained a place in a department store where she worked up to the year she was married.

Stella's education, begun in Europe along the most old-fashioned orthodox Jewish lines, was continued in this country in the public schools. From the beginning she not only displayed a great fondness for study, but also gave every evidence of possessing more than average intelligence. Throughout her school days she worked hard and almost invariably led all her classes. Her education was not extensive, however, for at thirteen and a half she had to stop school "because her mother needed her help with the housework."

Her religious ideas were in her early years a replica of those of her parents. She prayed and worshiped in the most orthodox manner, and, in addition, accepted without question the beliefs in magic, witches, the evil eye, and similar superstitions which prevailed in the town of her birth. After passing her fifteenth year, however, she went rapidly to the opposite extreme and, soon abandoning both religion and superstition, professed herself to be an absolute atheist and materialist.

Her infatuation for Max was her first love affair of any importance. She had always been popular with the young men, and she liked them, but at no other time had her affections become seriously involved.

Stella's affair with Max, her visit to the fortune teller, and the immediate sequelæ of this visit are of so much importance that I must take up the history of these matters in considerable detail.

In the early summer of 1910 Stella went to a country boarding house for her vacation. There she first heard of Max. He had been at the place the previous summer and made himself a general favorite. All spoke with enthusiasm of his intelligence, his refinement, and his good looks. He was to arrive shortly, and on the day he was expected, Stella, whose curiosity had been awakened by the praise she had heard of him, went to the railroad station in order to get an early glimpse of the paragon. Catching sight of him just as he stepped from the train, she felt, from that very instant, that she loved him. Immediately and with a sense of deepest conviction she said to herself, "Here is the man I must marry."

He was introduced, and appeared to like her at once. Soon, to her joy, it became evident that he preferred her society to that of any of the other girls, and in a short time her love became an all-consuming madness such as she had previously never dreamed of. She was in the most tensely excited emotional condition imaginable. She could neither eat nor sleep. At night, or whenever she was alone, she cried continually. She lost weight rapidly and to such a degree that her friends began to comment upon her appearance.

Max, though by no means in a condition of equal distraction, was to all appearances in love. From morning to night he was in her company, paid her every attention, and showed the utmost jealousy of every look or word she bestowed upon possible rivals. All the guests at the boarding house were sure that a proposal was imminent. Nevertheless it did not come. On the contrary, Max maintained a most inflexible reserve. Not the slightest hint of love passed his lips; never did he attempt even the most fleeting and noncommittal of caresses.

When their vacations ended and they both returned to the city, Max called on Stella frequently, took her to various places of amusement, and, as far as his acts were concerned, gave every evidence of love and devotion. But, in what he said, he was as reserved as ever. On no occasion did he let fall a single word that could be construed to mean anything more than that his feeling for Stella was the most ordinary unromantic sort of friendship.

This paradoxical attitude on the part of Max struck me as being so singular that I at once asked Stella if she knew the reason for it. "Yes," she replied, "Max was not a marrying man. I know that because he said so to a friend of mine, who told me all about it. But he assured my friend that if he were to marry anybody he certainly would marry me, and I know that is so."

When I asked *why* Max was not a marrying man, Stella explained that he was very ambitious, but had only a small salary, and, as he felt that an early marriage would seriously handicap him in business, he had decided to forego that pleasure. But this explanation, though seemingly plausible enough, left me with the vague suspicion that perhaps Stella was not telling all she knew.

Stella's disastrous visit to the fortune teller occurred in August of the same year she met Max. She had continued in a state of mad infatuation all summer, and, when she confided her condition to her cousin Rose, the latter immediately suggested magic as a way of inducing in Max a like state of mind, and ultimately bringing about a wedding. Rose, who was superstitious and credulous to the highest degree, supported her recommendation by relating a great number of instances of maidens (with whom, she said, she was personally acquainted) who had resorted to such methods with most remarkable and gratifying results. But Stella scoffed at these stories, as she did at all the rest of the wonder tales Rose was continually telling, and at first refused to have anything to do with magic and fortune tellers.

Some days later, however, when Stella had accompanied Rose, who had some eye trouble, to what we will call St. Christopher's Clinic, she said suddenly as they were walking home, "Rose, I think I would like to go to a fortune teller after all."

This suggestion Rose received with much enthusiasm, and, informing Stella that she had only recently heard of a man reputed to possess truly extraordinary powers, she proceeded to conduct her to him without delay.

The fortune teller, magician, or *Mahoshef,* as they called him, proved to be a fat, dirty, and ignorant Austrian Jew who inhabited a greasy tenement in the neighborhood of Canal Street. Rose was ushered into his presence first, while Stella waited in a room outside where the Mahoshef's wife entertained her with tales of his prowess.

Soon Rose returned in great excitement. "He's a *wonder*, Stella!" she cried. "He knows everything! He knew what your trouble was the minute you came in. He said right away that you were very nervous over a love affair. What do you think of that!"

Stella replied to this somewhat sarcastically, but she arose and went into the Mahoshef's room. She was already a little afraid of him. In spite of the fact that his wife's recital of his achievements had excited her profound contempt, and that the man's appearance and behavior, once she was in his presence, served to increase this feeling, she had, nevertheless, a vague fear of him all through the visit.

The first thing he did was to offer to tell her, without asking any questions, her own name and the name of her sweetheart, and though he succeeded in doing so by means of a somewhat clumsy trick, Stella immediately saw through it and jeered at him for his pains. But the Mahoshef, not in the least discouraged, wormed out of her the story of her affair with Max, and promptly assured her that by means of certain powers of which he was master he could not only obtain Max for her as a husband, but, if she preferred, any other man she would name, regardless of what his race, creed, color, or social position might be. As evidence of his ability in this line he showed her a book wherein, so he said, were written the names of many of the most prominent and wealthy women of the city, for all of whom he assured her he had performed similar services.

"I can do everything!" he cried boastfully. "For me all kinds of *Kishef* (magic) are easy!"

It was just about this point, however, that in spite of her contempt, in spite of her full appreciation of the grotesque incongruity between what the man professed to be and what his manner of living indicated, Stella began to believe him. She therefore directed him to proceed with his Kishef and bring Max to her feet at the earliest possible moment, while she permitted him to collect in advance the fee of fifty cents which he demanded for this important service. Her belief in him was so strong that when she left him—after he had urged her to buy an infallible cure he had invented for rheumatism and she had politely declined on the grounds that she was not at the time afflicted with that malady—she returned home in the most cheerful state of mind she had experienced in some months.

"I'm *so* happy," she said to Rose; "now I know I can marry Max."

There followed two days of joyful expectation. Stella and Rose talked continually of magic and witches, and of the pleasing results they expected from their venture. And all the while Stella's faith in the Mahoshef seemed unshaken; yet, paradoxically enough, her skepticism appeared to be almost as strong as ever. "It was all Rose's fault," Stella complained to me afterward; "she talked so much superstition into me that finally I got to believe it, although I really knew better."

On the evening of the second day after their

visit to the magician the two girls were lying in bed discussing the usual theme. Stella again said, "I'm so happy—now I can marry Max"; but after a pause she continued, "I'm sorry, though, to have to get him in this way. I don't like this magic business—I'd rather get him in the right way. I wonder what he'd think if he knew. I'm afraid I'm going to worry—I think that after we are married I'll tell him all about it—I'll worry myself sick if I don't."

"You're a fool," returned Rose. "Why should you worry about *how* you get him as long as you *do* get him? You're too honest! You make me sick!"

This matter was soon dropped and Rose went on to tell the story of a young woman who had caused a man to fall violently in love by secretly putting some menstrual blood in his tea. "It worked wonderfully," concluded Rose. "The man was crazy about her, but all the rest of his life he was never very well." "Oh, by the way," she went on, "did you know, Stella, that if Max has magic done to him he'll be weak and sickly all the rest of his life? He can't live to be older than fifty at the very most, and maybe not even that long."

Immediately upon hearing these words Stella was seized with terrible fear. "Oh!" she cried, "isn't that awful! I can't have a man's days shortened for my pleasure! I can't have him lose his life on my account."

"You are so stupid," replied Rose in great contempt; "why should you care? I wouldn't let the lives of fifty men stand in the way of my happiness.''

But this lofty sentiment had no effect upon Stella. Almost the very instant she heard the words, ''if Max has magic done to him he'll be weak and sickly all the rest of his life,'' the terrific fear had come upon her that the Mahoshef was exerting magic upon *her* and that *she* was going to die. All the rest of the night she spent crying and screaming in constant terror.

Early the next morning she went back to the Mahoshef, told him she did not want the young man after all, and begged him to stop the Kishef at once. He immediately and repeatedly assured her that she had nothing to fear, but this did not help her, and, returning home, she told her family that she was going to die, ordered her clothes to be given away, and indicated where she wished to be buried.

On the following day, although she was as much alive as ever, her fear was unabated, and she returned to the fortune teller to renew her entreaties, but, as before, without relief. For several days she continued to visit him, but, finally, as his assurances brought her not the slightest comfort, she told him she was going to see a doctor. He was evidently alarmed by this, and threateningly forbade her to do anything of the kind.

Eventually of her own accord, she went to the Broadway Clinic. There one of the clinic physicians became much interested in her case, and, as I have said, she finally improved under the hypnotic suggestion which he administered. But before this improvement took place she spent five days as a voluntary patient in a hospital for the insane and a week or so in a neurological hospital.

With the onset of her obsession, her attitude toward Max underwent a peculiar modification. Up to that time, although apparently she was madly in love with him, she had maintained the most perfect maidenly reserve. As soon as the obsession came on, however, her love for him seemed to diminish, but, singularly enough, her reserve diminished also. Though she had invariably been anything but forward in her relations with men up to that time, she now began to pursue Max in a most vigorous and aggressive manner. She continually pressed him to come to see her, hinted most broadly at the state of her affections, and used every means at her command to bring him to the point of proposing. But in spite of all her efforts he remained as noncommittal as ever—indeed, if anything, he became more reserved.

At last, driven to desperation by this Fabius of the affections, she adopted tactics which not only forced the issue, but, from the point of view of decisiveness, left nothing to be desired. Thus, one day in November, when Max was calling upon her, she said to him, "If a young man loves a young lady, and wants to marry her, he should say so. Otherwise, she might learn to love some one else."

Max, doubtless feeling unable to attack this obviously unimpeachable precept, replied, "If a young man were in love with a young lady, and felt that he was in a position to marry, he *would* say so."

And to this highly abstract proposition, which Stella apparently found to be quite as unassailable as her own, she made no reply.

Max then changed the subject, and, after discoursing for a short time upon the weather and other matters of equally profound public and private interest, politely wished her good evening and withdrew. Except for one occasion, when she happened to meet him on the street, she has never seen him since.

It was shortly after Max's final visit that she began to improve. From the time her obsession began she had been so sick that work was out of the question, but now she felt so much better that she became anxious to earn money again, and, in December, she went back to her old place in the store.

Her acquaintance with Barney began in November, soon after her friendship with Max ended. Previous to this time Barney had been living in another city and Stella had never seen him. However, she had heard of him frequently through his sister, Esther, who was one of her closest friends. Barney appeared to like Stella from the first, and, as time went on, his feeling rapidly became warmer, so that by the end of three or four months they reached a secret understanding and still later announced themselves as engaged.

For a while things went fairly well with Stella after she returned to work. Her fear of the fortune teller had almost disappeared, and she seemed to be in very good spirits. Then, in March, the fear suddenly returned and she was as sick as ever.

The revival of the obsession occurred under the following circumstances. Just before Saint Patrick's Day Stella heard some of the girls in the store talking of the coming celebration and asked one of them what it was that gave the Saint his particular claim to distinction. "Oh, don't you know that?" returned the girl. "Why, he was the one who drove the snakes out of Ireland."

Stella became fearful immediately. "Oh, that must have been magic!" she said to herself. "I'm afraid—if that could happen, maybe the Mahoshef can do magic to me!"

All the rest of the day she felt anxious and uneasy and kept thinking about magic and witches. The next morning when she awoke the old fear was upon her, in all its original fury.

She went to work, however, but in the store she was so overwhelmed by fear that she lost all control of herself, fell to the floor crying and screaming, and had to be taken home in a taxicab.

As soon as she was able to do so, she again went to the Broadway Clinic, but the treatment she received there helped her no longer. The fact of her approaching marriage added to her perplexities, and she felt her condition to be most desperate. Finally, she took some of the money she had saved for her wedding finery and went to see Dr. Dana, hoping that he could either convince her that she had nothing to fear, or else show her some way out of her difficulties.

She gave him her history, telling him particularly of her great fear that she ought not to marry, because, as it seemed to her, she might go insane at any moment.   Dr. Dana stated in most positive terms that she was not going insane and that she need have no fear on that score of making her husband unhappy.   This comforted her for perhaps an hour, but no longer, so in a few days she returned for further assurances.   Dr. Dana then referred her to me.

After this, as has been said, Stella came to Cornell Dispensary for nearly a year without obtaining any particular relief from her fears.   To be sure, she was no longer subject to the wild attacks of crying and screaming which occasionally had taken place during the first few months of her illness, and certain minor obsessive ideas connected with her major fear had apparently disappeared, for she ceased to talk of them.   On the whole, however, she had made no real improvement. These transitory obsessive ideas should be mentioned, for they will be of interest later.

When Stella first came to me she feared not only that the fortune teller was able to do Kishef to her, but *also that people he knew—his friends or acquaintances—likewise had this power.*   For this reason she was afraid to go to the neighborhood in which he lived.

In this same early period, Stella was also afraid of any one who looked at her fixedly, particularly strangers.   Thus, if she were on the street and saw some one staring at her, she would immediately fear that this person was performing magic on her and that she would become insane as a result.

In a similar way she was afraid of the doctor who had hypnotized her at the Broadway Clinic. Whenever she thought of him she feared that he was doing Kishef to her. He was in Europe the first summer she came to me, but the fact that she knew he was thousands of miles away from her did not diminish her fear in the slightest.

All these ideas were never very prominent, and, as I have said, Stella ceased to refer to them after a short time.

But her main obsession, the fear of the fortune teller, was remarkable for its intensity. Apparently she was in constant terror throughout all her waking moments. There was practically nothing that would interest her or take her mind away from herself more than momentarily. Over and over again she would say in a certain stereotyped way, "He has power over me—I'm afraid he's doing me harm—I feel I'm not safe—he bosses my thoughts—he's making me insane."

She continually questioned me about magic and similar matters. "Are you sure there isn't any magic?" she would ask. "How do you know there isn't—have you studied it? Is it a scientific fact that there can't be any? There were great men in the Bible, and Shakespeare was a great man, but they believed in magic and witches—how do *you* know they were wrong? If such bright men believed in those things there must be *some* truth in them—it makes me afraid—I think the *Maho-shef* has power over me," etc.

Any attempt I made to reassure her on any of
these points usually ended in making her feel
worse rather than better. For she would invariably corner me in some way, and, as soon as I
failed to give a satisfactory answer, she would be
in a panic.

Before her illness began Stella had always appeared to possess a very sunny, fun-loving disposition.   Even during it at times she showed a keen
sense of humor and talked in a very witty and
amusing way, but usually she was greatly depressed and ready to cry at a moment's notice.
Her depression, however, was as nothing when
compared to her fear.   Indeed, I recall no other
case of neurotic fear which so deeply and vividly
impressed me with the terrible reality of the patient's suffering, or in which the familiar hypocritical note of satisfaction was so conspicuously
absent from the patient's complainings.   There
was no doubt whatever that Stella was really and
honestly sick.

.   .   .   .

There are many other suggestive circumstances
which I could have included in this record of historical data, but I will omit all but three which
seem most significant in furnishing the back-
ground for the problem at the time of beginning
the analysis. The first of these was Stella's
intense and lasting rage when she discovered,
after her illness began, that at the time they first
went to him Rose and the Mahoshef were not total
strangers but had known each other some time;
the second was that for some time Stella concealed

from me her civil marriage which had taken place
a week before she first consulted me. (Jewish
people often have a civil ceremony performed by
a city official some little time before the religious
ceremony.) These two facts will be accounted
for later. (Pages 403 note and 424.)

A third matter which in part was equally mysterious, while at the same time another part gave
some hint of the nature of Stella's unconscious
psychic process, was her evident belief that if
Max had Kishef done to him he would be weak
and sickly all the rest of his life, and could not
live to be over fifty. Such credulity was entirely
inconsistent with her attitude toward all other
superstitious ideas. Though her obsession, and
certain compulsive thoughts connected with it,
represented a sort of belief in superstition, yet in
all these instances her "belief," if it may be so
called, was accompanied by an even more positive
disbelief, so that she would say in speaking of
these things, "I *fear* this or that is so, but I *know*
my fear is perfect nonsense," whereas in respect
to all superstitions not related to her morbid fears
she showed not a sign of credulity. But she never
said that she thought the prediction that Max
would be weak and sickly was perfect nonsense,
while her whole attitude, in ways I cannot describe in detail, thoroughly convinced me that she
had accepted this prediction as the absolute truth.
In short, her (apparently real) belief that Max
would be sickly was not, as in the case of her compulsive superstitions, accompanied by the simultaneous opposite feeling of disbelief.

But, although I could not explain *why* Stella did believe that Max would be weak and sickly, yet some of her remarks in this connection disclosed the existence of a conflict, and brought to light one of the several wishes or impulses which furnished the motive power of her obsession. Thus, she once remarked, "The thought that Max would be a sick man made me doubtful about marrying him. I was crazy to have him, but I didn't want to marry a man who was going to be ill for years and unable to support me. I felt that if I married him, and that if he was sick and had to die anyway, I wanted him to do it soon, and not to wait until I was so old I would have no chance of marrying again."

Here, obviously, was a distinct conflict. Stella was unwilling to give up Max, but she was apparently almost unwilling to be burdened for years with an invalid husband, which, for reasons not yet explained,[1] she believed Max would be. Under such circumstances she desired a compromise —namely, that Max's life would be short, for if she could look forward to this, she would neither have to forego the pleasure of marrying him, nor would she have to bear indefinitely the burden of an invalid husband.

But we can hardly suppose that Stella could have entertained a wish for Max's early decease without having a certain feeling of guilt. And guilt demands punishment. It seems, then, not unlikely that the obsession served this purpose, among others. She had wished for the Mahoshef to do magic to Max, and she had wished for Max's

1 See page 368.

death. What finer example could be desired of "that even-handed justice which commends the ingredients of our poisoned chalice to our own lips" than that as a punishment for these wishes she should have to fear that the Mahoshef was doing magic to her, and that she, too, was in danger of death? The fact, then, that the obsession was so well suited as a punishment for what Stella must have felt guilty of, makes it not unreasonable to suppose that an impulse to penance and self-punishment formed the first, though by no means the most important, of its determinants.

(c) *Preliminary Survey*

Before proceeding to report the results obtained during the period in which Stella was under analysis it may be well to state the problem as I saw it at the beginning of this treatment.

To those who hold to the suggestion-theory of the genesis of obsessions, this history, as I have related it, presents no conspicuous problems. A young woman of neurotic and presumably impressionable temperament, brought up among extremely fanatical and superstitious people, develops a neurosis during the strain and excitement incident upon an unsatisfactory love affair. This neurosis, judging from its content, is simply a re-awakening of a belief in magic which she entertained as a child. The visit to the fortune teller and the various remarks of the superstitious cousin—occurring, as they did, when the young woman was in a very excitable condition—would be looked upon as sufficiently influential to bring about the reawakening, and thus cause the neurosis. From such a viewpoint the case is little more than a simple equation. Neurotic predisposition, environmental influences, an event of presumably high suggestive value—all three factors tending in the same general direction—produce, when added together, an obsessive fear. What could be plainer? The case explains itself!

The psychoanalyst, however, would see in this history many points that call for extensive and careful investigation, and would feel utterly at a loss to explain the obsession without knowing a great deal more about the patient's life than has yet been recorded. Nevertheless, he might readily find in the material at hand matters which would lead to interesting speculations as to the etiology of the neurosis, and would give some hints both as to the nature of the problems confronting him and as to the sort of causal factors which he might expect to find.

For instance, it appears that the patient became sick in the midst of a love affair, improved as soon as it ended, but again became sick shortly after entering into an experience with another lover. Is this correlation between romance and illness to be looked upon as accidental or as causal? And if the latter, what sort of causes might be at work?

On theoretical grounds we may give partial and tentative answers to these questions. A neurosis, as Jung has said, invariably expresses some trend of thought and feeling away from, or hostile to, the individuals who stand in closest psychological re-

lation to the patient.[1]   Such a position was once
occupied by Max, later by Barney. We may therefore infer that some sort of emotional conflict
existed in the mind of the patient in regard to
these two persons—that for some unknown reason
it was impossible for her to adjust herself perfectly to either one of them, and that this non-
adjustment had to do with the outbreak of the
neurosis.

And this view is supported when we come to ex-
amine certain facts already at our command. For
example, Stella's love for Max was apparently
pathological. It began as a typical case of "love
at first sight." Although this phenomenon is perhaps normal enough in stories, it is seldom so in
real life. The condition, judging from the few
cases I have had a chance to study, is always a
compulsion. The patient has formed a strong
love-fixation—usually upon some individual of
high significance in the years of childhood—but
this fixation becoming for some reason offensive
to the patient's conscious personality has been subjected to repression and driven more or less completely from consciousness. The phenomena of
love at first sight represent either a transference
—usually incomplete—of this love, now partly or
wholly unconscious, to some new love-object,
against whom there are no particular conscious

[1] "Analytical Psychology," p. 129. As a matter of fact the persons to whom Stella stood in closest psychological relation were
her parents, and her neurosis showed that she was as poorly
adjusted to them as she was to Max and Barney. But the matter
of her adjustment to her parents is one that for the moment we
need not consider, although we shall take it up later.

resistances, or else a flight from the old love-object, or a combination of both transference and flight. In any case, the person apparently loved is not the person actually loved, though in time, in some cases, a complete transference may take place.

If we now apply these principles to Stella's case, our conclusion would be that Stella *seemed* to love Max so much, *simply because, in some unknown way, he represented a substitute for, or a flight from, some one else with whom she was actually in love, although probably she would not permit herself to realize it.*[1]

Incidentally, if the foregoing conclusions are correct, certain other features of her affair with Max become comprehensible. Thus, though ladies in story books are supposed to lose flesh and appetite, and to spend long hours in weeping whenever they fall in love, we cannot regard these manifestations as normal accompaniments of love in real life. If, however, we are right in supposing that Stella's love for Max was either an imperfect transference or a flight, these morbid phenomena are not so difficult to understand. That is, if, while she was consciously scheming to marry Max, she was unconsciously in love with some one else she had good reason to be depressed.

Other signs indicated a lack of adjustment in Stella's relations with Barney. It did not require a long acquaintance with Stella to convince me

---

[1] This does not mean, of course, that *all* her seeming love for Max had this origin—merely that a part of it did, particularly at first.

that she felt toward Barney none of the mad infatuation which she seemed to have experienced for Max. For instance, whenever she talked of Max her face would light up, and, for the moment forgetting her fears, she would plunge into the most vivid and enthusiastic description of him imaginable. "Oh," she would say, "he was *so* refined! How I loved him! I thought I'd die if I couldn't be his wife. If I could have married him I would have been contented to live in only one room all the rest of my days."

But when she spoke of Barney there was a great difference. "*Of course* I love Barney," she would say in a somewhat argumentative tone, as if expecting immediate contradiction from some invisible hearer: "I love him *as a friend*. My feeling for him is *geistliche Liebe*—not *Leidenschaft*. He is intelligent and refined and I respect him— yes, I have the *greatest* respect for him." But these protestations were accompanied by none of the enthusiastic animation that characterized her references to Max.

It was quite evident, then, that she felt for Barney a much less intense love than she appeared to feel for Max. But a still more positive conclusion in regard to this matter could be drawn. If an emotional, neurotic girl, on the very eve of her wedding, cannot work herself up to the point of saying of her betrothed something more enthusiastic than, "I love him *as a friend*—I *respect* him," one need have little doubt as to the true state of her feelings—in all probability she does not love him at all.

In full accord with this conclusion is another
matter that has already been mentioned. Stella
felt that she was doing wrong in getting married,
and that she was almost certain to make her husband unhappy. To be sure, these ideas *appeared*
to be a logical result of her *fears*. Seemingly, she
thought, "I am going insane, and *therefore* I ought
not to marry—*insanity* will be the means of my
bringing trouble upon my husband." But psychoanalytic experience shows quite conclusively
that a compulsive idea, or any similar symptom, is,
generally speaking, never the cause of *anything*
—it is always an *effect*.[1] We may conclude,
therefore, that, in Stella's case, her feeling that
she ought not to marry, and that she would make
her husband unhappy, depended not upon her obsession, but upon some other, concealed factor,
which adequately justified this feeling. In other
words, there must have been some good reason
why she should not marry Barney, although apparently she would not frankly admit this to herself. This reason was, perhaps, that she did not
love him, but did love some one else.

But if we continue these speculations we are
in great danger of falling into the error of feeling
that we understand the case when we have only
begun to study it. Let us, therefore, enter as
soon as possible into an examination of the ma-

---

[1] If, for example, a man develops a neurotic symptom which
apparently causes him to be unable to continue his business, we
are likely to find upon analysis that for some reason the man
wanted to give up his business, and that this wish was the immediate cause of his doing so.

terial brought out by my analysis, for by this means any danger of our feeling prematurely that we understand the neurosis will soon be effectually dispelled. Incidentally, it should be remarked at this point that thus far I have given Stella's history *as I received it—not as I know it now*—and that we may be prepared to find it in many respects erroneous, misleading, and incomplete.

PART II. ANALYTIC

(a) *The Father-Complex*

When I had finally decided to begin the analysis I informed Stella that I wished to try a new treatment—one which would require her fullest coöperation to be a success—and that her part would be to perform the difficult task of following a very simple rule, viz., to tell everything that came to her mind, whether or not the thought seemed to her pleasant or unpleasant, important or unimportant.

Having heard this solemn injunction, Stella began to laugh.

"That's silly," she said. "That will never cure me. Anyway, you know all about me already. What more can I tell you?"

But, after a few moments, she began to talk about her mother.

"My mother," she said, "is a very nervous woman. She is just like I am; she isn't well. I am more fond of my mother than of any one else in the world. Whenever she is out of my sight I worry about her and fear something will happen to her—that she may get sick or be killed in an accident.''

I felt that my acquaintance with Stella had lasted long enough to allow me to venture some comment on these remarks. I began by saying that not all that goes on in our minds is accompanied by consciousness; thus, we could have various impulses or wishes of quite considerable strength without being clearly aware of them. Such wishes sometimes presented themselves in consciousness in the shape of fears.

But at this point Stella interrupted me. ''What!'' she cried excitedly, ''do you mean that I *hate* my mother, that I *want* her to die?''

I said I was not able to deny that such a condition of affairs might exist and asked her what she thought about it.

''Oh, I know you are wrong,'' she exclaimed; ''I love my mother and always will. If she died, I would want to die, too.''

To this I replied that the existence of a very great love would not necessarily disprove the co-existence of an opposite feeling. Stella paid no attention to this, however, and in a somewhat illogical way continued her protests. At this point we were interrupted and had to defer the discussion to the next setting.

At the next visit she immediately began with the question, ''What could make me hate my mother?''

''I cannot say,'' I replied; ''what do you think about it?''

She answered that she could offer no explanation; but, after a considerable pause, she suddenly said, "Doctor, there is something I think I ought to tell you. My father used to touch me."

When I asked her to explain this remark she finally furnished me with the following information. When she was about twelve years old her father began a practice of coming to her bed at night, fondling and caressing her quite amorously, and placing his hand upon her breasts and genitals. This, Stella frankly admitted, had excited her greatly; and, though she had protested against these practices, she had always enjoyed them. She added, in explanation, that up to the time her obsessions began she had always been extremely passionate and easily excited.

Her father's visits had continued two or three times a week until she was somewhere between sixteen and nineteen years of age, when they ceased, but exactly when or under what circumstances Stella professed to be unable to remember. I can, however, supply the missing information from what I learned much later in the analysis. When she was seventeen and a half years old a number of friends were staying at her house, in consequence of which Stella slept in a different room from her usual one. In the middle of the night she was suddenly awakened by her father's standing over her bed and fumbling with her bedclothes. Not recognizing him for the moment, and being confused at not finding herself in her own room, she was very much frightened; but, when she did realize who it was, her fear was changed to anger

for the fright he had given her. "Why can't you
leave me alone!" she said indignantly. "Don't
ever do that to me again! I've had enough of
your nonsense."

"Can't a father kiss his own daughter?" he replied. "Anyway, I was only trying to see that
you were covered warmly enough."

"That is not so," returned Stella. "If you
must amuse yourself, why don't you go to my sister? If you ever try to touch me again, I swear I
will tell my mother!"

This threat seemed to have its effect, for her
father never ventured to resume his visits. Stella
had often protested against them before, but this
was the first time she had threatened to tell.

I trust that it is now plain that Stella had answered the question of why she "hated" her
mother. This hate, if it may be so called, depended upon her attachment to her father. The
fears that her mother would die, etc., were part of
the wish phantasy, which, as I later learned, she
had often entertained consciously, that her mother
would die, in order that she might assume the
mother's place with the father. These death
wishes and feelings of hate existed in spite of a
well-developed love for the mother. Let me again
emphasize that the ability to entertain simultaneously the two opposite feelings of love and hate,
with a high degree of intensity and toward the
same person, is one of the prominent characteristics of compulsion neurotics. In them love and
hate may coexist indefinitely, instead of one drowning out the other as would normally be expected to

occur. The opposed feelings in these cases are
not as a rule simultaneously conscious. The hate
is usually confined more or less successfully to the
unconscious, and the conscious and foreconscious
love becomes overdeveloped to serve as a reaction
and a cover for it.

A great deal more could very well be said of
Stella's father-complex, which, it should be evident to any one, must have been extremely strong.
I will not pursue this subject, however, simply for
the lack of space, as there is so much else that requires discussion. We shall later hear more of
the effect of this complex.

(b) The Separation-Complex

The next matter that came into prominence in
my talks with Stella was the question of her feeling and attitude toward her husband. Even before beginning the analysis I had come to the conclusion that she cared little for Barney and had
asked myself why she had married him. The
question became even more puzzling, for I learned
that while she had been receiving attention from
Barney, Stella had had still another suitor, upon
whom she had looked with much more favor. This
man, whom I will call Lehmann, was not only
much better looking than Barney, but, in addition,
he was a manufacturer in most comfortable circumstances, while Barney was practically penniless. Lehmann was madly in love with Stella,
and his family would have looked with favor upon
the match. And so I felt sure she would have
much rather married Lehmann than Barney, though

whether she would have preferred Lehmann to Max I was not certain. The question of why she married Barney was, then, greater than before.[1]

Early in the analysis Stella had a dream, which, although throwing some light on the problems in the case, seemed at first to add to them rather than otherwise. The dream was simply that a certain recently married woman had left her husband, then residing in Boston, and come to New York.

This dream was a reproduction of an actual fact that had occurred in Stella's experience. The woman referred to, after living with her husband only a few weeks, had run away from him and returned to her parents in New York.

We are familiar with the observation that the chief actor in the dream is practically always the dreamer. With the woman of the dream Stella could readily identify herself, for both had worked in the same store and both had been married for only a short time. One could suppose, then, that the woman represented none other than Stella herself. Stella dreamed, then, that she followed the example of her friend; and this could only mean that she, too, had a wish to leave her husband and return to her parents.

[1] I should, perhaps, state at this point that this and similar questions that came up in the analysis I submitted to Stella in the hope that she would answer them. It was quite useless, however, for she would either reply that she "did not know" or else would give some evasive explanation which it was quite impossible to accept. For instance, many times she maintained that she had married Barney for love alone, whereas at other times her own admission, as well as many other indications, showed that this explanation was entirely incorrect.

Hoping, however, to find some more significant source of identification than that just mentioned I asked Stella to tell me more about the woman. She responded by informing me that the woman was very fat, while her husband was quite the reverse; and then added this most singular remark, *"I think she was too strong for him."*

What Stella meant by this I had not the slightest idea, so I asked at last if she had used the phrase in some sexual sense, and to this she assented with such alacrity that I was quite sure she had meant nothing of the kind—that is to say, I felt she was unwilling to explain exactly what she had in mind, and so when I had suggested that it was something sexual she readily agreed, thinking this would satisfy me and that I would press her no further. Being now quite convinced that there was some really important reason for Stella's identifying herself with the woman, and that it probably was contained in her relations with Barney, I asked, "Did you ever feel that you were too strong for Barney?"

"Yes," she answered rather reluctantly and would say nothing more.

I kept on questioning her and finally brought to light, first, that Barney suffered from *ejaculatio præcox*, and, second, the following matter, which seemed even more important. Barney had suffered several attacks of gonorrhea before his marriage. A short time before I began the analysis he, discovering what he believed to be a returning gleet, had consulted a doctor, who for some reason examined his semen and told him, in

Stella's presence, that in all probability he was sterile and would remain so. This was very painful to Stella, for, as she then told me, she was extremely anxious to have children, not only because she was most fond of them, but also because, as she expressed it, to have them would make her marriage stronger.

I was not at all convinced that the information I had obtained had exhausted the significance of the dream, and I was even in doubt as to whether all of it had to do with the dream, because, as I had broken in with questions, I could not regard all of Stella's statements as free associations. At any rate, whether connected or not, both the information I brought out and the dream were evidently of no small importance. The dream showed plainly enough that Stella had a wish to separate from her husband, but whether this arose from the mere fact that he was sterile, or whether there were other reasons for it, could not at the time be determined.

I told Stella that I interpreted the dream as an expression of a wish on her part to leave her husband, but she promptly disputed this, saying, "I will never want to separate *so long as we are both alive.*" But, as this sounded to me as if she had an alternative in mind, I said, "Do you mean that you would like him to die and free you?"

"No," she replied instantly, "I do not wish him dead"; but, after a pause, she suddenly said, "I am not going to lie to you; I have wished him dead, often. This morning when I was washing his clothes I swore to myself and said that I wished they were his death clothes.''

She went on to say, however, that she did not feel this way all the time. ''When he is nice to me, and when I think we can go ahead and make money, keep up a nice home, and maybe have children, I feel that I can love him and I do not wish him dead; but, when he is mean, I hope he will die right away. Usually, when I wish him dead, I am sorry afterwards and think maybe I will be punished for such thoughts.''

It was not until after this communication that Stella told me of a new detail of her fears. It seemed that before her marriage she was afraid to let any one know about her illness for fear that it would come to Barney's ears and he, thinking her either insane or about to become so, would withdraw from the engagement. After her marriage she was even more afraid that, as a result of magic, she would become insane and he would then be able to divorce her. After she had once told me this detail, it became one of the most frequent themes in Stella's conversation. She continually asked me to assure her that she was not insane; she did all sorts of things for fear people would think her so; she would never admit to any one that she felt ill in any particular for fear they would immediately conclude that she was losing her mind; and she was never tired of questioning me in regard to the laws relating to insanity and divorce. She was particularly distressed by the fact that her history was on file at the Broadway Clinic and similar places.

"I know," she would say, "if that history, in which it is written that I went to a fortune teller and then *thought* I was insane, was brought into court, the judge and jury would surely believe I really *was* insane and give Barney a divorce in a minute."

When I reminded her that all the doctors she had consulted had instantly told her she was not insane or ever likely to be, she would reply, "I am afraid if it came to court they would change their minds." "I don't believe they would stick to what they said." "I am afraid they would go back on me." "Maybe they were afraid to tell me the truth, anyway," etc.

I noticed that she talked more about her history at the Broadway Clinic than about any of the other histories and seemed ever so much more anxious over it. She was continually planning to go to this Clinic and, on pretense of requiring treatment, get hold of her history and tear it up, but she never planned to do this with the history at the neurological hospital or at Cornell. Indeed, many times she started for the Broadway Clinic, intending to do away with the record, but on the way would come the reflection, "Maybe it would look worse if I did tear it up—maybe people would think I did it because I knew I was insane and was trying to destroy the proof," etc., and thus she never got to the point of putting her plan into execution.[1]

[1] This element of her fear, namely, that by means of the history at the Broadway Clinic it would be proved that she was *insane,* etc., is what I had in mind particularly when, in the introduction,

Two sets of reproaches, quite similar in content to the obsessive fear that she would be divorced she frequently made against her husband. The first originated in the fact that he had once lived in the same house with a young woman named Ada, who apparently would have liked very much to marry him, although there is no reason to suppose he reciprocated this feeling. That he was in all probability utterly indifferent to Ada, Stella in her "sober moments" seemed to know as well as any one. Nevertheless, the greater part of the time she was loud in her complaints that Barney cared nothing for herself but was only waiting until she should become insane so that he could divorce her and marry Ada.

"He is no man!" she would cry. "Anybody else would stick by a wife if she got sick, but he wouldn't! As soon as he found he could prove me insane he would do it, and get rid of me as quickly as possible."

These complaints, uttered in the most spiteful, angry tones imaginable, Stella repeated hundreds of times; and, when she was in the mood for complaining, no argument could make her see what at other times she freely admitted, viz., that her accusations were entirely without foundation.

Another set of reproaches against Barney referred to his attitude in money matters. She continually complained that he was mean and stingy,

I spoke about displacement as shown by this case. We shall see eventually that her anxiety about her history at this clinic was indeed well founded, but that the foundation for it was something entirely different from what appeared in her obsession.

that he insisted on her working at the store when she should have been caring for things at home. She was particularly venomous over the recollection that one time he made her go to work in a snowstorm, when, in her opinion, the weather was so bad that she should have stayed at home. "I might easily have caught pneumonia and died from being out on a day like that," she said, "but he wouldn't care. A few pennies are more to him than my health and life. The only thing he married me for was that I should work for him."

As a matter of fact, her husband did insist upon her working at times, but, apparently, not from choice. Financial conditions were bad; he had little work; and what she could earn was not only a very acceptable addition to the family income but at times an absolutely necessary one. He, as in a way she really well knew, did not demand of her anything that other men in the same walk of life did not expect from their wives.

That Stella's complaints were absolutely unfair and unreasonable no one was in a better position to know than herself. Why, then, could she not take a reasonable view of the situation and give up her unjust complaining? The obvious explanation that she *wanted* to think her husband at fault in these matters—that it gave her some sort of comfort or satisfaction to be able to accuse him in this wise. But why should this sort of thing give her satisfaction? This question, to any one with a little analytic experience, is not difficult to answer. She must have felt herself guilty of the same things for which she reproached her hus-

band. This defense mechanism is a very familiar
one and has been referred to earlïer in Chapter IV.
Stella's reproaches against her husband could,
then, be applied to herself; and this means, first,
that she had the intention of getting rid of her
husband and marrying some one else, and, second
(since she reproached her husband with being too
interested in money matters), that some financial
or economic condition must have interested her
more than she felt was right. This interest perhaps, in some unknown way, had been a factor in
bringing about their marriage; possibly she had
married Barney merely to have some one to support her.

It is to be observed that Stella's complaint that
her husband wished to get rid of her is quite in
harmony with the dream just analyzed. Both
indicated that Stella wished or intended her marriage to Barney to be only temporary. She would
not admit, however, that she wished for a separation, although, as the analysis progressed, she
showed little hesitation in confessing that the
greater part of the time she most heartily wished
her husband was dead. That she really did wish
for a separation, perhaps as an alternative less
acceptable than her husband's death, I firmly believed in spite of her denials. Indeed, I was disposed to think that this wish was a determinant
of her fears that through the fortune teller's Kishef she would become insane and be divorced.
But as I was in no position to prove my point I
had to let the matter drop for the time.

Before leaving the theme of Stella's reproaches

against others, I must take up her attitude toward
her husband's sister. This girl originally had
been one of her closest friends, but Stella had not
been married very long when they began to quarrel most frightfully. It was plain to be seen, however, that these quarrels were really Stella's fault.
They usually originated from her making without
the slightest provocation some unreasonable and
unjust accusation against her sister-in-law. One
thing which seemed to be concerned with Stella's
inclination to pick these quarrels, and to which
she frequently referred during her visits to me,
was this. It seems that shortly before her marriage, Stella on the advice of some doctor and
contrary to her own inclination, had told Barney
of the obsession from which she suffered, and he in
turn had told his sister. (I should add here that
Stella promptly repented of her confession and
soon after her marriage told her husband the obsession had entirely disappeared.) Some time
after they were married Barney was out of the
city for a few days, and, as it so happened, his departure had followed closely upon an argument in
which Stella, his sister, and himself were all involved. During his absence his sister wrote him
a letter which Stella, prying through his things
upon his return, found and read. This interesting document contained among other matters the
following words: "That girl (Stella) was insane
when you married her. Maybe she isn't exactly
insane now, but just the same she will always
have a crazy head. She knew she was a sick girl

when she married, but you were an easy mark and let her rope you in.''

Stella's rage upon perusing these amiable sentiments should have found adequate expression in her having torn her clothes and hair, yelled, screamed, rolled on the floor, and ornamented with her nails the faces of her husband and his offending sister; still all this by no means removed the memory of the incident from her mind nor served to prevent her from bearing a lasting resentment. Indeed whenever she thought of the matter she would immediately become incoherent from anger and excitement. ''Roped him in!''; she would cry. ''A nice remark for a friend to make! The mean, low, false thing! Could any *decent* person say a thing like that? There isn't a more false and tricky girl in the world. I'd like to scratch out her eyes and wring her neck,'' etc.

Again applying the principle of interpretation already described, one would have to conclude that Stella thus reproached her sister-in-law because she herself felt guilty of being a false friend. In just what respect she had been false remains to be seen, however.[1]

The fact that Stella found the accusation, ''she roped you in,'' so painful has to be explained in another way. The reason this remark so aroused her anger must have been, I concluded, that it contained a very considerable element of truth. If the accusation had been *entirely* unjust, I felt, she would not have minded it nearly so much. ''It's

[1] Page 423.

only the truth that hurts." But, having come to such a conclusion, I was no better off than before, for, as far as I was aware, Stella had never done anything that could well be described as "roping in" Barney. To be sure, she married him without caring particularly for him, but, even so, it was Barney who had been the aggressor, and if any "roping in" had occurred he himself had done it. In spite of these facts, I could not reject my original conclusion that in some sense Stella had "roped in" Barney and that she felt guilty about it, but the only course left for me was to wait in the hope that in the course of the analysis new material would be brought out to confirm my views.

Let me now sum up what has been learned in regard to Stella's feeling and attitude toward her husband. First, the conclusion that Stella married Barney caring little or nothing for him, which was reached before taking up the analysis proper, has been fairly well confirmed. Second, from analyzing one set of Stella's reproaches against Barney there has been furnished reason to suppose that some unknown economic conditions caused her to marry him. At the same time, this was hard to understand, since she had another suitor, Lehmann, whom, apparently, she preferred to Barney, and who was better off financially. Third, we have reached the conclusion that Stella wished to be free again either through Barney's death, or, possibly, through divorce or separation. Fourth, we have two other pieces of information which are as yet of uncertain significance; viz., that somehow or other Stella felt guilty of roping Barney in, and that, whatever it might mean, she felt that she was "too strong for him."

(c) The Assault Obsession

Let us now leave for a time the subject of Stella's relations with Barney and take up another matter which at first seems to have no connection with the first. Stella had been coming to me some considerable time when one day she said suddenly, "Doctor, the Kishef obsession is not the only one I ever had. Several years ago I had another that I have been afraid to tell to you."

The complete history of this first obsession I was a long time in learning. I will, however, give it here without going into the details of how I acquired my information. Stella, when about seventeen and a half years of age, had once taken supper at the house of a friend of hers, a young married woman named Mrs. Denzer. Mr. Denzer was not present at this meal, but considerably later in the evening he came in accompanied by two other young men, who boarded in his household. For some unknown reason Stella began to have a certain fear of these men, although in her previous acquaintance with them nothing had occurred to justify such an emotion. But, in consequence of this feeling, she soon arose and, putting on her hat, announced that it was time for her to go home. But Mrs. Denzer would not hear of her departure and insisted that Stella must spend the night. This made Stella more anxious than ever, and she protested with no little vehemence that for her to

remain all night was impossible. Mrs. Denzer
was deaf to these protests, and finally settled the
matter by locking the only door of exit and putting the key in her pocket, so that Stella had to
stay whether she liked it or not. By this time
Stella's anxiety had shaped itself into a definite
fear, viz., that after she had retired for the night
one of these men would attempt to assault her in
her sleep. That such a fear was utterly absurd
she was quite well aware, for none of the men
had ever betrayed the slightest inclination to do
anything improper either to her or, as far as she
knew, to any other well-behaved young woman.
But, in spite of this, she was unable to drive the
fear from her mind. She decided, therefore, that
after going to bed she would try to remain awake
all night, while as an additional precaution she
took her underskirt and bound it over her genitals,
so that, should she fall asleep in spite of herself,
any evilly intentioned person would have difficulty in carrying out his purpose. However good
her intentions may have been, she did fall asleep
eventually, and when she awoke an hour or two
later she found herself possessed by the horrible
fear that while she slept the dreaded occurrence
had actually come to pass, namely, that one of the
men—she knew not which—had assaulted her
while she was unconscious. After a hasty self-
examination for evidences of such a happening
she was momentarily relieved to find that the bandage she had made of her underskirt was undis-
turbed and that such signs as genital soreness,

drops of blood, or any of the similar phenomena which she had been led to expect were accompaniments of the first coitus, were entirely absent. The relief following upon this examination was short-lived, however, for it occurred to her that while she slept any blood stains might have been removed and the bandage readjusted or that her imaginary seducer might have known of some method of performing the act without leaving any painful results. Thus, her fear persisted, and she said to herself, "Since I was asleep, I have no *absolute* knowledge or proof that it didn't happen."

At any rate, she left the house of her friend as quickly as possible and in a most distracted condition hurried home. Arriving there, she threw herself upon a bed, crying and screaming. Her mother, attracted by the noise, came in, and Stella soon told her what she feared and insisted upon being examined then and there for evidences of defloration. Her mother promptly complied with this request and assured Stella that there was absolutely nothing the matter with her except "Mushagahs im Kopf." [1] But this did not satisfy the young lady, and in a day or two she had herself examined by a doctor, but with the same result. Her fear remained unabated in spite of the doctor's assurances. In the next few weeks she went to one doctor after another, receiving from each assurances that everything was as it should be, but without gaining any relief from her fear.

[1] Craziness in the head.

Why these assurances did not assure her will later become clearer. They did not touch the right spot.

All this time she was extremely anxious to obtain a certificate to the effect that she was a virgin, but she hesitated to ask for it for fear that the doctors would suspect her of "something queer." At last, after returning home from having been examined by a woman doctor, who, by the way, had hurt her considerably, Stella found a drop or two of blood on her underskirt. This discovery greatly excited her, for she felt that even if up to this time she had been wrong in fearing her hymen was ruptured, there was no doubt of its being ruptured now, as the result of the doctor's examination. Hence, she returned to this physician, demanding a certificate which should state either that her hymen was entirely intact, or else that it had been ruptured accidentally during examination. Such a certificate, somewhat ambiguously worded, she did finally receive.

The assault obsession lasted without abatement for some eight or nine months, but then it gradually cleared up. After this it reappeared occasionally even up to the time the Kishef obsession began, though never with any great severity.

Naturally enough, Stella told of this obsession to very few people. One she told was her mother, who, much to Stella's real or assumed dissatisfaction, told it to her father. The only other person to whom Stella spoke about it was Rose, the same cousin who was connected with the Kishef incident. To Rose she did not speak frankly, however.

Rose had observed that Stella seemed to have something on her mind, and questioned her as to the nature of the trouble. Stella at once began to cry, saying, ''Rose, I am afraid something awful has happened to me—something that has made my body different than it was. If what I fear is really true, it would be wrong for me to get married, and I ought not to do it.''

I should, perhaps, state that the question of marriage had come up at this time, for Stella had a suitor, a young man in good circumstances, who was highly favored by her parents, although not, if we are to believe her, by Stella herself. But, at any rate, his attentions lasted only a short time, and he soon passed out of her life.

Now, toward understanding the motivation of this obsession the following matters can be produced. First, it is to be noted that the obsession came on only a short time after the incident I have described and which put an end to her father's masturbatic visits to Stella's bedside. One might suppose, then, that her libido, thus cut off from its earlier outlet, had found a new channel of expression in the shape of the obsession. Incidentally, Stella, ill with an obsession, was in a position (of which, I may add, she took every advantage) to demand more in the way of sympathy and attention from her father than she would have been able to secure under ordinary circumstances. Thus, she received a sort of compensation for the loss of the more physical form of gratification which was no longer forthcoming. Furthermore, the illness, which gave her father an enormous

amount of trouble and distress, served as a
weapon with which she revenged herself upon him
for taking her too readily at her word and stopping his visits.[1] It also seems probable that the
self-reproach connected with the idea of assault
represented a displacement of the guilt which she
had felt for allowing her father to touch her and
for wishing he would continue to do so.

But there is also reason to suppose the obsession represented a direct fulfillment of certain
wishes that Stella had previously entertained.
For both in day dreams and in night dreams she
had frequently imagined herself to be the subject
of an assault, and she was perfectly conscious of
having had a wish that through no fault of hers
such a thing might happen to her. For, as she
explained, though she would never part with her
chastity *voluntarily,* yet, if in spite of her best en-
deavors to the contrary it was taken away from
her *by force,* the situation would then be quite different. Her virginity once lost, the chief motive
for remaining in the paths of virtue would have
been done away with, while, on the other hand, she
would feel almost justified in compensating herself for the catastrophe by indulging in intercourse, a form of pleasure which, as she was of a
very erotic nature, she was extremely desirous of
having.

[1] The relation between the obsession and a wish on Stella's part
to be masturbated by her father will be referred to again in connection with the analysis of the Kishef obsession, where at the
same time the significance of Stella's repeated visits to doctors
will be given further consideration.

That some erotic wishes were in her mind the night the obsession came on is not to be doubted, for she distinctly remembers that all the evening she was at Mrs. Denzer's she had been occupied in comparing, with a certain envy, her friend's situation with her own. Thus, she not only reflected on the pleasures that were accessible to her friend upon retiring, but also indulged in certain erotic fancies in which she occupied her friend's place in the domestic relation, or passed through similar experiences with a husband of her own. It seems highly probable, then, that Stella's erotic wishes formed one of the determinants of the obsession; that is, as she herself summed up the situation, "What I imagined that evening at first for pleasure soon became a fear and finally an obsession."

But the obsession probably corresponded to the imaginary fulfillment of still another wish, namely, a wish for pregnancy. I have already stated that Stella's menstruation had always been irregular. During the period of her father's nocturnal ministrations, and on such occasions as she did not become unwell when she expected, she was always terrified by the thought that she was pregnant by him. (It should be added that this fear, which, of course, can be readily translated as the fulfillment of a wish, is not as absurd as it seems, for her knowledge of how impregnation is effected was at that time very vague.) A wish to be pregnant by her father as well as by others had even entered her consciousness at times, for she well remembered that she had frequently indulged in day phantasies having such a content. That the wish to be pregnant was uppermost in Stella's mind on that particular night can hardly be doubted, for Mrs. Denzer had two children the possession of which Stella greatly envied her and which she at times took pleasure in imagining were her own. An additional fact which I learned much later was that Stella was expecting to be unwell on the night the obsession appeared. But, since she had this expectation on the fateful night, her bandaging herself on retiring was not so entirely without reasonable motivation as it at first seemed. This act was in part prompted by the reflection that the flow was due to appear, and when on the morrow it had not done so, she had a sort of confirmation of the idea she had been assaulted; that is, she found herself displaying one of the symptoms of pregnancy.[1]

To sum up, then, our present knowledge of the obsession, it formed an imaginary fulfillment to two wishes, one to be assaulted and the other to be pregnant and to have children. The wish to be assaulted, as Stella pointed out, was not so much a desire for the act itself as a wish that through no fault of hers she would be placed in such a position that she would have nothing further to lose by illicit sexual relations. The obsession also served as a means of obtaining compensation for the loss of her father's sexual attentions and for denying herself the pleasure of marrying the young man who was then courting her. Just why

[1] An additional fact in regard to the delay of this period will be produced later. Page 387.

she did not take advantage of this opportunity to gratify her desires in a normal way by marrying him will become clearer as we go on with the analysis.

But, before temporarily leaving the subject of this obsession, as we will have to do now, let me express a hope that no one will be hasty in judging the interpretation offered as fanciful and absurd, for at a later stage in the report of this analysis, material is to be produced, which, to my mind at least, forms most adequate and surprising confirmation.

(d) The Main Sources of Resistance against Marriage

We shall now again occupy ourselves with the theme of Stella's relations with her husband. The analysis had been in progress, if I remember correctly, between two and three months when a very serious occurrence took place. Barney, who, without my knowledge, had for some little time complained of a cough and a tendency to become easily tired, finally presented himself at a public clinic, where, after being examined, he received the depressing intelligence that he suffered from pulmonary tuberculosis. This diagnosis was soon confirmed at other clinics, and, consequently, preparations were immediately made for sending him to a sanitarium in the country.

When Stella, who for a few days had been so fully occupied that she did not present herself at the dispensary, resumed her visits and communi-

cated to me this distressing information I was
surprised to observe that there apparently was not
the slightest change in her mental condition, either
for the worse or for the better.   One would naturally expect a crisis of this sort to have produced
some exacerbation of her symptoms or, possibly,
the reverse, and the fact that nothing of the kind
occurred arrested my attention immediately, although at the time I could think of no way of explaining it.   I did arrive at an explanation, later,
however, upon the basis of the facts which I shall
now present.

The first fact which upon analysis seemed to
have a bearing on the question in hand was this.
Stella had once told me that some time in the first
three or four months of her coming to the clinic
she had conceived the idea that I was an Irishman,
and that this thought had caused her to feel a certain aversion or resistance toward me.   That she
did feel so surprised her considerably, for she had
never before been conscious of any prejudice
against the Irish; and, in addition, her reason told
her that, despite her peculiar feeling to the contrary, I was not Irish.   I learned eventually that
she first felt this aversion toward me one morning when she noticed a spot of blood on my lip,
where I had cut myself in shaving.   We shall defer for a moment the analysis of this peculiar idea
in order to take up the presentation of another.

One day, some weeks *before* the matter of her
husband's tuberculosis came up, Stella inadver-
tently addressed me as *Mr.* Frink.   This particularly impressed me because in our acquaintance

of over a year she had not done so to the best of
my recollection. I immediately asked her to explain her mistake, and she replied that she could
not, adding, however, that there came to her
mind the thought of a certain Mr. Schermer.
Asked for some information about this man, Stella
told me that she had made his acquaintance a few
days before under the following circumstances.
A certain relative of her husband had had the misfortune to be arrested for the violation of some
sanitary law and at the moment of our conversation was languishing in jail. Stella had been
detailed to interview Mr. Schermer, the head of a
certain lodge to which the incarcerated one belonged, in the hope of invoking some financial and
political aid in that gentleman's behalf. Mr.
Schermer had listened to Stella's representations
with many expressions of sympathy, but it soon
became apparent that his position in the matter
could be summed up in the words, ''I am sorry, but
I can't do anything.''

Having concluded the description of her visit
to Mr. Schermer, Stella paused. Urged to give
further associations, she stated that there came
to her mind a certain Mr. Frank, but immediately
explained that this association was of no consequence, for she had thought of him merely because
his name was so similar to mine.

We are accustomed to find that when two idea
groups are connected by a superficial association
—one of sound, for instance, as in this case—they
are also connected by some deeper, more important, but concealed association. With this in mind,

I asked Stella to tell me what occurred to her about Mr. Frank. And, since her association concerning Mr. Schermer had contained the idea, ''he couldn't do anything,'' I was not surprised when Stella told me that there had been confided to her by Mrs. Frank the information that Mr. F—— was impotent. My explanation of Stella's slip of speech was, then, that she had identified me with some other individual who in some undiscovered particular resembled Mr. Frank in being sexually weak and Mr. Schermer who, in another sense, ''couldn't do anything.''

Now, I happened to know that, at the time, Stella was identifying me with both Max and Barney, for she frequently took occasion to remark that in our looks and manners she perceived many points of resemblance. But, feeling that there was some basis of identification deeper than mere similarity in appearance and manners, I asked of Stella, ''Did you think Max was sexually weak?''

''I did,'' she replied, after a moment's hesitation.

''And do you think me so?'' I continued.

''I hope you will excuse me,'' she replied, laughing, ''but I think you are weak, too.''

Upon considering this information, however, it at first did not seem very illuminating, after all. I had supposed that Stella had in some way identified Max, Barney, and me; that is, that there was some unknown common factor which she ascribed to us all. The associations just recorded seemed to indicate that this was sexual weakness, and she had already told me that Barney suffered from premature ejaculation. Yet the view that she ascribed *to all three of us* some sexual weakness was difficult to accept, for by what conceivable process of reasoning could she have formed any opinion in regard to the sexual power of Max and myself? Furthermore, something in Stella's tone made me suspicious that the phrase, "sexually weak," did not comprehend all she had in mind, but merely served as a cover for something else she was not ready to betray. The phrase must have had some significance, however, for it had come up in connection with the dream already related when it was associated with the idea that she was "too strong" for her husband.

It occurred to me that sterility might be the concealed common factor, for Stella supposed her husband to be sterile and knew that I had no children. But here again arose the same difficulty. Though she might suppose two members of the triad to be sterile, how could she have formed any opinion about Max in this particular?

I had, then, either to abandon my hypothesis that some reproductive weakness was, in her opinion, common to the three of us, or else conclude that she had in mind some other sort of deficiency, possibly related to sex, and that it was this that she supposed to be common to Barney, Max, and me. This latter conclusion seemed to me the most acceptable, for there had been a hint of this same elusive deficiency, whatever it might be, in the results of the analysis of the dream.

There soon came to light another transference phenomenon, which proved to be the key to a solution of the mystery. Stella began to manifest a considerable anxiety about my health. She would tell me I smoked too much, that I should spend more time in the open air, and that I must be careful about my diet. These remarks usually ended in her laughing at herself and saying that, since I was a doctor, I must think her very presumptuous in advising me on matters of health. But, in spite of this, as likely as not at the next visit she would repeat the whole performance.

This anxiety about my health might very well indicate that she suspected or feared that I had some malady of a general nature and not primarialy sexual. But some essentially nonsexual illness might have, secondarily, an injurious effect upon one's potence and reproductive ability. Thus the hints that had come up to the effect that Stella thought Barney, Max, and me deficient in the sexual sphere might really have had an origin in her thinking that all three of us suffered from some nonsexual physical malady. Upon analyzing Stella's peculiar notion that I was an Irishman, not only is the hypothesis confirmed but the analysis also discloses what physical illness she supposed we had.

It will be remembered that her thought that I was Irish came on when she saw a spot of blood upon my lip. Blood upon the lips might well suggest hemoptysis, and, hence, tuberculosis. Now, Stella was accustomed to refer to tuberculosis as the "Con" and to a person suffering from that disease as a "Conner." But Connor is a familiar Irish name. I am thin and quite subject to colds;

hence, when Stella saw a drop of blood upon my lip there could easily have started in her mind a train of thought having as its theme a question as to whether I were not a consumptive. But, if for any reason Stella had a resistance against the theme of tuberculosis, what more natural than that, if she began to suspect that I was a "Conner" in the sense of being consumptive and to feel a certain aversion to me on that account, this affect of aversion should be displaced by way of the other meaning of the word (Connor) and so appear in her consciousness attached to the thought that I was an Irishman? In this way it becomes clear how Stella could feel a repugnance to me as being an Irishman and yet at the same time be convinced that I was not Irish.

This interpretation, I confess, might easily be regarded as rather fanciful were it not for the fact that the thought that I was Irish had such a significant starting point, viz., the spot of blood upon my lip. This, it seemed to me, placed my interpretation practically beyond question and justified my forming the hypothesis that the defect which Stella had supposed to be common to Barney, Max and me was, in fact, pulmonary tuberculosis.

Let us now see how this hypothesis fits the facts at our command. The supposition that Stella thought—or perhaps I should say knew—that Max had tuberculosis explains, in part at least, several important things which at first were most mysterious.

The first one is the fact that, although Max appeared to be in love with Stella, he made no definite advances and did not ask her to marry him. This attitude was quite natural if he really had tuberculosis, for under such circumstances, no matter how much he cared for the young lady, he might well have hesitated either to make love to her or to ask for her hand.

Second, Stella's remark that she knew Max was not "a marrying man," which I had never been able to get her to explain satisfactorily, is now easy to understand. If she thought he had tuberculosis she would suppose that he would on account of it not intend to marry.

Third, it no longer seems utterly incomprehensible that Rose's remark concerning Max, "he'll be weak and sickly all the rest of his life," should have had such a profound effect upon Stella and have formed the starting point of an obsession. If Stella believed that Max had consumption, this remark, coming as it did from some one who had never even seen him, might well have startled Stella and filled her with a superstitious dread.

Fourth, the fact which at first seemed so singular, viz., that Stella seemed to believe in Rose's prophecy that Max would be sickly all his life, no longer appears strange. If Stella believed Max had tuberculosis, she had good reason for accepting Rose's prediction that he would never be strong.

Fifth, the doubt in Stella's mind as to the advisability of marrying Max, which we concluded existed, without knowing its exact cause, we can now explain. Presumably it was her belief that Max was tubercular that was the source of the conflict which resulted in her wishing that if she married him his life would be short.

Sixth, the idea that Stella was "too strong" for Barney, which was met with in analyzing the dream already recorded, and which, although Stella said the phrase had a sexual meaning, I thought represented some other sort of deficiency, can now be explained. The deficiency was tuberculosis, and Stella felt that she was too strong to be married to so weak a man.

Seventh, assuming that the idea of deficiency met with in analyzing the dream really referred to Barney's being tubercular, it is possible to explain why Stella showed no particular reaction and experienced no change in her symptoms when Barney went to the clinic and the diagnosis of phthisis was made. That is, the dream occurred *only a short time after I began the analysis of her case* and if, as it seems, the weakness on Barney's part, at which the analysis of the dream hinted, was really tuberculosis, it is clear that Stella suspected Barney had this disease *when she first came to me and long before he was examined by a doctor*. This explains why the report of the doctor's findings failed to affect her—she was entirely prepared for it; the fact that her husband had tuberculosis was to her an old story, and the doctor's assertion of what she already knew of course produced no reaction.

It is clear, then, that the hypothesis that the weakness or defect which Stella apparently supposed to be common to Max, Barney, and me, was in reality tuberculosis, not only is perfectly har-

monious with the facts that have been brought out,
but it enables us to explain very readily many
previously baffling things—things which, it seems
to me, could be explained by no other hypothesis.
For these reasons I felt perfectly justified in looking on it not as a mere hypothesis but as an exposition of actual fact.[1]

I therefore began to lay before Stella the explanations just set forth, with expectation that
she would confirm me in every point.   But she
did nothing of the kind.   I asked her if she had
ever thought me tubercular, and she admitted that
such an idea had once or twice crossed her mind.
She also admitted that shortly before Barney was
examined she had wondered if perhaps he had not
some lung trouble, but in regard to Max she would
make no such admission, saying, ''Do you think I
would have been such a fool as to want to marry
him if I had suspected that he was sick?''   To this
I replied by calling her attention to the fact that
by her own admission she *had* wanted to marry
Max in spite of the fact that she supposed he
would be ''weak and sickly all his life.''   But this,
instead of making her agree with me, had just the
opposite effect.   She at once retracted her former
admissions, disagreed with everything of any sort
that I undertook to tell her, and so clearly manifested an inclination to combat at all costs my attempts to explain her neurosis that I stopped with-

[1] My belief was that Stella in some way knew that Max and
Barney had tuberculosis—in the latter case independently of the
doctor's report—and that because I am thin and have a smoker's
cough she had transferred to me the idea that I too suffered from
the same malady.

out having told her of all the conclusions that have been set forth.

But though Stella had not confirmed me in words, I looked upon her quite obviously unreasonable opposition as an involuntary confirmation. That is, I thought that she knew me to be right, and was, in fact, surprised to find how much I had been able to learn of what she wished to conceal. Her vigorous opposition was then determined, I believed, by the fact that there were other things she did not wish to disclose, for she now felt she could not keep them from me and concluded that her greatest safety lay in disputing every conclusion I made and making no admission whatsoever.

I explained this to her without materially decreasing her resistance however, and there followed a very long period in which I made practically no progress in the analysis of her obsessions. She had no dreams, would give but few associations, ''nothing came to her mind,'' and she was late for every sitting. The only themes that she was always ready to talk about were the hopelessness of her case, the futility of psychoanalysis, and the impossibility of her being able to respect me either as a physician or a man after I had made against her such stupid accusations and persisted with them in such a stubborn and unreasonable manner.

All this I could interpret as an effort to avoid facing the perception that it was very largely her own fault that we were not making better progress—that is, she endeavored to believe me and my method of treatment at fault as a defense against the feeling that she herself was to blame in not doing her part by disclosing all she could.

I was soon convinced that there was something in her life that was so painful to her that she would almost rather remain sick than have it known, and on this account I would have given up the treatment had it not been for two reasons: first, the hope that in spite of her resistance I would some time find out what she was concealing and so gratify my very considerable curiosity as to what made her sick; and, second, that a set of anxiety hysteria symptoms came into prominence at this time and that I had no great difficulty in analyzing them. These kept up my interest and prevented me from giving up the work. I will not refer to these symptoms here, for they represent a sort of digression from the theme of the main obsession which is already long enough.

The long period of intense resistance was finally brought to an end in the following way.

Stella came one day and began immediately: "I've been awfully sick, Doctor. Last night I had a terrible attack of fear—the worst I ever had, I think."

"What were you afraid of?" I asked.

"Of the fortune teller, of course," she replied; "I thought surely I was going insane right away. I don't see how my mind can stand such terrible fear."

She went on with her usual complaints, "I'll never get well," "I'm lost," "I have no future," etc., but I interrupted her by asking: "Don't you know what made you afraid? What happened to bring on the attack?''

''That I'll nev—nothing happened—I don't know what brought on the attack,'' she replied.

But she did not interrupt herself soon enough to prevent my realizing that what she had started to say was, ''That I'll never tell you!''

I had already become convinced that there was something of importance in Stella's life that she was concealing from me. I now had confirmation of this belief, for it seemed plain that Stella knew very well what had occasioned the severe attack she spoke of. I therefore said to her that I was sure she could explain why this attack occurred, but she insisted that this was not so and that there was nothing she could tell me. I replied that I could not believe her, and also said that, since it seemed to me that she was intentionally concealing something important, I was unwilling to exert myself any longer unless she would do her part—in short, unless she told me the cause at once I would give up the treatment, for I felt that as long as it was concealed my efforts would do her no particular good, and that for me to continue would be simply a waste of time. [1]

She protested that I was very unjust, that she was concealing nothing, and ended by saying, ''How can you think there is anything I would

[1] Although it had some results in this case, the use of threats is not a technical procedure that can be recommended. The physician should try to understand the patient's resistances against disclosing information and overcome them by explaining them, rather than, so to speak, by using force.

keep back after all the embarrassing things I have told you?''

I replied that I was satisfied I was right, and that at any rate, right or wrong, I was no longer willing to treat her unless the important piece of information I expected was immediately forth-coming.   She knew that I meant what I said.

At this point I was called out of the room for a few minutes.   When I came back she said, ''Well, doctor, I've been thinking it over and I've made up my mind.   I know I shouldn't take up your time unless I let you know everything.   At last I'm going to tell you my secret.''

''Well,'' I asked, ''what is your secret?''

''Con,'' she replied briefly; ''I've had tuberculosis.   I've been in two different sanitariums.''

Then followed a story which gave an entirely new insight into Stella's psychic conflicts and soon proved to be the key to the solving of many of the mysteries of her neurosis.

Stella's tuberculosis began when she was thir-teen and a half years old, manifesting itself by cough, marked loss of weight, and severe and re-peated hemorrhages. [1]

The diagnosis was made by several private phy-sicians and also at the Broadway Clinic, from where after a little delay she was sent to a sani-tarium in the country.   There she remained for about five months, improving considerably, but finally she ran away and returned to New York

---

[1] It was on account of her lung trouble that Stella had to leave school at an early age rather than, as she stated at first, that her mother "needed her to help with the house work."   Page 315.

because she was "so homesick." After remaining in New York for a few months her symptoms returned to such an alarming degree that she again applied at a dispensary and was sent to a second sanitarium. In this place, which we may call Oakwood, she remained for several months and improved a great deal. But she was again overcome with homesickness and finally left the institution in spite of the fact that the doctors advised her to the contrary. Having returned home, she continued to improve, so that before long she was entirely free from symptoms, and at sixteen years of age she was able to begin work in the store, apparently in the best of health. Unfortunately, this was not the end of her trouble. Later she suffered two distinct relapses, both of which as will shortly be seen, gave rise to most important problems in her life and played a highly significant rôle in the development of her obsessions.

The history of her tuberculosis is what I referred to in the introduction as the important set of facts I was able to corroborate by outside evidence. And one of the instances of undoubted affective displacement which I had in mind was the incident which occasioned the severe attack of fear just referred to. On the day in question a nurse from the Board of Health had called at the house during Stella's absence, in regard to something in connection with Barney's case. But Stella's mother, who can not speak English, did not understand just what was wanted and so when she told Stella about the nurse's visit Stella got the impression that inquiries were being made in

regard to her own tubercular history. She reacted to this—a thing, as we shall see later, which
might well have been the occasion for some alarm
—by anxiety *not* about the tuberculosis problem
but *about Kishef*. In short, she displaced her
emotions from the thoughts with which they really
belonged and attached them to an associated idea,
the fear of the fortune teller. Just why she selected this particular idea as the one to which
to make the displacement will be explained later.

The knowledge that Stella had had tuberculosis
already begins to throw a new light on certain dark
problems of her history. Thus, it is to be seen
that the onset of her lung trouble coincided with
that mysterious "nervous illness" in her childhood which followed the death of her beloved Aunt
Ida, and in which she suffered from depression,
anæmia, and loss of weight. In short, it is now
evident that this early illness was at bottom not
nervous at all, but physical. The anæmia, loss of
weight, etc., were due to the tuberculosis directly.
Nevertheless, Stella was not altogether wrong
when she stated that this nervous illness was a
reaction to her Aunt Ida's death, as we shall see
in a moment. There was a "nervous" element
in it.

In the first place, Stella, after admitting that
she had had tuberculosis, soon disclosed the fact
that Ida had died of the same malady, instead of
"from worrying about something" as she had at
first alleged. A fact of some significance is that
Ida's death had followed very shortly after she
and Stella had had a terrible quarrel. Stella,

though extremely fond of her aunt, had nevertheless, in the heat of this quarrel, wished that Ida
would die. When, then, Ida did die, Stella more
than half believed that this murderous wish had
killed her. And when still later Stella found that
she too had the same malady of which Ida died,
she felt that this disease had come upon her as
a punishment for her evil wish. This doubtless
had something to do with her depression. Incidentally this sequence of wish, wish fulfillment, and
punishment no doubt had a considerable effect in
fixing in Stella's mind a belief in the power and
in the punishment of evil wishes, and this belief
was apparently a factor in the development of the
Kishef obsession.[1]

The most important consideration in connection with Stella's neurosis was not so much that
she had had tuberculosis, but that people knew, or

[1] The fact that Ida died of tuberculosis did not dispel Stella's
belief that a wish had killed her. It was not known that Ida was
tubercular until a very short time before she died; not, in fact,
until after the quarrel that has been spoken of. Stella's idea was
that her wish had caused Ida to become infected with tuberculosis.
There is a Jewish superstition with which Stella was familiar
that in each day there is one minute during which whatever wish
a person expresses will be omnipotent. When Ida died Stella
thought that she had "hit the minute"—that her wish for Ida's
death at the time of their quarrel had happened to come at just
the fateful moment. Just which minute of any given day was
the fateful one no one, according to the superstition, ever knew.
On a number of occasions when she wanted something very badly
Stella made the ingenious experiment of trying to wish for it
every minute of the day so as to be sure to "hit" the particular
minute that conferred omnipotence. Unfortunately, on every occasion she eventually went to sleep or allowed her attention to
wander so that the minute theory was never conclusively proved
or disproved.

might know, that she had it. As she herself said, "I never worried so much that I had T. B.—I wasn't afraid of dying. What I did fear was that other people would find out that I was sick and that this would prevent me from getting married." In fact, when Stella first developed tuberculosis she was rather proud of it and liked the sympathy and attention it brought her. Soon, however—at least by the time she was sixteen—she took a very different view of the situation and would never admit to any one that there had been anything the matter with her, while she instructed her parents and relatives to follow her example. Her reason was, as she said, that if it were known she had once had lung trouble no one would want to marry her. Economic conditions are so strenuous in the sphere in which Stella lived that the young men cannot afford to let sentimental come before practical considerations in choosing a wife. Thus, if a girl had a tubercular history, she would not be likely to have any suitors, for, no matter how attractive she might be, none of the young men would care to marry her and run the chances of being burdened with an invalid. That this is so, Stella knew from painful experience. In more than one instance some young man who had been paying serious court to her had suddenly ceased his attentions and avoided her thereafter, while investigation revealed that the knowledge of her history, conveyed to his ears by some busybody, was the cause of his sudden change of front. In Stella's own words—which, I think, are not a great exaggeration—"Among the Jews on the East Side, it could be known of a girl that she drank, that she stole, or that she'd had a dozen illegitimate children, and she'd still have *some* chance of getting married. But if it were known she had T. B., then as far as marriage is concerned she might as well be dead—if she lived for a hundred years no one would ever believe she was really strong and no one would marry her. You can't convince an East Side Jew that any one ever recovers from tuberculosis—unless, perhaps, he has it himself."

Now, in spite of the fact that as she grew older Stella did everything in her power to conceal her tubercular history, there was always danger of its being found out, and under the most inopportune circumstances. Through her visits to various clinics and during her sojourn in the two sanitaria, she had met a great many people—patients and others—who, of course, learned that she had tuberculosis. On this account her secret was never safe and the tuberculosis problem consequently remained a constant source of anxiety and dread because it threatened to destroy her chances of a satisfactory marriage. At the same time she rebelled against the idea of concealing her history from the man whom she would marry, as well as that of becoming a burden upon him should her lung trouble recur. These conflicts and the part they played in producing the neurosis we shall take up in the interpretation of her earlier obsession.

(e) *Analysis of the Assault Obsession*

This obsession came on at a time of great conflict and difficulty. In the first place, Stella had recently been deprived of a source of sexual gratification through the incident which put an end to her father's nocturnal visits. From one standpoint she was glad these visits had ceased, for she no longer had to reproach herself for permitting them. But, on the other hand, she felt a certain regret, for, in spite of herself, her father was in a way more attractive to her as a sexual object than any one else she had ever known, and the pleasure of his visits was not easy to renounce. She knew, furthermore, that with merely a look or a word she could give him to understand that he was welcome to resume his attentions, and that he would not long delay in taking advantage of the hint. One conflict, then, concerned her feelings for her father and the question of what her attitude towards him should be in the future. That is, on the one hand, she wanted to get completely away from his influence, while on the other she was strongly tempted to give the signal that would restore the same conditions that formerly existed.

A still greater conflict arose in another connection. The fact that she was at the time deprived of her old source of gratification, as well as her wish to break completely away from her father, predisposed her to welcome some new sexual object as a substitute for him. It so happened that such a substitute was offered. A suitor had presented himself and was highly favored by her parents. She was not in love with him, it is true, but he was a manufacturer and in most comfortable circumstances, and this was a matter to which she was by no means indifferent. It is possible that despite her strong father complex a marriage might have resulted had it not been for a complication that had arisen. Stella had begun to feel ill, to cough, and to lose weight. These symptoms gave her good reason to fear that her old tuberculosis was active again. This made the question of marriage a most perplexing one. From one standpoint, a return of her lung trouble was in itself an argument in favor of marriage, for marriage offered a most favorable opportunity for recovery from the disease. If she were to accept her suitor she would be sure of more leisure, more comforts, and better food than had ever been her lot before, or than she could obtain in any other way, and she knew that all these things, in view of her health, were of great importance. Marriage too would not only give her certain advantages in the fight with disease, but would also remove her from a position of great disadvantage which she might otherwise occupy. Unless she married she would have to work, and if she kept on working her condition was almost certain to become worse, so that sooner or later she would have to give up and go to a sanitarium. This latter possibility was something she could not face. Comparatively few people knew of her first attack of tuberculosis, but, if she had to go to a sanitarium again, practically every one of her acquaintances would know it, she would be branded as a consumptive for many years to come, no matter how fully she recovered, and her chances of making a suitable marriage in the future would consequently be reduced almost to zero.

In spite of the arguments in favor of accepting her suitor there was much to be said against such a course. In the first place she did not love the man. In the second, she was convinced that if he knew her past history, to say nothing of her present fears, he would drop her instantly. If, then, she were to marry she would have to conceal everything pertaining to her tuberculosis and to do this was most repugnant to her. Not only was she reluctant to make false pretenses in such a matter as matrimony, but, in addition to this, she would always be in danger of having her husband find out that he had been deceived, either through her developing active symptoms of the malady, or from some one who knew of her earlier attacks.

It is to be seen that her immediate problems at this period centered upon the question of whether or not she was really having a relapse. To be sure, she had symptoms of apparently serious import, but they did not settle the matter beyond all doubt. Thus, she could say to herself, "I feel badly, it is true, but how do I *know* that this is tuberculosis? I am no doctor, so I can't be *sure*. Maybe I only imagine that I don't feel well." Under such circumstances the logical course would have been to go to a doctor and have her lungs examined. This would have settled the question immediately. If her lungs were found to be normal she could have obtained a certificate to that

effect and married with a relatively clear conscience. But as a matter of fact she was unwilling
to have the question settled. In her inmost self
she was practically certain that her lungs would
not be found normal, and she was not disposed to
exchange what opportunity she had of doubting
the return of her malady for the cold reality of
knowing it. On the other hand, she had certain
resistances against marriage which were derived
from her father complex. Though of course had
she been examined and pronounced normal by a
physician she would have been glad, nevertheless
these resistances gave her a tendency to welcome
any excuse for not marrying. An excellent excuse would be removed if she were examined and
her lungs found normal. As was pointed out
much earlier, she had a wish to return to her former relations with her father, but the fulfillment
of this wish was opposed by her ethical self. In
the event of her being deprived by tuberculosis or
anything else of all opportunity to marry, the wish
for her father would take advantage of such a
situation and make out of the deprivation an
excuse for a return to him.

All these conflicts and difficulties had been in
existence before Stella's fateful visit to Mrs. Denzer's, without, however, bringing forth a neurosis. We should suppose, then, that something
in this visit must have reënforced these conflicts
and thus given rise to the obsession. And such
was actually the case. As has already been indicated, Stella's immediate problems were, first,
had she tuberculosis? and second, if she had it

should she conceal it and marry in spite of her feeling that this was not honest? If some evil genius had set out to lead her into this particular kind of wrongdoing it is doubtful if he could have devised anything better suited to his purpose than simply taking her to Mrs. Denzer's at that particular time. Nowhere could he have found an argument in favor of dishonesty more subtle or better calculated to appeal to Stella than that presented by Mrs. Denzer's life. Like Stella, Mrs. Denzer had had tuberculosis as a girl—in fact, it was in a sanitarium that they became acquainted. Like Stella again, Mrs. Denzer had had a suitor—in the person of Mr. Denzer—at a time when she was none too sure of the soundness of her health and whom she felt she would lose if he knew her history or her condition. But at this point, unlike Stella, Mrs. Denzer had not hesitated. On the contrary, she had accepted him instantly and married at the earliest possible moment without giving the least hint that she had ever had trouble with her lungs. Her marriage turned out well. Thus, on the fateful evening of the obsession, Stella beheld her in possession of a nice home, a devoted husband, and two fine children, to say nothing of the best of food to keep up her strength and a competent maid to relieve her of all occasion for spending it. And when before the eyes of sick, tired, and penniless Stella there was displayed this so seductive spectacle which seemed to say to her, "If only you would be dishonest, you too might have all these things," it is not surprising that something extraordinary happened.

Let us now consider just what this happening was. What, in other words, was the relation of the obsession to Stella's various problems? It will be remembered that Stella's first fear began when Mr. Denzer and the two other men returned to the house, and that it consisted in the feeling that she must remain no longer or one of these men would assault her. As has also been said, she had no actual reason to fear these men. All three of them were attractive to her. Mr. Denzer made a great pet of her, one of the men had told Mrs. Denzer that he would like to marry Stella, and the other was a medical student of that refined type that always excited her interest. Under ordinary circumstances each might have been expected to excite *desire* in some form, rather than fear. In fact, this was the very reason that Stella felt herself to be in danger. The situation was one which, even before the coming of the men, presented colossal temptations. The arrival of the men, all of whom were attractive to Stella, reenforced the temptations to such a degree that she was no longer sure of herself. She could scarcely avoid thinking, "Oh, if I were not so honest! If only I had no conscience, what advantages and what pleasures would be mine!" That is, if it were not for her moral inhibitions she could either enjoy the sexual, hygienic, and economic advantages of marriage after the manner of her friend, or, throwing to the winds all thought of marriage, go to a sanitarium, resolved that upon her recovery and return home she would indulge herself without limit in the erotic pleasures afforded by

the paternal finger.   Her fear, then, was a fear of
temptation, and expressed a wish to be robbed of
her virtue, and to be "dishonest" in one or both
of the ways indicated.

This fear took the form of a dread of assault
for two reasons.   The first was that an assault
would, through no fault of hers, place her in a position where she would have comparatively little
to lose by further sexual activity—would, in other
words, fulfill her wish to be robbed of her conscience, or as nearly so as such a wish is possible
of fulfillment.   The second reason was that the
words "honest" and "dishonest" had for Stella
a double meaning.   She was accustomed to speak
of a virgin as an "honest girl" (apparently a direct translation of "ehrliche Mädchen"), and thus
"honest" meant to her chaste, "dishonest" signified unchaste, although these words in addition
had for her the same meaning that is usually given
to them.   Thus her wish to be, or her fear of being, "dishonest" in the usual sense of the word—
which here referred to her inclination to conceal
her tuberculosis and marry under false pretenses
as Mrs. Denzer had done—was represented in the
focus of her consciousness as a fear of becoming
dishonest in the other meaning of the term.   "Dishonest" was thus a common term which expressed
both types of the temptation to which she was
subject.

During the night the fear that she *would become*
"dishonest" changed to a feeling that she *was*
"dishonest"—that she had been assaulted.   This
was brought about by a feeling of certainty that

had come to her that she really was again suffering from tuberculosis. The absence of menstruation she had found to be a symptom, in her case at least, indicating that an active pulmonary process was going on. For several days before going to Mrs. Denzer's she had been expecting to be unwell, and had the flow appeared she would have been relieved. When, in the morning, she awoke to find that it was still absent her fear that she had suffered a relapse changed to a conviction that such was the case and thus dispelled all expectation that she would be able to lead the life that her conscience dictated.

Stella's obsession that she was assaulted in her sleep represents, then, among other things, a downward displacement of her tuberculosis complex. Thus the fear she expressed to Rose that something "awful" had happened to her and had made her body "different" was fundamentally correct, but she located the trouble in the wrong region— in her genitals instead of her lungs. Also when she went from one doctor to another to be examined for a rupture of the hymen she was carrying out the perfectly logical impulse to go to a doctor for an examination of her *lungs*. Her wish to be examined was entirely right—the only thing wrong was that she had displaced the examination several bodily segments downward.

In the same way the obsession, by means of displacement, gave outlet to another impulse. Stella had threatened to tell her mother that she had been "touched" by her father, but this threat she had not carried out. When she developed the obsession she did tell her mother that she had been "touched" (to be touched is a slang phrase for intercourse—a virgin is a girl who "has never been touched") but the ambiguity of the word "touch" allowed her to discharge her impulse to tell, but without disclosing just what had occurred.

This obsession lasted some months. Fortunately Stella was able to get together enough money so that she could give up her work and go to the country for a time. This change gave her the start she needed, so that when she came home her physical symptoms eventually disappeared, and after a time she was able to return to her work in the store. Her obsession cleared up after the symptoms of lung involvement had disappeared, but not until she had at last decided to refuse the young man "because," she told herself, "she was not a virgin." The obsession reappeared from time to time up to the beginning of the Kishef fear, though never with any great severity. These recurrences coincided with those times in which she had some reason to doubt the soundness of her physical health, or was confronted with some sexual temptation or the problem of marriage.

(f) The Rôle of the Tuberculosis Complex in Determining Stella's Love Choice

When Stella had once admitted that she had had tuberculosis her resistance diminished enormously and it was possible to work out many things that had previously been inexplicable. Thus, I was able eventually to discover the reason for her sudden infatuation for Max and to answer

the extremely baffling question of why she married
Barney. Once she had confessed the great secret
of her tuberculosis, Stella not only ceased to deny
that I was correct in my conclusion that she had
supposed Max, Barney, and myself to be tubercular, but she corroborated me in every particular.
Thus, she confessed that she felt Max was a consumptive from the *very first instant she saw him,*
and that she was confirmed in this belief, first, by
the fact that, although apparently in love with her,
he was so paradoxically reticent, and, second, by
her learning that he, like herself, took a six weeks'
vacation every summer. For, said she, when poor
people take long vacations it means they have to
—they cannot afford it unless it is a question of
health.[1]

Now, the singular fact that Stella's infatuation
for Max and her belief that he was tubercular
began *at the same instant* was paralleled by a
similar occurrence in her affair with Barney.
Now that her resistances had diminished, Stella
not only agreed that I was right in thinking that
before he was examined she believed that Barney

[1] With the knowledge of tuberculosis which she had gained by
the observation of her own case, and through being in clinics and
sanitaria, Stella was a diagnostician of no mean skill. Her ability to detect tuberculosis from the general appearance of a person
was such that a physician might envy her. But a fact that is
of more importance is that she had absolute confidence in her
powers in this line and once she had made up her mind that a
person was a consumptive she would have been slow to change
her opinion even if a physician skilled in physical diagnosis had
disagreed with her. I mention this in order to make it plain that
though it might seem that she had insufficient grounds for being
certain that Max and Barney had tuberculosis she *was* certain,
nevertheless.

was a consumptive, but she also told me that even *before she married him* she was convinced he had the disease.   In fact, her family also suspected the same thing, and, calling him "der tote Mann," did everything in their power to prevent the match.[1]

Now, it may be added, that sometime earlier in the analysis Stella told me she first felt that she wanted to marry Barney just after he had told her he had been giving some lectures at the Y. M. H. A.   The fact that he lectured, she said, gave her the impression that he must be very intellectual, and for this reason she felt she would like to marry him.   When, after her confession, I happened to ask what first made her suspect that Barney was not well she answered that while he was telling her about the Y. M. H. A. lectures she noticed that he was very hoarse and that this immediately aroused her suspicion.   In other words, in her affair with Max, and again in her affair with Barney, a desire to marry had arisen *exactly at the same moment as the suspicion that the object of this desire was tubercular*.   This looked to me very much as if a causal relation had existed between the two phenomena—I mean to say, that apparently Stella had wanted to marry Max and Barney *because* she thought them tubercular.   This sort of desire, at first thought, seems a very

[1] It may be noted at her first visit to me Stella said, in response to my suggestion that she put off her marriage for a time, that neither her own nor her husband's parents would listen to any proposal of delay.   As we have learned, quite the reverse was true, at least so far as Stella's parents were concerned.   They not only would have been glad to have her put off this marriage, but would have done almost anything in their power to prevent it.

strange one, yet there were reasons enough for its existing.

In the first place, Stella felt that if she married a well man without having sound health herself she would be doing wrong to her husband. But if she could pick out a tubercular husband she would in a way be doing him no greater wrong than he was doing her, and, thus, in a sense, they would be quits. Again, if she married a well man she would have to reproach herself for exposing him to infection, whereas if her husband were already tubercular this occasion for self-reproach would not exist.

In the second place, she could look upon a marriage with a tubercular man as a temporary one. That is to say, she could expect that her husband might die, and with that superstitious faith in the omnipotence of her wishes which is so common among neurotics, she had a sort of belief that he would do so when it would most suit her convenience. Another reason for a belief that such a marriage would be a temporary one was this. At the time she married, Stella knew practically nothing of the laws of divorce, and she thought that if she wished to be free from a tubercular husband, particularly if he were not well enough to support her, all she would have to do would be to state the case before the nearest judge, and, provided she successfully concealed the fact that she too had had the disease, he would give her a divorce instantly.

The chief advantage of a temporary marriage was that it would give her a chance for comparative rest from her work in the store, to build up her health, and thus get into condition to make a permanent marriage should the right man come along.

Another element in the case was her family. Because she had had tuberculosis they were very anxious to have her married and off their hands. In a way she wanted to assist them in this endeavor, for she realized that at times she had been a great burden. But, on the other hand, she resented their anxiety to get rid of her, and especially so because they made it pretty plain that on account of her history they felt any husband who could support her was good enough and, consequently, never made the slightest effort to get her one that would be really worth while. Consequently, Stella felt that it would serve her parents right if she contracted a second-rate marriage, and, as a result of her husband's inability to support her, soon had to return to the parental flat. In other words, it would give her a certain spiteful satisfaction to make an unsuccessful match.

But there was still a more important reason why Stella wished to return home to her parents, namely her attachment to her father, which, it need hardly be said, was a very strong one. As is well known even quite ordinary family relations between a father and daughter are not infrequently sufficient to produce such a fixation of the child's love upon the father that she is never able—or willing—to transfer it to a more suitable object. But where, as in this case, there had been actual physical sex-relation between parent and child the tendency to develop a fixation that would form a permanent obstacle to normal transference is of course very great. In fact, it is by no means impossible that even if there had not been the difficulties in the way of marrying which tuberculosis created, and even if Stella's suitors had been much more numerous and desirable than was actually the case, she still might have been unable to break away from her father and fall in love in a normal way. At any rate, since Stella's feelings toward her father amounted to her being consciously in love with him—not even stopping short of the wish to bear children by him—it is clear that, however strongly she felt that she ought to break away from him and form a more normal attachment elsewhere, she was incapable of a thoroughly sincere effort in that direction, for the wish to succeed in it was constantly opposed by an equally strong, even though less clearly perceived, hope that she might fail and so retain her original state.

If then we bear in mind that because of her love for her father, Stella was reluctant to take any step that would mean a permanent separation from him, we are better able and understand why she chose a consumptive for a husband and to comprehend the analysis of the Kishef obsession, upon which we are about to enter.

(g) The Affair with Max and the Analysis of the Kishef Obsession

In this obsession Stella's tuberculosis played the same rôle as it had in the assault obsession.

The prime object of her vacation in the country which led to her acquaintance with Max, had been the restoration of her heath. For again the hard work in the store had been too much for her, and she had perceived signs of returning lung trouble. It is to a recurrence of her tuberculosis rather than to the kind of love described in story books that the loss of weight and similar symptoms which accompanied her infatuation are to be attributed.

The infatuation itself was determined very largely by the elements we have just described in discussing the influence of tuberculosis on Stella's love-choice. That is, although she would not have admitted it, she was already alarmed about her health and worried by the knowledge that soon her vacation would be over and she would have to go back to work in the store. When with her first glance at Max she saw he was tubercular and at the same time attractive, she felt that marriage with him represented a way out of her difficulties, and this thought, though not clearly perceived by her consciousness, made her say to herself "Here is the man I must marry," and was largely responsible for her seeming infatuation. That over and above considerations of mere expediency Max was extremely attractive to her can hardly be doubted.

When her vacation ended and she returned to work in the store she knew that the rest had done her comparatively little good and not only that she was still far from well but also that she had a good prospect of becoming worse if she kept on working. Naturally she began to feel that she should consult a doctor, and possibly go to a sanitarium, but here again, as at the time of the assault obsession, she could not bring herself to face this painful necessity, or, indeed, to admit that it really existed.

When, earlier in the day of her first visit to the Mahoshef, she accompanied Rose to St. Christopher's Clinic, thoughts about tuberculosis and the need of consulting a doctor must have been in her mind. To visit any clinic would have inevitably brought up such reflections, but St. Christopher's was particularly well suited to have this effect, for Stella had been told there by one of the clinic physicians, when several years earlier she applied to be treated for nasal catarrh, that he found signs of active tuberculosis in her lungs.

Now that we know that Stella's tuberculosis complex must have been stimulated by the visit to the clinic, it is easy to explain her sudden change of front in regard to consulting a Mahoshef. Before going to the clinic with Rose she had scoffed at all that lady's suggestions of magic, but immediately after the visit she veered about and expressed a desire to see a fortune teller after all. The reason is plain enough. The need of going to a doctor for an examination and treatment was brought forcibly to her mind by going to the clinic. She could not bring herself to face the ordeal of an examination, however. What she did do, then, was to make a compromise. Instead of going to a doctor she decided to visit some one like a doctor—in short, a magician—for she had often heard from Rose and others that these individuals could cure all the ills that flesh is heir to. Thus her visit to the Mahoshef was really a substitute for a consultation with a physician—and the motive for it was a wish to get rid of that great obstacle to marriage, tuberculosis, rather than a desire to have Max's state of mind changed by supernatural means. Without doubt she thought his *mind* was in the proper state anyway—that he would marry her if his body were sound.

Some time before making this visit Rose had said to Stella, "You are so much in love with Max that you'll make yourself sick worrying about him. You know you once had hemorrhages, and you can't be very strong now. If you let yourself get so worked up the old trouble may come back." Stella replied to this that she never really had tuberculosis and tried to convince Rose that this was so without being at all satisfied that she had succeeded, although Rose did not dispute the point and pretented to be convinced.

When, then, at their first visit to the Mahoshef, Rose, having preceded her into his presence, re-turned crying, "He knew what your trouble was right away!" Stella, demonstrating the truth of her own proverb, "Auf dem Gonef brennt die Hüttel,"[1] began to feel uncomfortable and to wonder if he could possibly have guessed that she had tuberculosis. But at the same instant it dawned on her that Rose might have given him some hint of her history, for, knowing that Rose was suspicious and feeling sure that she had not

[1] On the thief the hat burns.

succeeded in convincing her that she had never had the disease, Stella thought it not unlikely that Rose, shrewdly suspecting that the problem of tuberculosis was worrying her a good deal, had communicated this suspicion to the Mahoshef with the kindly intention of giving him every possible advantage. The vague fear of the Mahoshef, which, as we have said, Stella felt all through her first visit, can now be accounted for by the fact that she suspected that he had some idea of her tubercular history.

It will be remembered that Stella began to believe in the Mahoshef when he boasted to her, "I can do *everything;* for me *all* kinds of Kishef are easy." This meant to her an implication that he could not only make love matches but also cure diseases, and it was the latter point that interested her, for this was just what she had hoped he could do. Her faith in him which then began was, in part perhaps, a remnant of the old superstition of her childhood, which had been reënforced by the wonder tales which Rose had told with such convincing sincerity, but more largely it was a wish product. That is, she believed because she wished to believe. Her faith was the ordinary *spes phthisica* which leads consumptive patients to put so much reliance on all sorts of outlandish remedies.

Finally, the idea that the Mahoshef possessed the powers of a doctor, or that he could be regarded as a substitute for one, was strengthened when, as has been said, he offered to sell her a cure for rheumatism. Thus, when Stella said to Rose after leaving the Mahoshef, "I'm so happy, now I can marry Max," her thought was "Perhaps the Mahoshef can cure Max and me of tuberculosis and thus make it possible for us to marry," rather than any idea that some change in Max's emotional state was to be brought about.

In her conversation with Rose two days later Stella said, "I had rather get him in the *right* way. After we are married I will tell him all about it." And what she had in mind was her tuberculosis history. Her words were clearly the result of a feeling that for her to marry without telling her suitor of her history was a "wrong way" of getting a husband.

At the same time, these remarks show that her faith in the ability of the Mahoshef to cure her was by no means absolute, for had she been positive that he could make her entirely sound and well she would have felt little guilt about marrying, no matter what her past history had been. When, then, Rose told the story of the man who by drinking menstrual blood was made to love, Stella's already overtaxed credulity gave way, for to be confronted with the task of believing a tale so utterly absurd and beyond the bounds of probability was the proverbial last straw. Thus, without clear consciousness of doing so, she had to think, "If Rose can believe a thing so foolish as that, how can I put any confidence in her when she tells me that the Mahoshef has such wonderful powers? What a fool I have been to think he could cure tuberculosis!" [1]

---

[1] Probably the essential nature of these thoughts is that orig-

It was natural, then, that when a moment later Rose said, "Do you know, Stella, that if Max has magic done to him he will be weak and sickly all his life and can't live to be over fifty, if even that long?" there should form somewhere in Stella's mind the ironical and contemptuous reflection which may be expressed as follows: "Indeed, you are more right than you realize, friend Rose; he *will* always be weak and sickly if he has magic done to him—and if he *doesn't* have it done to him! He has tuberculosis, and, in spite of what any Mahoshef or doctor can do for him, he will always be weak and sickly, and of tuberculosis he will die." [1] But, naturally, there also came the thought "The same thing, I fear, is true of me," which was formulated in the same ironical way, "Just as truly as Max is going to die *of Kishef*, so truly I am going to die of it. The same sort of magic that will cause his death will also cause mine (that is, what we will die of will be tuberculosis). This thought, then, "I am going to die of the fortune teller's Kishef (*in the same way as is Max*)," which is *simply another way of saying,* "I have tuberculosis, and I will never be cured of it," formed the starting point of her obsession.

To gain some understanding of why this thought became obsessive, that is to say, why all the affects belonging to the tuberculosis complex were trans-

inally they were wordless, although I am here obliged to express them in words.

[1] This pessimistic reflection corresponds to the opinion regarding the curability of tuberculosis which is held by the old-fashioned Jews of Stella's acquaintance. Most of them believe that real consumption can never be cured.

ferred to it, we need only to represent to ourselves
what must have been the state of Stella's mind
at that time. The theme of tuberculosis was one
that for a long time she had not faced squarely.
As soon as she began to realize, in her girlhood,
that tuberculosis would diminish her value in the
eyes of men, she not only denied to others that
she had had the disease but refused to admit even
to herself that she had ever had it. Thus, she disputed the significance of repeated hemorrhages,
loss of weight, cough, and similar symptoms, and,
although all the doctors who ever examined her at
the times she showed symptoms had made the
same diagnosis of tuberculosis, she always told
herself that as the result of prejudice or some
other influence they were mistaken, basing this
contention on the fact that she had never had a
positive sputum, and that for the greater part of
her life she had maintained fairly good health
though working in an unfavorable climate and
under unfavorable conditions.

But for Stella to maintain a conscious belief
that she was not and had never been tubercular
would mean simply that she repressed and refused
to admit to her consciousness various perceptions
that would inevitably lead to the formation of a
directly opposite opinion. In other words, even
supposing that she could believe *consciously* that
she never had had the disease, yet unconsciously
she entertained an entirely different conviction.
Thus, though at the time of her affair with Max
she knew in a way that she was having a relapse,

she would not admit to herself that such was the case.

The concern consequent upon her unwilling and unadmitted knowledge of her condition was temporarily diminished by her visit to the Mahoshef, for, with a faith like that which a drowning man has in a straw, she had hoped that he would be able to do away with her malady. But in a mind so shrewdly materialistic as Stella's any belief in his powers was of necessity short lived. The absurdity of Rose's story of menstrual blood as a love potion was enough to swing her back to her normal position of incredulity. Thus as her transitory faith in the Mahoshef gave way she was plunged into a state of despondency in which she was on the point of admitting not only that she really was sick but that perhaps she might always be so, but Rose's remark, which caused her to think, "I am going to die of Kishef (in the same way as is Max)," supplied at the critical moment a euphemistic phrase with which to make the admission. To say, "I am going to die *of Kishef*," since Kishef was a thing she really neither believed in nor feared, was less painful than the bald, cold statement "I have tuberculosis, and it is of *that* I must eventually die." But no matter how delicately expressed, a thought having such a meaning, and coming as it did at the moment when a forlorn hope had just been destroyed, was inevitably accompanied by intense and disagreeable emotions. The thought "I am going to die of the fortune teller's Kishef" appeared in Stella's consciousness as something unmotivated, strange, and foreign to the rest of her thoughts—in short, as an obsession—*because it was there construed literally,* rather than in the figurative sense in which her unconscious employed it. The reason for this misconstruction and misunderstanding was, as I have tried to show, her reluctance to realize and admit a painful fact.

The emotional accompaniments which made this obsession so compelling did not all have origin in the way just described. As we shall see, once the obsession started, the affects belonging to other painful thoughts were transferred to it, and at the same time reënforcement was received from certain *wishes* which however manifested themselves in the shape of fear.

One displacement came about as follows: Since Rose had never even seen Max and could have had no reason for supposing him tubercular, her remark, "He will be weak and sickly all the rest of his life," etc., might well have startled Stella by its uncanny accuracy. Naturally she thought something like this: "What a coincidence! It is almost as if that she-devil Rose were reading my mind." But, since Stella's thinking was habitually done in a mixture of Yiddish and English, the place of the phrase "that she-devil" was taken in her mind by another phrase, viz., "that Machseveh," "Machseveh" being a feminine form of what would in English correspond to "rascal" or "devil." But it so happens that the word "Machseveh" is not only used to denote a rascally person but signifies also *a witch*—in short, "Mach-

seveh," a witch, *is the feminine of "Mahoshef,"*
a magician or wizard. Furthermore, the powers
which a Mahoshef and Machseveh are reputed to
possess include not only those of making love
matches and curing diseases but also that of reading minds—telepathy is thus a variety of Kishef
—so Stella's reflection "Rose is guessing my
thoughts" naturally took the form "That Machseveh (that she-devil, Rose) is doing Kishef to
me," a phrase which, *but for the mere difference
of masculine and feminine word forms, is identical
with the wording of her obsession.* It is easy to
understand, then, how affects arising from disagreeable thoughts with which Rose was connected, especially such thoughts as could be figura-
tively expressed in terms of Kishef, could become
displaced in Stella's consciousness via "Machseveh" to "Mahoshef" and thus merge with the
already existing fear of the fortune teller.
Such a substitution of the fortune teller for Rose
was further facilitated by the fact already pointed
out that Stella suspected that Rose had made a
confidant of him; that is, she could say, "Whatever
Rose knows, *he* knows. To tell Rose a thing is the
same as telling it to the Mahoshef." [1]

[1] There can be introduced here the explanation of Stella's anger
upon discovering that Rose and the Mahoshef were already acquainted at the time of their first visit to him. We have already
seen that Stella suspected at the time of this visit that Rose had
told him of her tuberculosis. This suspicion was strengthened
when he said to her, "I can do everything!" and when he attempted to sell her medicine, for she wondered if this did not
mean he was hinting that he knew of her lung trouble and that
he would try to help her if she cared to be frank with him. The
discovery some days later that Rose had known the Mahoshef

The thoughts from which affective displacement came about by this route arose as follows. Not only did Rose divine the facts with Kishef-like accuracy in her prediction concerning the health of Max, but also, it seemed to Stella, in another connection. It will be remembered that early in the analysis we learned that Stella wished that, if Max turned out to be a helpless invalid after she married him, his life would be short. Because of these wishes she could regard herself, as far as her thoughts were concerned, as a murderess. It was also pointed out that in connection with Ida's death

before they went to him changed what had been in the first place only a vague suspicion into a practical conviction that Rose had betrayed her. For the fact that Rose had seen fit to conceal this acquaintance indicated a certain duplicity on her part, while the existence of the acquaintance, implying as it did that Rose had confided in the man and had some secret understanding with him, made it seem highly probable that she had told him all she knew about Stella. Thus, it is to be seen that the reason Stella became angry at Rose when she discovered the old acquaintance between her and the Mahoshef was that this discovery, to Stella's mind, represented quite positive evidence that Rose had betrayed her. She was angry at Rose's seeming untrustworthiness, for she felt that if that young lady could so readily betray the great secret to the Mahoshef she might just as readily betray it to almost any one else, and where such a betrayal would be much more serious. Another element was the fact that Stella felt no small resentment toward Rose because the latter had apparently refused to be convinced that Stella was not a consumptive. Stella's wish to convince Rose of the soundness of her health was at bottom a wish to convince herself. Her resentment at Rose's apparent skepticism thus corresponds to that familiar phenomenon known as the projection of a reproach.

It must be added, however, that Stella's anger at Rose was not quite as real as it seemed. That is to say, it served as an over-compunction for a feeling of a different sort—a matter which will be clearer when we take up the wish element in the obsession.

Stella did regard herself as a murderess not only in thought, but also in fact, for she believed that she had killed Ida with an evil wish. Stella could think of herself as, potentially, a murderess for still another reason, for she was not sure that she would not adopt some means of hastening Max's departure more material than mere wishes if after she married him he became incapacitated and lingered on a hopeless invalid unable to support her. Indeed, the fact that she had something of this sort in mind explains her exclamation, "I can't bear to have a man's days shortened for my pleasure! I can't have him lose his life on my account!"[1] But it is clear that though Stella had a certain basis for saying to herself, "I am a murderess," it was an admission that she would have been very reluctant to make; and, consequently, her mind would automatically take advantage of any mechanism representing an escape from a thought so painful. Such a means of escape was provided in this way. When Rose had said of Max, "If he has Kishef done to him he can't live to be over fifty," Stella of course thought, "Whenever Max dies, *no matter of what cause,* Rose will think that it was Kishef that killed him; and, since I am the one who caused the Kishef to be done, Rose will look upon me as a murderess." And, as we have just shown, Rose, in Stella's opinion, would be right in thinking her a murderess. Here

[1] After she married Barney and it became evident that his health was failing she often had impulses to choke him or poison him and was by no means always sure that she would not act upon them.

again Rose, though through wrong premises, would reach a correct conclusion in a way so remarkable that it could be thought of as mind reading or "Kishef." Of this figurative way of expressing the disagreeable fact that Rose's estimate of her would be in a way true, Stella's mind took instant advantage. Hence, instead of saying to herself, "Rose will be right *if she thinks I am a murderess*," or, in other words, instead of putting the psychic accent on the last part of the ideas represented by the above sentence, where it belonged, her mind accented the first part, the idea "Rose guesses my thoughts rightly," which as she thought in Yiddish would have the form, "That Machseveh is doing Kishef to me" (Die Machseveh tut mir Kishef); and this thought, construed *literally* by her consciousness, and further distorted by the condensation whereby the masculine "Mahoshef" was substituted or merged with the feminine "Machseveh," bore with it all the affects of displeasure and self-reproach originating from the unwilling knowledge of her murderous tendencies.[1]

But still another group of ideas came to be represented in Stella's consciousness by her fear of the Mahoshef. Not only in the two connections just spoken of but in still another Rose had seemed to divine what Stella was thinking; for as has already been said, Stella thought that Rose guessed that she was worrying about tuberculosis. She felt sure that when they discussed the matter of

---

[1] Compare the discussion of thing-ideas and word-ideas in Chapter IV.

hemorrhages Rose, though pretending to be impressed by her protestations, was really not at all
convinced that Stella had never had the disease.
And Rose's warning, "If you worry so about Max,
T. B. will come back on you" had made Stella wonder if Rose did not suspect that this had already
occurred and that it was a return of the T. B. more
than any thoughts about Max that was the real
source of her worry.   So, too, when they went to
the Mahoshef Stella thought it not improbable
that if Rose told him anything about her history
she had added, "and very likely she is not feeling
any too strong now, which may be the reason she
seems so worried." [1]

[1] It is perhaps true that Stella's grounds for thinking that Rose
had divined and perhaps disclosed to others that her tuberculosis
had recurred were not particularly good ones. As a matter of
fact, for Stella to fear that another had guessed her secret—a
secret, be it remembered, which she hardly admitted to herself—
did not require sound logical grounds. It is well known a
guilty person fears in a characteristically illogical way that his
guilt is suspected by others, even by those who cannot possibly
know anything about it. In the same way it often happens that
a person thinks that another suspects him of something that he
consciously believes he is not guilty of but of which he is actually
guilty, though unconsciously. One of my patients, for example,
who developed a neurosis shortly after he became engaged, told
me he believed a friend of his suspected that he became ill only
as a means of backing out of his engagement; and, as it turned
out eventually, a wish to withdraw from the engagement actually
was one of the chief determinants of his illness. But at the time
he became ill this wish was a totally unconscious one. Phenomena of this sort are well known under the term, "the projection
of a reproach," and that the existence of this mechanism is well
recognized is evidenced by such familiar phrases as: "A guilty
conscience needs no accuser." "The wicked flee when no man pursueth." To some extent, then, Stella's thought that Rose and the
Mahoshef knew she had tuberculosis depended upon a projection

At any rate, for Rose to guess that Stella was having a relapse—for in fact Stella was fat and looked perfectly well—was remarkable enough to be expressed in terms of mind reading or divination. Hence, whatever affects belonged to the idea "That I have tuberculosis is known to others" could be displaced in Stella's consciousness to the idea "The Mahoshef is doing magic to me."

This point, that magic meant among other things *to have knowledge of the secret of her tuberculosis,* has been emphasized because upon it depended some of the minor fears from which Stella had suffered. Since for her to think a person was doing magic to her could be a substitute for the thought that that person knew of her tuberculosis, one can understand why she had fears of friends of the Mahoshef, of people who stared at her on the street, and of the doctor who hypnotized her at the Broadway Clinic. All of these persons she had reason to think knew or might know that she was a consumptive. She feared friends of the Mahoshef, and under this guise friends of Rose also, because she thought Rose and the Mahoshef were untrustworthy persons and might betray her secret to their acquaintances. She feared the doctor at the Broadway Clinic because her old tuberculosis history was there on file, and he might have seen it or have learned of her story from some of

of the repressed thought "*I* know I have it." This thought, "I know I have tuberculosis," then, contributed to the obsession through two mechanisms: first, identification with Max; second, that of projection. In addition, as we shall learn shortly, there was a wish element in the case that made Stella exaggerate any real likelihood of her tuberculosis becoming known to others.

the men in the department for tuberculosis. (This particular physician served also as a substitute for *several* physicians, at this clinic and elsewhere, who might know of her lung trouble.) The reason that she feared that people who stared at her on the street were doing magic to her was this. Any one is apt to think when he sees another person staring at him, ''Is that some one who knows me but whom I do not recall?'' but Stella would add to such a thought, ''Is that some one who knows me *from having seen me in a sanitarium or T. B. clinic,* and so is aware that I am a consumptive?'' a thought which, because of her resistances, reached her consciousness as a fear of divination or of magic.

But there remains still another determinant of Stella's obsession to be considered. We have seen that, according to the wording of the young lady's obsession, the source of all her troubles was the Mahoshef. It was he and his influence which, it seemed to her, menaced her mental integrity and after her marriage threatened to bring about a divorce from her husband. The rôle which the Mahoshef played in her obsession was, then, quite analogous to that occupied by the arch persecutor in the delusions of a paranoiac. But we have come to believe that in paranoia and allied conditions the person hated and feared as the arch persecutor either is, or represents, some one whom the patient, usually without realizing it, actually loves.[1] It is not unreasonable to conclude, then,

[1] Freud—Psychoanalytische Bemerkungen über einen autobiographisch beschriebenen Fall von Paranoia. Jahrbuch für Psy-

that a similar state of affairs must have existed in this case. But, since there is no reason to think that Stella loved the Mahoshef, it would seem that he must have stood as a representative of some one whom she really did love.[1] The power which to Stella seemed to emanate from the Mahoshef we may suppose, then, was really her love for this person whom the Mahoshef represented. Thus, as we might naturally expect, magic or Kishef was a symbol for love, for in the figures of ordinary speech love is spoken of as a *magical power,* a form of *enchantment,* the lover is said to be *bewitched* by his mistress, and she to have *cast a spell* over him, etc. ''The Mahoshef is doing magic to me'' means then, among other things, ''I am in love with *him,*'' *i. e.,* with some person whom the Mahoshef represents.

But who was the person loved by Stella and represented in the obsession by the Mahoshef? There seems to be little room for doubt on this point. All the evidence indicates that Stella's father was the person in question. As has already been said, she was in love with him in the fullest sense of the word. She wished to remain with him, to assume the place occupied by her mother, and to be sexually gratified by him.

choanalytische und Psychopathologische Forschungen, Bd. III, Hft. 1, 1912.

[1] This line of reasoning has brought us to a conclusion almost identical with that reached when before beginning the analysis we were considering the question of love at first sight, namely, that Stella must have been in love with some person, then unknown to us, and that presumably this love was an important factor in the development of the neurosis.

These wishes were opposed and to some extent obscured by others of an ethical order which impelled her to marry and leave home. But the conflict of these forces, reënforced by the conflicts arising out of the tuberculosis problem, eventually resulted in a sort of pseudo-marriage—a marriage with a consumptive. That is to say, her love for her father led her to contemplate and eventually to take a step which must lead to infinite trouble, anxiety, and unhappiness. It is evident, then, that if all of Stella's troubles could be attributed to the influence of any one person, that person was not the Mahoshef, but her father. From the standpoint of harm done he was the *real* Mahoshef. He, and not the fortune teller, was the one who "bossed" her thoughts, had "power" over her, and was "driving her crazy," or as we can better express it, to do "crazy" things. "The Mahoshef is doing magic to me and I am going to die—or go crazy" is then a substitution for the thought "I am in love with my father, and this love is leading me to do insane things that will lead to my destruction."

In addition to the factors just mentioned there were still others which had some influence in causing Stella to identify the Mahoshef with her father. The fact that the two men were of about the same age and appearance, and that they were both obviously old-fashioned and superstitious, without doubt had some significance. Furthermore, both were in some degree deserving of the term Mahoshef in its colloquial significance of rascal. But a more important factor was this. It will be remembered that Stella's visit to the Mahoshef was really a substitute for going to a doctor. Now, the idea of visiting a physician had for Stella a peculiar significance. As a little girl of nine or thereabouts she and other little girls had been wont to amuse themselves by "playing doctor." They examined one another, pretended to deliver each other of babies, administered enemas, etc. But the most interesting form of "treatment" which took place in these games consisted in the masturbation of the "patient" by the pretended medical man. Thus, the idea of going to a doctor for examination and treatment was always associated in Stella's mind with some thought of sexual gratification by means of masturbation. For the same reason a doctor, or more especially a person who, though *not actually a medical man assumed the rôle of one,* as did the Mahoshef, could stand as a dispenser of masturbatic gratification, and, consequently, as a substitute for her father, who had afforded her pleasures of that sort.[1] The starting point of the identification seems to have been the moment when during her first visit to him the Mahoshef took Stella's hand and so held it that his thumb was interlocked with hers in a peculiar way, of which she says, "It made me think of sexual intercourse."

[1] This same idea of playing doctor obviously had to do with the assault obsession. Her repeated visits to physicians at that time signified among other things a wish to have restored the masturbatic visits of her father, which had terminated just before this obsession began. She wanted to be "examined" or "treated" in the earlier sense of the words, but her father, the "doctor" she really wanted, she would not go to for the purpose directly.

Up to this point the ideas which determined Stella's obsession have been considered purely as painful ones and little has been said about *wishes* having anything to do with it. We are taught, however, that the wish element is invariably present in any neurosis and, as will shortly appear, this case was no exception to the general rule.

Stella was of a very passionate nature and had possessed almost from her girlhood an intense longing for sexual intercourse. But though at times she had been sorely tempted to do otherwise she had resolutely deferred any fulfillment of this wish, partly on account of moral considerations, but more largely, as she was well aware, because she expected to marry eventually and felt that it would be highly inadvisable for her to be lacking in the physical evidences of virginity when that event should take place. But she could expect to marry only if she preserved good health—or at least the appearance of it—and succeeded in keeping her tubercular history more or less secret. If it were evident that she was a consumptive or if her history became widely known, then the chances of her making a satisfactory marriage would be reduced to a practical zero, and consequently the consideration which had been most potent in withholding her from gratifying her desire for intercourse would no longer exist. And she felt—or feared—that if there were no *practical* advantage in keeping her hymen intact, then mere ethical considerations alone would be insufficient to prevent her from yielding to the temptation to have

sexual intercourse.[1]   Furthermore, she had often
said to herself that a girl who through such a
stroke of ill fortune as having tuberculosis was
deprived of an opportunity to secure the advantages of marriage was on the whole morally justified in compensating herself for such a hard fate
by taking advantage of any opportunity for enjoyment that was presented to her, whether sanc-
tioned by convention or not.   It is to be seen, then,
that for Stella to say to herself, ''You are never
going to be well, and there are so many people who
do know, or through Rose, the Mahoshef and
others, will know of your trouble that you will
have no chance of marrying a desirable man'' was
practically the equivalent of saying, ''There is no
longer any particular reason, moral or otherwise,
why you should not have sexual intercourse if you
want it.''   The fear of the Mahoshef then both
from the point of view of its face value—since it
represented her as being ''bossed'' by some one
else or about to be deprived of her reason and consequently as not responsible for her acts—and
in view of its inner meaning, ''I am going to die
of Kishef in the same sense as is Max; my tuberculosis is divined by so many that my chances of
marriage are spoiled,'' *was a wish-fulfillment in
the sense that it represented various excuses for
doing as she pleased,* particularly in matters of
sex.

---

[1] That the temptation was a real one is indicated by the fact
that she had a great many dreams which upon analysis proved
to be prostitution fantasies. The financial as well as the sexual
element played an important rôle here.

It must not be thought from this that Stella ever ceased to want to be well or to have other people think her so. She wanted these things very much and the thought that she might not get them was indeed painful. And she was on the whole willing to lead a moral and virtuous life as long as she could think it probable that in the end she would be rewarded by securing the sort of husband that would suit her. At the same time, the more the probability of her getting this reward was decreased the greater was the tendency for her libido to revert to former interests within the family, and to fantasies of prostitution. That portion of her libido that was directed progressively toward the goal of a suitable marriage, impelled her to repress or belittle any indications that she was not or could not be physically well, while the portion directed regressively towards her father or towards immediate and financially profitable gratification had just the opposite effect, and impelled her to exaggerate the obstacles in the way of matrimony. Thus when circumstances were such that she had definite reasons for saying, "There isn't *much* use in my being good, for the chances of my getting a *suitable* husband are *small*" there was always an impulse to think "I have *no* chance of getting a good husband, there is *no* use in my being good—hence I no longer have to control myself," thoughts which of course were apt to come to her consciousness in a more or less distorted form. The various obstacles to marriage represented in her obsession were *painful* in so far as she desired a suitable marriage and the eventual sexual outlet it would represent, but *pleasing* in so far as she desired an excuse for returning to her father and for gaining a sexual outlet immediately.

One reason that she sought to make a temporary marriage instead of gratifying herself without any formality was in part because she was not sure that she would not eventually recover and have a chance to make a satisfactory marriage. A temporary marriage allowed her to mark time until she could know more definitely whether she was going to recover fully or not. If she should regain her health she could then decide either to remain with her husband or else seek to make a permanent marriage elsewhere, while on the other hand, if she found herself getting worse it would be time enough to return to her father or indulge with other men who took her fancy. In the meantime she could get what sexual gratification her husband might be able to give her, though she did not expect that it would be very much.

This meager expectation was realized, for coitus with Barney rarely gave her pleasure, though it was her resistances just as much as any weakness on his part that was responsible for this. That is to say she would not allow herself to love him or to enjoy herself with him. To love him meant to be in a state where she would *want* to be faithful, unselfish, and devoted, but the prospect of being faithful, unselfish, and devoted to a penniless consumptive, especially when she herself was one, was so uninviting that her mind automatically resisted whatever tendency she had to make the transfer of libido that would result in her wishing to do these things. Thus, though she was bound legally she was not bound emotionally. Her attitude on the whole was one of waiting for the time to arrive when either she would be well—when she would want to get rid of Barney and make a better marriage—or when she would know positively that she was not going to recover, at which time she would think about promiscuous gratification.

We can now understand why she was afraid that if the Mahoshef was making her insane Barney would divorce her. This fear can be translated as follows: "If it is true that like Max I will always be a consumptive, and consequently cannot look forward to a satisfactory marriage even if I am moral, I will cease to be a responsible person—in short I will lose control of myself and do things which will give Barney full grounds for a divorce." That the sort of "Kishef" her father exerted upon her was also an element in this fear need hardly be said. The ideas represented by her obsession (namely: that she was incurably tubercular and that too many people knew of her condition for her to have a chance to make a suitable marriage), all of which amounted to the thought that there was no particular use in her being moral, and also the thought that she was in love with her father, corresponded to the main sources of her resistances against Barney. Her love for her father gave a motive for not loving her husband and the fact that her own health was poor she used as an excuse for not making the best of things after he became an invalid.[1]

The Significance of the Return of the Kishef Obsession, and Further Details of Interpretation

When, shortly after the Kishef obsession first appeared, Stella of her own accord went to the Broadway Clinic for treatment, her action was altogether similar to that of her making repeated visits to doctors at the time of the assault obsession. In both instances she felt that there was something wrong with her lungs and that she should be examined. But in the one case she directed the examination to her genitals and in the other to her mind, carefully avoiding the critical region of the thorax. But though when she went

[1] The fear of insanity and divorce had a further determinant than the one just mentioned. When the obsession first developed she feared that as a result of the fortune teller's magic she would *die*. When she first met Barney he happened to speak one day of Harry Thaw and stated (incorrectly, but Stella did not know this) that Mrs. Thaw divorced her husband, when after the murder he was declared insane. It was then that Stella feared that through Kishef she too would become insane, and that when she married her husband could divorce her on that ground. This fear obviously corresponds to an identification with Thaw—or in other words, with a murderer, who, however, was excused by the law. The reason for this identification was that she thought that if she got well and Barney did not, she would wish him dead or perhaps kill him, while if she didn't get well and had no chance to make a better marriage her love would then revert to her father and she would wish her mother dead. (If she had a satisfactory husband she would not have been jealous of her mother nor had the fears to which, at the beginning of the analysis, we referred as manifestations of a desire to replace her mother.)

to the Broadway Clinic she entered the wrong department yet she was in the right clinic for a lung examination to be made. For this was the clinic at which she had been examined, and from which she was sent to a sanitarium when she suffered from tuberculosis as a child. Her old history was still on file there, and some of the doctors who attended her in that early period were still connected with the clinic. She did get into the tuberculosis clinic eventually and received treatment there up to the time, when, after Max went out of her life, she became well enough to work again in the store.

The return of her obsession in the spring coincided with a renewal of conditions practically identical with those under which it first made its appearance. Barney came into Stella's life about the time Max went out of it, but naturally it was some little while before she began to think of him seriously as a possible husband. But at the time she met Barney she was being courted by another man, Lehmann. We have already said that as time went on Stella became secretly engaged to Barney. But as I eventually learned, Stella, as if to make assurance doubly sure in respect to getting a husband when she wanted one, became at the same time secretly engaged to Lehmann. She remained engaged to these two men until, shortly after her obsession returned, she suddenly married Barney at the City Hall. Not until after this event did she inform Lehmann that she was not to be his. As has been said much earlier, I was convinced that Stella would have greatly preferred

Lehmann to Barney. I did not understand why she married Barney until the following information came to light. Lehmann went South in the fall of 1910 and expected to return in January. Later he wrote Stella that he had been delayed by business matters and his return was postponed indefinitely. For a time, however, he kept up an active correspondence with her, but then suddenly his letters ceased. Almost simultaneously, his sister who had made it a point to call upon Stella every week suddenly ceased her visits. As Stella learned eventually the reason for this was that Lehmann and his sister had both been taken seriously ill, but this she did not know *until after she married Barney.* In other words, she of course thought that the sudden cessation of Lehmann's letters and his sister's visits had only one cause —namely that some one had told the Lehmann family that she was a consumptive. Her sudden decision to marry Barney was in part a reaction to the reflection that Lehmann was out of her reach.

But a more potent reason for this sudden marriage was the fact that the symptoms of active tuberculosis which had subsided in December were again returning. In fact she gave up her work again and went back to the Broadway Clinic where she was under treatment up to within six weeks of her marriage. Her decision to marry Barney was then in some degree a result of the reflection that he was a last resort. She felt if she did not take him she might never get another chance to marry, for if she got much worse she would have

to go to a sanitarium, and with that she thought
her morality would come to an end.

The return of her obsession just before St. Patrick's Day was a reaction to the conditions just
described. When the girl in the store said of the
Saint, "He was the one who drove the snakes out
of Ireland" Stella thought something of this sort,
"That is a likely story! If I could believe *that*
(viz.: that one man could rid a country of snakes)
I could believe the impossible." But the impossible seemed to her, about that time, to be a complete recovery from tuberculosis. She was sufficiently discouraged by the return of her pulmonary symptoms to be on the point of saying, "There
is no use deceiving myself any longer—I'll never
be really well." Hence the impossible story of
St. Patrick and the snakes could connect with her
tuberculosis complex. Her thought was something like this, "Yes, if St. Patrick could drive the
snakes out of Ireland (a thing which I believe impossible) then the Mahoshef could do magic to me
—that is, could cure my tuberculosis, which also
I believe to be impossible." Thus the return of
the obsession corresponded to an ironical comment on the hopelessness of her disease, or in
other words, to the same sort of thought, occurring under similar discouraging circumstances as
that with which the obsession started in the first
instance. And just as the idea "My tuberculosis
is known" was one of the important determinants
at the time the obsession first appeared, so it was
now; in this case it referred primarily to the

events which had led her to believe that the Lehmanns had learned of her malady.

In the light of our knowledge of the motives which led Stella to marry Barney and of the circumstances under which the marriage took place, we are able to understand a number of the minor features of the case the meaning of which has heretofore not been apparent. At her first visit to me, Stella expressed the fear that the Mahoshef was making her insane and that consequently she ought not to marry for by doing so she would inevitably bring trouble and unhappiness upon her husband. As was pointed out, her belief that she ought not to marry could not be regarded as merely a logical deduction from her obsessive fear of the Mahoshef, but must have depended on other considerations which adequately justified it. We now know what these considerations were. She married knowing that six weeks earlier when she last visited the Broadway Clinic signs of tuberculosis were present in her lungs, she believed Barney was also a consumptive, she was not in love with him, and she did not intend that their marriage should be a permanent one. In short, she had the best of reasons for feeling she ought not to marry, and that trouble and unhappiness must inevitably result if she did. Her fear of the Mahoshef might therefore from one point of view be regarded as an *explanation* of these feelings which she had accepted because it was less painful to her than the true one.

Her desire to have Dr. Dana and me assure her that her fears of insanity were groundless and

that there was no reason why she should not marry
amounted to a wish to shift to some one else the
responsibility of her doing something she felt to
be wrong. But under the circumstances it is easy
to understand why any assurances she received
gave her no permanent satisfaction and failed to
do away with her feeling of guilt.

It was her perfectly well founded sense of guilt
which caused her to make against Barney and his
sister the reproaches to which reference was made
early in the analysis, and which we have concluded could be turned against herself. She accused Barney of having married her only to have
her work for him, because one of the chief reasons
she had married him was to have him work for
her—she wanted some one to support her in order that she might have an opportunity to recover
her physical health without going to a sanitarium.
But as she had not intended to remain bound to
Barney after that end was attained, or in the event
of his lung trouble depriving him of the ability to
support her, she brought against him the reproach
that if she became ill (insane) he would instantly
get rid of her and marry Ada. Her bitter resentment at being required to work after she married
him—which was particularly venomous upon that
occasion when she had to go out in a snow storm
—was peculiarly significant in view of the fact
that one of her chief reasons for marrying was her
wish to be relieved of the menace to her health involved in having to work and the exposure to in-
clement weather which this had necessitated.

She reproached Barney's sister with having

424 MORBID FEARS AND COMPULSIONS

been a false friend because she herself had been false. If she had been a true friend to the girl, she would not have married her brother under circumstances that could mean nothing else than ultimate disaster. In truth, she had "roped in" Barney, and it was because the accusation to that effect which Barney's sister Esther made was, in substance, true, that Stella so deeply resented it. In the same way, another of Esther's statements, "She was a sick girl when you married her" enraged Stella because of its essential correctness.

The fact that Stella must have been sure that at the time of her wedding her tuberculosis was still active—she could hardly believe that in the six weeks that elapsed between her last visit to the Broadway Clinic and the day of her wedding she could have made an absolute perfect recovery —accounts for her having concealed from me the fact of her civil marriage to Barney which took place at the City Hall. That is, the reflection that she could not have been well when she married made her overcautious, and, as the probability that she still had pulmonary signs at the time of her marriage varied inversely as the length of time that elapsed between her last examination at the Broadway Clinic and the day of her marriage, she was anxious to represent this time to be as long as possible and so she concealed from me the fact of her first wedding ceremony.

The reason Stella seized every opportunity to quarrel and find fault with Barney in the few days that preceded his departure for Oakwood was that this was a time when she was especially conscious

of a sense of guilt. For Oakwood was one of the
two sanitaria in which she had been a patient in
her girlhood. The thought that he was going to
an institution where she herself had stayed
brought vividly to her mind the deceit she was
practicing upon him, and especially so since she
felt that he might meet some patient or attendant
who would remember her and accidentally disclose
her history. (As a precaution against any such
misadventure she secretly removed from Barney's
suit case a photograph of herself he had intended
to take with him, for she was afraid that some one
might see it and exclaiming, "Oh, I know that
girl, she used to be a patient here," thus disclose
the secret of her history.) But as a defense
against the guilty feeling which then possessed
her she reacted by trying to find Barney guilty
of something and by blaming him instead of herself.

Conclusion

After Stella had confessed to me that she had
had tuberculosis, some six or eight weeks were
spent in working out and discussing with her the
various explanations that have been here set forth.
Her fear of the Mahoshef and of Kishef then disappeared entirely and has never returned since.
A minor obsessive idea relating to morality, which
she had had throughout the greater part of the
time she was coming to me, still persisted, so that
even though she had improved remarkably she
was not entirely well. (This minor obsession has
not been mentioned here.)

At this point the analysis was interrupted and I have done no work of any consequence on the case since. As soon as Stella told me that she had had tuberculosis I of course sent her to be examined by an expert internist. He reported that though it was evident she had once had active tuberculosis the process appeared to be entirely healed and there was nothing to be feared at the time. Eight weeks later she had some bloody expectoration, and upon examining her again he reported that she did have a few signs. But she began to lose weight, so as soon as possible I sent her to the country, where in a comparatively short time she gained thirty pounds. Her mental condition remained exactly the same as it had been when she left. When she returned from the country, her husband soon joined her and they departed for a place where they thought they could make a living and at the same time be benefited by a more favorable climate. Soon after reaching this new home, however, Barney began to drink heavily—this he had never done before. His health immediately showed the effects of the dissipation and he died in about a year. Stella kept her physical health and on the whole has been very well mentally. She writes me that occasionally she has fears "about morality" but that they are neither constant nor very distressing.

Lest the reproach be made against me that in the beginning I neglected the physical aspects of this case, I wish to state that I made a careful examination of Stella's heart and lungs when she first came to me, but found nothing pathological.

She was distinctly fat all through the period I knew her, and there was nothing in her appearance or—save a slight anæmia in her blood examination —to suggest that she was tubercular. The anæmia was no more marked and in no way differed from that often found in women with severe neuroses. I may add that she was examined by a number of neurologists about the time she came to me and that they too failed to find anything in her lungs. But in view of what she eventually told me of her physical symptoms during this period, and of the findings of the physician in the tuberculosis department of the Broadway Clinic, I think it highly probable that she did have signs at the time I first examined her, but that they were so obscure that to detect them it would have required some one more skilled in making pulmonary examinations than is the average neurologist.

I am surprised not that the patient failed to become entirely well after the analytic work, but, on the contrary, that she improved so much. Though she gained a considerable understanding of why she was sick the analysis stopped before the resistances were sufficiently overcome for her to set about making the adjustments in her life that should follow upon a complete understanding of the mechanism of the illness. It is, I think, now quite generally understood that psychoanalysis cures not so much through its leading patients to know in detail why they are sick, but through the changes and readjustments in their lives which they are enabled to make in the light of this knowledge. Beyond the fact that Stella eventually told Barney of her tubercular history she made no definite attempts at readjustment or toward improving her life with him.

The history of Stella's tuberculosis is of course the set of facts which in the introduction I referred to as having been established by external evidence. On reading over what I have written, it appears to me that in my desire to make the confirmable facts conspicuous I have made them seem unduly important—or rather, that their conspicuousness has overshadowed and obscured the importance of the wish element, and particularly the sexual wish element in the case. Despite the fact that the problem of tuberculosis, as such, was very important to Stella, nevertheless it alone would have never given rise to an obsession. It was from her unsatisfied desire for sexual gratification that much of the real driving force of her obsessions was derived. Both obsessions tended to fulfill this wish by representing that that consideration which made for chastity had ceased to obtain. In the one case she feared—wished—that through no fault of hers she had lost her chastity, a state of affairs which appealed to her because she could feel that by sexual indulgence she had nothing further to lose. In the other case, she felt that she was "bossed" by an evil person, that her mind was leaving her, and that, consequently, she would not be to blame for whatever acts, sexual or otherwise, she chose to perform.

By way of emphasizing these facts it may be well for me to include here a piece of information which, among many others, I had intended, for the sake of brevity, to leave out. At the time of the assault obsession Stella, though apparently in an extremity of fear that her hymen had been ruptured, *made repeated attempts to rupture it with her finger*, and was deterred from accomplishing her purpose only by the pain that these efforts involved. She continued these attempts until, after having visited the woman physician who has been spoken of, she finally obtained a certificate to the effect that her hymen had been ruptured by vaginal examination—*i. e.*, in a perfectly legitimate way. Such seemingly paradoxical behavior on Stella's part can be understood only if we remember that her *fear* that she had been robbed of her chastity was really a *wish* for such to be the case. Clearly enough, what she really wanted to get rid of was not her hymen but that ethical part of her personality which withheld her from sexual gratification. But since her ethical self was not done away with, neither fears, certificates nor any other of her justification mechanisms ever resulted in her doing what she wished to do.[1]

[1] For the sake of accuracy I should perhaps say that what I have spoken of in this chapter as Stella's desire "for intercourse" could really be separated into several constituents. Curiosity, a wish to experience everything her mother had experienced, and certain perverse tendencies corresponding to childhood conceptions of the sexual act composed a large part of this desire. (See the further reference to Stella in Chapter VIII.)

CHAPTER VIII

MORBID fears of psychoneurotic origin (i. e., those not belonging to psychoses, to toxic deliria, etc.) come under the head either of the compulsion neurosis or of anxiety hysteria. The latter term, as we have said before, now includes the condition called the anxiety neurosis, i. e., those cases in which the physical factors are in the foreground in causing the damming up of the libido.

Anxiety hysteria is the commonest of all the psychoneuroses. It may occur at any time of life, and is common in childhood, while the compulsion neuroses rarely develop in any obvious form until after the attainment of puberty. It is the neurosis most frequent in women, while the compulsion neurosis occurs most often in men. The vast majority of cases carelessly called "neurasthenia," "nervous breakdown" or just "nervousness" are really examples of anxiety hysteria.

While in conversion hysteria the symptoms are chiefly somatic, and in the compulsion neurosis a mixture of various emotional and volitional disturbances appears, the chief manifestation of anxiety hysteria is morbid fear and the physical accompaniments thereof. These fear symptoms may be divided into two sorts, the "phobia" and the "panic."

For instance, a woman suffers from the fear of being on the street alone. While she is at home she is comparatively though not absolutely free from anxiety. Also, she can go walking upon the street that leads from her home to her husband's office, and for a certain distance on some of the side streets, but outside of this very limited orbit she is afraid to venture unaccompanied. If she tries to do so, she is at once seized with a spasm of most agonizing fear, accompanied by tachycardia, dyspnœa, cold perspiration, vertigo and faintness, and the idea that she is about to have a stroke of apoplexy. This attack of acute fear is the "panic." The deterring fear is the "phobia." As long as she obeys the limitations imposed by the phobia, and does not attempt to venture alone beyond certain specified regions, she rarely has panics, and suffers relatively little active fear.

Another woman has a phobia of dogs, thinking one may bite her and she will have hydrophobia. She never leaves her house without wondering anxiously if she is going to meet a dog. If she sees one approaching, the typical panic ensues. Whenever possible she rides in cabs in order to be safe against the animals. If she goes walking with her husband, she insists that he carry a heavy cane in order to protect her. The mere mention of dogs, particularly if anything is said about their going mad or biting any one makes her very nervous.

A third patient has a phobia of knives. If she sees a sharp knife, she becomes afraid that she may use it to injure herself or some other person. She cannot go into a butcher shop, a hardware store or any other place where she is likely to see knives or other sharp instruments exposed. She will not be left alone in her house until she is assured that the carving knife, scissors, and all such instruments are put away and locked up out of her reach. If she were ever left alone in a room with an open pen knife lying on a table, she would have a panic at once.

The three special features of anxiety hysteria are then the attack or panic, the phobia, which serves to keep the individual away from such situations as lead to the development of the panic, and the ideational element—the notion of what it is that is feared. In addition to these typical symptoms the patient also suffers in varying degrees from minor ones such as restlessness, indigestion, flatulence, insomnia, depression, etc. In not all cases are the symptoms developed to typical phobia formation as described here, but in mild ones may be limited to a diffuse uneasiness or anxiousness, or a tendency to unreasoning worry.[1]

---

[1] Worry is often spoken of as a cause of insomnia, of depression, and in fact of almost any sort of psychoneurotic state, particularly among those all too numerous non-medical writers who flood the popular magazines with shallow articles on medical subjects. "Don't worry," they glibly advise, "and then you won't have insomnia or depression or nervousness or whatever it is you may be suffering from." They might just as well say: "Don't have insomnia, and then you'll sleep," or "Don't have de-

What then is the relation of the typical symptoms to the processes of the Unconscious and what are the mechanisms by which they are formed? The fear, the impulse to run away from something, is conditioned, as was said before, by a damming up of libido which threatens to break through the repression. What the patient fears is his own unconscious sexual impulses. But in place of the ideas corresponding to these impulses there appear in his consciousness some substitute ideas, bearing, to be sure, a certain relation to the repressed ones, but generally referring to some possible external danger. The inner menace is represented through projection by an outer one, and, by taking care to avoid this outer one, the patient is really attempting to escape from a part of himself. The essential process of the symptom formation is that of a *displacement* of the anxiety affects into which the repressed libido has been converted.

There is a story of a farmer who, when driving slowly along the road leading to the town, was met by a neighbor who asked him: "Well, Cy, whar ye goin'?"

"I'm a goin' down to the village to get drunk," replied Cyrus, gloomily, "and, Gosh, how I dread it!"

pression and then you'll be cheerful." For, generally speaking, "worry" is not a *cause* of the neurotic state, but a *symptom* of it. The worry which these writers would regard as a cause of insomnia, nervousness and so on, is really a *morbid anxiety* which, in common with the insomnia, depression and other symptoms in the case, results primarily from conflicts, resistances, and a damming up of the libido.

This story impresses us as funny, for we are not accustomed to think of people looking with dread upon the fulfillment of their own wishes. We should be tempted to say to the farmer: "Well, if that's the way you feel about getting drunk, why do you do it? You don't *have to* get drunk if you don't want to." Yet such a remark would show a lack of appreciation of the situation. For Cy *did* want to get drunk. On the other hand he wanted to avoid it, or at least its unpleasant consequences. He had in short, two perfectly incompatible wishes, one just as real as the other. His state was that of conflict—a conflict which resembles those that cause a neurosis, save for the fact that both sides of it were conscious. We are not accustomed to think of people dreading the fulfillment of their wishes, because ordinarily when there is a conflict between two conscious wishes, we cast up accounts between them, and fulfilling the more urgent one, tend to overlook the fact that the other existed. For instance, a man sees a fine looking runabout and says: "My, I want a car like that." But then, when he has inquired the price and finds it to be two or three times what he expected, he then says, "No, I don't want it" just as if the wish for it had suddenly evaporated.

The wishes which give rise to the neurosis are those which behave just as the farmer's wish to become intoxicated. They persist in trying to fulfill themselves in total disregard of all possible unpleasant consequences of this fulfillment and of the existence of other wishes incompatible with their being fulfilled. The individual fears them as he might fear bad companions whose demoralizing influence would lead him into forms of indulgence whose consequences would not be a source of pleasure but of pain.

It is clear that if the farmer had no objection to getting drunk, or to the consequences of so doing (if he had no *resistances* against this form of wish fulfillment) his desire for alcohol would not have been a cause of "dread." Let us imagine that he did go to town and that his worst fears were realized, that his getting drunk had more painful consequences than ever before, that he was robbed of a large sum of money, got into various scrapes, and finally landed in jail. Let us further imagine that while he was thus incarcerated and had time to meditate upon his sins, an eloquent preacher visited him, and not only succeeded in convincing him of the error of his ways, but converted him to religion, and made him firmly and sincerely resolve never to touch alcohol again. In short, let us suppose that his resistances against drinking were enormously increased. At the same time we shall suppose that his craving for alcohol (which, to make the point clear, we must conceive to be a very intense one) remained as strong as ever (as it very well might) and continually assailed and tormented him. Under such circumstances as these, we might very easily conceive that the farmer would be *afraid* to go into saloons. This would be a very real and reasonable fear *caused by desire*.

Now let us go further and imagine that through

some miraculous process his craving for drink is transferred from consciousness to the Unconscious, but without in the slightest degree diminishing its vigor. The desire is just as urgent as ever, though the farmer no longer knows that it exists. Under such circumstances we can easily conceive that if he went into a saloon, say to collect a bill, he might very well experience a sense of uneasiness, of impending evil, of fear, *without being aware of the cause of this fear,* since the craving on which it depends is an unconscious one. Such a fear would be just like those which exist in anxiety hysteria. This attack of fear would correspond to the panic.

When the farmer first experiences this fear, he says to himself: "What's the matter? I feel frightened. Why am I so scared?" He cannot say to himself: "You are afraid you will break your pledge, and get drunk again and shortly go to the dogs," which would be the correct explanation, because his desire for drink is now an unconscious one, and to get drunk is the very last thing in the world he ever expects again to do. Nevertheless he is seeking for an explanation of his fear. We will suppose that at this point he looks up and sees scowling at him an evil-looking, blear-eyed, ragged, dirty and villainous old alcoholic who is leaning against the bar. Here is presented an opportunity for rationalization of the anxiety. The farmer thinks: "Maybe it's that man I'm afraid of. He looks mean enough to murder somebody. Perhaps he is planning some harm to me!" And we can imagine that this rationalization is accepted as the true explanation, particularly as the evil looking alcoholic might become connected in the farmer's mind with the unconscious desire for drink, through some such train of thought as: "There, but for the grace of God, stands myself!" In this way what is really a fear of drinking could become what *appeared* to be a fear of evil looking men. Then, if the matter developed along the lines of an anxiety hysteria, the farmer would thereafter have panics when he found *other* villainous looking alcoholics in his vicinity, for they would serve as a reminder of his danger, and he would develop phobias concerning places in which they might be found. Perhaps he might even become afraid to leave home alone. Yet these fears would at the same time protect him against the *real* cause of his anxiety by keeping him at home or out of saloons and similar places where *alcohol* as well as evil looking men are to be found. This feature would also be very much like what often happens in anxiety hysteria.

This may all seem very fanciful, but nevertheless it gives a good picture of the way an anxiety hysteria develops. The essential differences are that in the case of anxiety hysteria the symptom-producing wishes belong to the holophilic impulses. (There is no such thing as unconscious desire for alcohol—rather the craving for alcohol itself results from unconscious desires, and several desires instead of a single one go to produce the symptom.) The first phase, as in the case we have imagined, consists in the appearance of

anxiety without the individual having any notion
of why it occurred (a phase, by the way, that is
generally overlooked). That is to say, some of
the libido of the wish-presentations, breaking
through the repression, is drawn off as anxiety,
while their idea-content remains repressed. At
the next discharge of this energy a substitute idea
from the foreconscious is found which serves to
rationalize or explain the anxiety, and at the same
time bears some associative connection with the
repressed ideas, just as the farmer's fear of villainous alcoholics connected with his unconscious
desire for drink. The energy of the wishes escaping repression is in other words *displaced* to a
substitute idea, which ordinarily corresponds to
some object or situation in the external world.
Attacks of anxiety may then be brought on in two
ways, one by an increase of the unconscious libido
tensions and the other by stimuli proceeding from
the feared object corresponding to the substitute
idea. The feared object is often a substitute for
the sexual object toward which the repressed
wishes are striving. Phobia formations then develop and tend to protect more and more against
the evoking of active anxiety by prohibiting the
patient from approach to situations in which stimuli from the feared object or condition are to be
received. Naturally even if the patient gives in
to the limitations which the phobias impose, he is
not totally free from anxiety. Flights from the
external stimuli of the substitute idea have no influence upon those attacks of anxiety which de-

velop through an increase of the libido tensions within.

Why the patient is absolutely unable to reason away these fears which he himself knows to be foolish, we can understand if we imagine our farmer trying to dispel his fears of evil looking men by carrying a revolver to protect himself from possible attacks, or by trying to assure himself that they mean no harm to him anyway. These measures have no effect for they do not bear at all on the real cause of the fear. A revolver is no protection against getting drunk! Those measures which in some cases *do* have some effect in reassuring the patient against his fears are found on analysis to have a definite bearing on the *real* cause of fear. For instance, if the farmer took some righteous person with him whenever he went to town, with the *conscious* idea of having protection *against the attacks of evil men,* this person might however give a *real and rational* sense of security, for he would be the sort to prevent, if he could, the farmer from indulging in alcohol.

It may be said that morbid fear generally, and in the anxiety neurosis in particular, is an expression of the essentially passive or feminine traits in the personality. The anxiety neurosis may then be considered as the negative of the masochistic perversion, though at the same time other perverse tendencies are expressed in the symptoms. The matter of pregenital organization or synthesis, such as we spoke of in connection with the compulsion neurosis, has not been as well worked out for the hysterical conditions.

To supplement what has been said as to the
mechanisms of the symptoms, I will now give some
brief extracts from the analysis of certain fear
symptoms which were at one time suffered by the
patient Stella, whose acquaintance we made in the
preceding chapter.

Several years before I first saw her she began
to experience a marked sense of fear if she were
left alone in the house. She felt a still greater
fear of having to pass through any hallway alone,
and if she were compelled to do so, she would
ordinarily have an intense panic, accompanied by
weakness, tachycardia, pallor and similar symptoms. It was not until I had known of these fears
for some time that she told me that in the panics
she had the idea that there was a ghost (a ''dead
soul'') coming upon her from *behind* to choke her.

She had panics not only in hallways but also
when she went to the toilet—unless her mother or
sister stood waiting outside the door all the while
Stella was within. On such occasions it would
seem to her that a dead soul was about to come
out at her from the hole in the closet seat. I
should perhaps say that Stella never really believed that she saw any of these ghosts, and was
perfectly well aware that her fears were utterly
unreasonable and absurd.

These fears were expressions of anal-erotic and
birth wish-phantasies. A hint that they had such
origin came while she was describing a particularly severe attack. She was leaving a certain
house at night and had passed through a door at
the bottom of the stairway. This door slammed

behind her before she had opened the outer one. Thus she was for a few moments shut in the entry- way between the two doors as if in a very small room. Before she could open the outer door and escape to the street she was seized with a terrible fear that some one was coming through the *back* (inner) door to choke her. *Concerning the door in front of her she felt no fear whatever.*

Immediately after telling me this, she made a rather suggestive slip of speech. She was speak- ing in German, and used the words *von dem Hin- terer* (from *the* behind, i. e. the gluteal regions) when she had intended to say *von hintern* (from behind). After this she told me that she felt no particular fear when alone in a house, *so long as she stayed in the front part.* She recalled at length that as a child she had entertained the usual theory that children are born from the rectum. Also she reproduced a great number of memories of phantasies of anal coitus, wishes for which she had even consciously experienced, at least momen- tarily, during most of her married life. As we already know, her great desire for children was left ungratified through the sterility of her hus- band. These wishes for children, expressed in the form of anal birth phantasies, together with anal- erotic desires, formed the basis for her phobias. Of the truth of this statement little further evi- dence is required than that furnished by a record of the occurrence of her attacks. This showed that panics appeared when she found herself in any situation suggesting *back* part, *back* entrance, *back* opening or *back* passage.

The idea of the "dead soul" or ghost, which was to come from behind to choke her, has the following explanation. The analysis revealed it as a condensation of phantasies of rectal coitus and births represented by a fusion of certain infantile sexual theories. An early notion among children is sometimes that the fertilizing element is either flatus or breath. This "vapor" is readily identified with the soul, for both the breath and the soul leave the body at death. But the souls of the dead are supposed to go to some mysterious region where they remain for a time and then return to earth as a new born child. In this way the ghost or soul of a dead person is the same as a yet unborn child. And when we alter the idea in Stella's fear according to the suggestion afforded by her slip of speech—i. e. that the dead soul was to come not so much *from behind* as *from the behind* (the anus), it is evident that we have represented a phantasy of birth by rectum. The toilet seat, from which she feared a ghost would come, is easily recognized as an external representative or symbol of the anus, a hole into which feces *go* in place of one from which they come out. Choking, in which the breath or soul *leaves* the body, in like manner stands for conception, in which a new soul *enters* it.[1]

What Stella really was afraid of was, then, her own wishes for children, and for what amounted

[1] The representation of an idea by its opposite is a common occurrence in symptom and dream formation. It is on about the same principle that a Negro is called "Snowball" or a fat man nicknamed "Skinny."

to a perverse method of getting them, anal coitus, which was one of her early conceptions of the sexual act. Against both of these wishes she had strong resistances. Before marriage, to have children meant to sacrifice her virginity; after it, to be unfaithful to her husband. Her objections to anal intercourse were more of the æsthetic than of the moral order. Consequently, in place of the ideas correctly representing these wishes there had entered her consciousness substitute ideas which, though closely resembling the repressed ones, not only concealed their meaning but allowed the developing affects to be referred to external situations from which escape could be made by flight.

CHAPTER IX

A CASE OF ANXIETY HYSTERIA

(THE CASE OF MISS SUNDERLAND)

THIS patient was an unmarried girl of twenty, born in America. At the time she became ill she was employed as secretary to a business man. Her previous history revealed nothing of importance. Except for the usual diseases of childhood she had always been in good health. The physician who referred her to me, a very careful internist, reported that he had examined her most thoroughly and found no organic trouble. Neurological examination was also negative.

Her nervous illness began seven or eight months before she came to me. One day while at work she was suddenly seized with a sort of fainting attack, which came on without any apparent cause. After five or ten minutes, she was revived through the efforts of some of the office force and was able to go home, though in a very weak and nervous condition. In a day or two she returned to work, but within the three weeks following she had two more of these attacks. The seizures were not convulsive. She appeared to be unconscious during them, but her loss of consciousness was not complete, for there was all the time before her

444

mind the idea that she was dying, that her end had come.

While out for her lunch one day shortly after her third experience, she was suddenly seized with an appalling fear of being alone. The idea had struck her that she might at any time have another fainting attack, in which she would die, or be run over, or meet with some other serious accident. This fear rapidly became so much worse that in a short time she was unable to leave her home alone, or to ride on the subway or street cars even if there were some one with her. Any attempt she made to go out unaccompanied or to ride in a public conveyance nearly always resulted in her developing a feeling of uncertainty and dizziness, with such an intense fear of falling in a faint and dying, that she would have to return home immediately.

In addition to these panics which appeared when she attempted to leave the house, attacks of fear occasionally occurred at home, though what brought them on or what she feared she was usually unable to say. Much of the time she was depressed and nervous. She slept poorly, and complained of palpitation and dizziness. Her fear, of course, had made it impossible for her to return to the office where she had been employed, so when I first saw her she had not worked for several months. A vacation in the country and various medical and dietetic treatments had had no effect on her symptoms.

The medical friend who sent her to me had explained to the girl and her mother that hypnotic suggestion might be of benefit, and she came to me to have it tried. At the first interview, as I started to explain to her something about suggestion, she interrupted me by saying she was very much afraid of that sort of thing and that she thought she might die if she were hypnotized. I attempted to reassure her, but she said, "Oh, it is a spooky thing! It is like this," (holding her arms above her head and waving her hands). "I am terribly afraid of it." After some more discussion she and her mother both asked if I could hypnotize some one else so they could see the process; and I therefore invited them to come to the clinic at Cornell, where I hypnotized one of the patients in their presence. After this demonstration, Miss Sunderland was even more afraid than at first, so that at last I explained to her that there was another kind of treatment that could be used in her case if she wished to try it, namely, psychoanalysis. She promised to think it over and in a week or so had decided to come to me.

Before the treatment was begun I had a private talk with the girl's mother, who assured me that her daughter was very innocent-minded, having been brought up with the greatest of care and shielded from all knowledge of evil. The mother shrewdly observed that the girl seemed to be afraid of men, adding that there was a very fine young man who had seriously courted her, but she seemed to dislike him and always appeared unhappy and ill at ease in his presence.

Another and rather surprising bit of information which the mother furnished was that the girl's first attack occurred on the day following a severe fright. Miss S—— had been walking through a lonely street, when a man some distance behind her suddenly shouted, and waving his arms, ran after her. She was very much frightened and tried to run, but she made little progress for her legs seemed heavy and she felt the same sense of inhibition or paralysis that is sometimes experienced in dreams. At any rate, the man who apparently was drunk or insane, soon gave up the pursuit, and the girl escaped seemingly none the worse for the incident, until there occurred the next day the fainting attack with which her illness began.

When the girl came to me for the visit which began the analysis her mother asked her in my presence if she had told me about this fright. The girl replied, "No," and when she and I retired to my office she seemed rather reluctant to speak about it and did so only after a little urging. As she described the behavior of the man, I was struck by the fact that she raised her arms and waved her hands with *exactly the same gestures that she had used in speaking of the "spookiness" of hypnotism.*

She then began to talk about the girl she had seen me hypnotize at the clinic, saying how afraid she would be to undergo anything of that kind. Then after a pause she asked, "Did you notice how that girl looked at you?" "No," I replied, "what do you mean?" "She looked as if she were in love with you," Miss S—— replied with a laugh. Miss S—— then with apparent irrelevance began to tell me that her brother was engaged to a girl

she disliked very much and that she hoped they
would not marry.   After this there was a pause,
and then she laughed, explaining again with apparent irrelevance that there had come to her
mind the recollection of how her sister, a very
amusing child of thirteen, had remarked after a
certain man had left the house, "Oh, I am *crazy*
about him!   I could love him to death!"

Then followed a still longer pause, after which
the patient begged me to tell her what she should
talk about.   I replied, of course, that she was to
tell whatever she wished me to know about herself.
At length she went on by saying, "I think one of
the things that made me nervous was reading the
newspapers."   Rather reluctantly she explained
that, some weeks before her first fainting attack,
she had read a number of reports in regard to an
investigation of white slavery which was then going on and that, partly through the reports and
partly through a talk with a girl friend she had
been led to believe that all young men were infected with "bad diseases."   This, she said,
troubled her a good deal.   She felt as if she
wanted to have nothing to do with men.   She was
afraid, also, to touch the straps in the subway, or
to handle money, fearing she might get some infection.   She added that a young man in the office
where she had worked (the same young man, I
learned later, that her mother had referred to) had
somewhat hairy hands and this made her think of
dirt and infection so that she could not bear the
thought of touching anything he had touched or
even of being in his presence.   She added, how-

ever, that while this man, whom we may call Mr. Densmore, had everywhere the reputation of being an exceedingly clean and straight person, this did not lessen her aversion to him.

These bits of information, which I have recorded, though at first glance seemingly irrelevant and disconnected, are when carefully examined, really reducible to one common element. The girl seemed to have a great fear of hypnotism. Now to most people, hypnotism means to be under the spell of another person, and hence it is a frequent symbol for sex attraction, as has often been shown through the analysis of neurotic symptoms, dreams and the delusions of the insane. That the fear of hypnotism in this case had such a meaning seemed to be true, inasmuch as the patient imagined that the girl I had hypnotized looked as if she were in love with me. Then, too, Miss Sunderland had used the identical gestures and expressions in speaking of hypnotism that she had later used in describing the actions of the man who had chased her. This would seem to indicate that in some way she identified hypnotism or the hypnotist with the man who had frightened her. And when it is remembered that in a woman's fear of an insane or drunken man there is usually, consciously or unconsciously, some thought of a possibility of sexual violence, it would seem that the sex or love element must have been the basis for the identification. Again, as the mother had remarked, the girl seemed to be afraid of men in general, and such a fear upon analysis usually is found to have origin in a sex conflict.

Further, the girl had mentioned, apparently apropos of nothing, that her sister had confessed to being "crazy" about some man. This association can be explained on the same basis. Patients who do not want to talk about their intimate lives are apt to talk about other people with whom they identify themselves. Hence one might suppose that the reason Miss S—— spoke of her sister was because of an identification based on the fact that she too was, in some degree "crazy" about some man, or was likely to become so.

The meaning common to all this material then, seems to be that the girl was afraid of love or sex.

We could suppose certain romantic or erotic impulses had begun to make themselves felt within her, but that she was trying to repress them, and in consequence they were distorted so as to be perceived by her in the shape of fear, instead of appearing in their true form.

But we can go still further. Since she was afraid she would die if hypnotized, and since hypnotism seemed to represent some sex influence, it would appear that death was a symbol for some result of sex influence both in this case and, presumably, also in connection with her symptomatic fear that if she went out alone she might fall in a faint and die. As Jung has remarked, young girls who speak of death think of love.[1]

That her fear of infection was connected with the sex problem, is obvious, but in just what manner it was connected will become more apparent later.

[1] "Diagnostische Assöziationsstudien," Bd. I, Beitrag VIII.

At the second visit, the subject of dreams came up, and Miss S—— remembered that some time earlier she had had a dream in which she was being pursued by a Japanese girl and from which she awoke very nervous and frightened. Mention of this dream will be made later.

For several succeeding visits our talk was of more or less superficial things and revealed little of the patient's unconscious processes. I learned that her family were very religious; that her mother, though very kindly on the whole, was somewhat strict and puritanical; and that her father was extremely indulgent and affectionate. He petted and made a great fuss over her, and she was devoted to him. On the surface at least Miss S—— and her mother were on the best of terms. Of her brother, who was a little older than herself, she was very fond, and she admitted that she was displeased and somewhat jealous when he began to pay attentions to the girl to whom he eventually became engaged. On the whole the patient's home seemed to be a very happy one. Mr. Libby, the man by whom she had been employed, had been an intimate friend of the family for many years; and, though not actually a relative, he had behaved as one. The patient was a great favorite with him; and, as he was very wealthy, he had been able to do a great deal for her. It was to gratify a whim of his, rather than that there was any need of her working, that she had taken a position in his office.

After several visits the patient had the following dream: She was struggling with a large, slim, long-nosed, gray dog, which was trying to bite her, while she endeavored to prevent it by holding his mouth shut with her hands. The dog finally did bite her somewhere in the thigh. She saw a little blood flowing from the wound, and then her body began to swell up to a great size, and she awoke terrified.

This is evidently a sexual dream. Its symbolism is very typical. Young girls are apt to conceive of sexuality as something animal-like and violent. When, therefore, a girl dreams of some violent attack or assault, one can feel quite assured that what she has in mind is something sexual. And, when this attack results in the shedding of a little blood and is followed by swelling of the body, the analogy to defloration and a resulting pregnancy is so striking that there need be little doubt as to what the dream means. In designating the thigh as the point attacked the dream employs the same symbolism that is familiar from the Bible, wherein the word "thigh" is often used when another part of the body is meant. In the case of a girl who, as this one, had been brought up in "innocence" and taught to regard sexuality as something sinful and dirty, to be avoided and feared, it is quite natural that dreams about sex should be accompanied by a sense of horror and fear instead of pleasurable emotions. Of all this, of course, I said nothing to the girl, but simply asked her to give associations to the dream, without in the least intimating that I suspected what it meant.

Though she said at first that the dream brought

nothing to her mind, after a little urging she admitted she had thought of something which she had felt ashamed to tell me because it had to do with sex. What she had in mind was this. Up to the time she read about the white slave investigations she had known nothing about sex and had felt no curiosity. [1] But these articles aroused her interest, and at last she went to a girl friend and asked for enlightenment. This girl gave with no little relish a description more vivid than accurate of prostitution, venereal diseases, the abduction of girls, and other matters of a similar character. The chief impressions which Miss S—— derived from all this were that the first coitus is a very terrible and bloody affair, in which a girl screams, faints, or even dies of pain, and that, when swayed by erotic emotion, men are little if at all removed from savages and wild beasts. Not unnaturally, Miss S—— was shocked and frightened, and she resolved to have nothing to do with men as long as she lived. At the same time, she had some dim suspicion perhaps things were not quite as terrible as they had been represented to her. In addition, the picture of the

[1] Before this, she said, she had had no knowledge of sexual relations and had not known how children came into existence. In fact, when she was nineteen years of age she had created some commotion by asking before a whole roomful of people why it was that widows did not have children. Knowing in a vague way that marriage had something to do with birth, she had not been able to understand why widows, since they had been married, did not continue to reproduce. She said she was not sure that she had known at that time that babies developed in the body of the mother. We shall see later that the patient's ignorance was not as profound as it seemed.

sexual act which her friend had painted had a certain strange fascination for her and kept recurring to her mind with annoying insistence in spite of the fact that she felt it wrong to have such thoughts and made every effort to banish them.

At any rate, these associations, which were brought to the patient's mind by the idea of violence, blood, etc., in her dream, show plainly her sado-masochistic conception of sexuality, and confirm my conclusion that her dream could be interpreted on such a basis. The dog in the dream may be regarded as a symbol for a sexually excited man, for as shown by her associations she had thought of men under such circumstances as being wild animals. The shedding of blood, the swelling of the body, etc., are details which complete the phantasy of defloration and pregnancy.

There now arises the question, Who is the man that the dog represents? Miss S——, when asked for associations concerning the dog, recalled that on the evening of the dream some young people had been at her house. She had shown them a set of snapshots, among which was a picture of herself with her arms around a large dog. The dog in the picture, however, did not look like the one in the dream.

After telling me this the girl stopped and said that she could give no further associations. But when I insisted that there must be something in her mind, she began to laugh and told me that Mr. Densmore, her "pet aversion," who was among those present on the evening of the dream, had said when he beheld the picture just mentioned, "My! How I'd like to be that dog!"

Our question as to whom the dog in the dream represents is now answered. It did not look like the one in the picture, but was slim, gray, and had a long nose. Mr. Densmore is slim, has a long nose, and on the evening in question wore a gray suit of the same color as the dog in the dream. Thus, the dream dog is a composite formed by fusing his image with that of the dog in the picture. It is he that the dog represents.

The analysis of this dream, which showed it to be a sexual fantasy with Mr. D—— as its object, on the one hand accords with the suspicions which have already arisen that the source of the young lady's fear was the sex conflict; but, on the other, it contradicts certain statements she had made. She had repeatedly asserted that she had disliked Mr. D—— intensely. If, as sometimes happened, some one jokingly accused her of liking him, she took the greatest pains to deny the accusation in most emphatic terms and to create the impression that her feeling toward him was one of boundless contempt. She had admitted that he had courted her and that she was convinced he would propose to her if she gave him the least encouragement. She never did encourage him, however, but, on the contrary, treated him as meanly as she could, tried to avoid him whenever possible, and spared no pains to prevent his rare visits to her house. All this is entirely at variance with what the dream seems to indicate, namely that Mr. D—— possessed

a strong sexual attraction for her. But we can
easily interpret her aversion, dislike, etc., as corresponding to the struggle in the dream against
the dog and to her efforts to hold his mouth shut.
("To keep his mouth shut" equals "to keep him
from proposing.")   The dream thus shows two
sides of the patient's personality, a concealed
phase upon which Mr. D—— exerted a strong sexual appeal, and the conscious phase which repelled
it.   In other words while hardly realizing it, she
had a certain wish that in spite of her protestations he would continue his attentions and that she
might eventually marry him, have sexual relations
with him, and bear his children, while her feelings
of dislike, etc., were really an overcompensation
for this submerged stream of feeling.

In the light of all this, the fears from which the
patient suffered can be interpreted as fears of
desire, or of temptation.   Thus, the reason she
was afraid to ride on the subway, etc., was that, if
she were able to ride, she would have no reason
for not going to the office, where she would see
Mr. D—— every day—a thing which she thought
would result in her eventually accepting him and
fulfilling her sexual wishes.   Her dislike of Mr.
Densmore and her fear were thus designed to
serve the same function of protecting herself
against her longing for him.   She tried to dislike
him in order to prevent herself from liking him
too much, or in a way that, in her opinion, was not
right.

I explained the dream to the patient, indicating
what wishes it seemed to fulfill and the reasons for

my conclusions, though without attempting to point out the relation of these wishes to her symptoms. (This, by the way, was the first reference on my part that had been made to matters of sex.)

She replied that although she regarded my explanation of the dream as a very ingenious and plausible one, it was entirely wrong. As far as Mr. D—— was concerned, she did not like him, never had liked him, and never would. In addition to this, she felt that it was depraved and sinful to have sexual thoughts. She never had sexual feelings and never expected to have them; her thoughts were always pure. She admitted that there were certain older men she had liked very much, but denied that in this liking there was anything sexual. I did not argue with her about these matters, but preferred to wait, feeling sure that sooner or later something would come up to confirm my interpretations.

After this the girl showed an increase of resistance, and for some time I could get little out of her. She said I was welcome to ask her any questions, but there was nothing more she could tell me. Of course I explained to her that there were no questions I wanted to ask and that the only thing expected of her was to tell what thoughts came to her mind, even if they did not appear to be of any great significance. She insisted that everything had been told and that nothing more occurred to her. At last I explained that this seeming absence of associations came about ordinarily when the patient was withholding something of which she was clearly conscious. I added later that this something not uncommonly proved to be the recollection of some definite sexual experience. As soon as I made this remark, I saw from the girl's expression that I had hit upon the truth, and I told her so.   She protested, but after a time she suddenly began to cry, and, saying that she was very miserable, ashamed, and unhappy, begged me not to ask her to tell any more.   I replied that I would not insist on her telling me anything she did not want me to know, but asked if she felt she could be really satisfied not to tell, now she had gone this far.   Finally, after imploring me not to think too hardly of her, she related the following story.

About a year previous to her illness, she formed a friendship with a girl a little older than herself and they had become very fond of each other. The older girl made a great deal of her and petted and kissed her continually, all of which she had enjoyed.   At length, they were invited to spend a night at the house of a friend, where, because there were other guests, it was necessary for the two girls to sleep together in the same bed.   After they retired they lay for some time in each other's arms, talking.   At length the older girl became very affectionate, kissing Miss S——, praising her beauty, stroking her face and arms, and pressing their bodies together.   After a time she began to stroke Miss S——'s thighs, gradually bringing her hand higher and higher until it reached the younger girl's genitals, where the stroking process continued.   Miss S—— lay perfectly still, half pleased and half frightened, until, when she began to experience sensations of an unmistakable character, she suddenly pushed the girl from her in anger and shame, protesting that they could never be friends or see each other again. The other girl tried to apologize and make up, but Miss S—— repulsed all these attempts, and lay awake the rest of the night tormented with guilt and humiliation. The next morning she left for home as early as possible, and strictly avoided the other girl thereafter.[1]

After this experience, she was greatly worried. Not only did she feel that she had committed a terrible sin in permitting such advances, but, when she noticed, on one occasion, a slight leucorrhœal discharge, she immediately attributed it to what had occurred, and was greatly in fear that she might have been seriously injured.

Soon after she heard a married woman of her acquaintance telling about a Catholic girl who had had a similar experience. The priest, this woman said, had told the girl that such occurrences were by no means unheard of, and that, if she was truly penitent, nothing further was required of her than to forget about it. Miss S—— had derived some comfort from this, but at the same time had never ceased to reproach herself. Of course I assured her that the incident was of very little significance and she need feel neither remorse nor alarm about it.[2]

[1] The other girl looked considerably like a Japanese and was often called "Jap." This explains the dream in which Miss S—— was chased by a Japanese.

[2] One usually has to give such assurances but can not rely upon them to remove the patient's self-reproach entirely. If the emo-

At the next visit to me Miss S—— said that she felt better and that she was glad she had had the courage to tell. At the same time she reproached herself a good deal and still seemed to take a very serious view of what she had done. I told her that such an experience was by no means unusual among girls—she had said that she could not believe any one else in the world had committed that sin—but she was by no means satisfied. In succeeding visits, it became apparent that her remorse though partly real was partly an exaggeration. She was serious in believing that she had committed a great sin, but at the same time she was overremorseful in order to compensate for the fact that in some degree the experience had been pleasurable and to assure herself that any longing for its repetition was absolutely foreign to her thoughts.

When we were discussing the homosexual experience, I took occasion to tell her a little of the significance of the sex instinct, saying that the impulse which led to her experience was primarily something perfectly normal and possessed by everybody and that the only thing to be criticized in her case was that it had been misdirected. I also remarked that the incident showed she was not so entirely devoid of a sex instinct as she had claimed at the time of the analysis of the dog dream. [1]

tion is strong it is dispelled only when the patient recalls and connects with it the corrective experiences of childhood out of which arose the ego-ideal specification or resistance applying to the immediate cause of the sense of guilt.

[1] It is to be seen that the resistances which began when the

In connection with our discussion of the homosexual experience, the girl remarked that ever since it she had felt a certain resentment toward her parents for not warning her that such things could occur. They had always been very zealous, she said, in cautioning her against allowing boys to kiss her or take any liberties with her, and these warnings she had heeded, and made friends only with girls. Her parents' warnings had, she felt, driven her from one danger into another, and perhaps worse one, where she had least expected it. She felt she had been rendered over susceptible to the possibility of homosexual experience by the fact that she had been led by her parents to so carefully avoid the heterosexual—a reproach that perhaps is not entirely without foundation.

She continued to dwell at considerable length on how profound her ignorance of sex matters had always been, until at last I remarked that such absolute innocence, as, for example, she had seemed to display by her question of why widows did not have children, was usually more apparent than real. A person of normal intelligence living in our environment would not reach the age of nineteen or more without divining more of sex matters than she had seemed to know, unless there had been produced by repression an inhibition of the thought process and an artificial blindness to

dream was analyzed were connected with the homosexual experience. The mention made of sex matter in connection with the dream of course brought to her mind the homosexual episode and made her afraid either that she would have to tell about it or that in some way I might find it out. The result was that for the time being her associations were blocked.

things sexual. In other words, such apparent ignorance as hers ordinarily denoted not a real ignorance of sex matters but rather an early acquaintance of some sort with them which was succeeded by a later repression.

After a time she admitted that perhaps there
was some truth in what I said, for she suddenly
remembered that when she was about thirteen
another girl had told her about intercourse, explaining that such was the way babies were made.
She could not believe what this girl told her, saying that she was sure her parents would never do
such a dirty thing. The next day this girl told
of her reply to a number of other girls, who
laughed so heartily over the patient's innocence
that she became convinced that what she had heard
was the truth. She felt shocked and frightened
that such a thing had taken place between her parents and thought them very hypocritical and dishonest to have kept up a front of smug morality
and virtue when all the time such awful things
were going on. These reflections, however, she
had put out of mind; and now, as she looked back
upon the matter, it seemed as if she had for a long
time really succeeded in forgetting what she had
been told.

Shortly after this visit she had a dream in which
she was a little girl and she lifted her skirts and
urinated on the ground. This dream led her to
remark that at five or six years of age she had had
scarlet fever, which resulted in "kidney trouble."
Upon questioning her I found that what she had
meant by kidney trouble was really nocturnal enu-

resis, a condition which had lasted for a year or more.

This bed wetting, since it came on so late, was in all probability a pollution-equivalent and connected with masturbation. Her connecting it with kidney trouble as a sequel to scarlet fever was a memory condensation serving to conceal the true nature of the condition.

The homosexual incident shows that the patient was not so utterly devoid of a sex impulse as at the time of the dog dream she had maintained, and the later recollection just narrated proved that she was equally incorrect with regard to her statement of absolute ignorance of sex matters, for she did have some knowledge of things sexual even from her early childhood. It may be noted incidentally, that in these early ideas the sexual was associated with the excretory processes, a fact, which together with the attitude of the parents toward sex, had to do with her strong feeling that the sexual was essentially "dirty."

In spite of the fact that the material just presented was contradictory to the statements made by the patient at the time of the dog dream, she was no more ready to accept my interpretation of it than she had been in the first place, and no essential change was produced in her attitude toward it. Fortunately, more corroborative material was not long in forth coming.

I was expecting that after the homosexual experience had been discussed, the analysis would progress smoothly for a while, but instead the patient began to show resistances of a new type.

She talked enough, to be sure, but what she said was obviously intended to be meaningless and misleading. She laughed a great deal and made many silly remarks. She showed a tendency to belittle everything I said, to be derisive and sarcastic, and to make fun of me. The motive for this soon became apparent, and in the following way.

In the early part of one visit, the patient spoke of a man much older than herself, whom she had mentioned on other occasions, and related that on the preceding evening, when she was at a theater party, he had begged for one of the flowers she wore but she was embarrassed and refused to give it to him. I noticed perhaps half an hour later that while we talked she was folding her handkerchief in some peculiar shape. As soon as she saw me watching her she laughed and covered the handkerchief with her hands. ''What were you doing?'' I asked. ''I was making a flower,'' she replied. ''And what had you in mind?'' I continued. She seemed embarrassed, but at last said, ''I thought if it was a real flower I would like to give it to you.'' ''Flowers are sometimes symbolic,'' I said at last (I had never told her what they symbolized). ''Is it possible the flower represents something else? What comes to your mind?'' ''Nothing,'' she replied; ''I don't think of anything—except, perhaps, the lamp on your desk.'' (Lamp is often a penis symbol.) ''Are you sure that is all?'' ''Yes,'' she replied; but after a pause she suddenly said, ''I have thought sometimes I would like to give you a kiss.''

I felt that the flower had possibly symbolized even more than a kiss, but thought it unwise to press the matter then; and the sitting ended. At the door just as she was leaving she said, "I was fooling; I didn't mean what I said. I would not want to kiss an old married man."

At the next visit she reported that she had felt quite badly during the two days that had intervened. As she was going up the stairs on reaching home from the last visit she had felt a pain in her heart, and this, with occasional dyspnœa, had persisted ever since. She had been very much frightened, fearing she had heart disease and might drop dead any instant. She had been very much afraid to make the next trip to my office, thinking she would die on the way; and she would have telephoned to break the appointment had not her mother insisted upon her coming.

The same night this pain began she awoke from her sleep saying over to herself, "And then we went to Asheville, but my cousin was there; and then to Palm Beach, but my sister was there," and possibly some other words that she could not remember. This dream, if it may be so called, has the following explanation. A few days before, Miss S—— happened to meet a girl of her acquaintance who had recently married, having eloped with a doctor. It seems that the eloping couple had wished to keep their marriage a secret until they had heard from the bride's parents, to whom they had telegraphed the news. The young woman gave an excited description of their difficulties, for there was some relative or acquaintance at nearly every place they went, on account of which they had to keep moving.   In speaking of this the young wife had used *the same words the patient was saying over to herself in the dream.*

The dream words can easily be interpreted as a part of a wish-phantasy in which Miss S—— has an experience similar to that of the young bride, a phantasy, in other words, that she had run away with a doctor.   The dream, then, is a continuation of the same trend which was responsible for the incident of the flower and for the wish to give me a kiss.   All of these were transference phenomena.   The heart symptoms and the anxiety which accompanied them belong in the same category. She had begun to think that she was developing a sentimental affection of the heart with regard to me, but this somewhat alarming reflection was substituted through conversion by what appeared to be an *organic* affection of the heart.

I explained to Miss S—— my interpretation of the dream and also of the heart symptoms.   She laughed very heartily at both but admitted I was right.   (The heart symptoms disappeared immediately after the explanation.)

She then confessed that she had entertained some more or less sentimental thoughts concerning me almost from the very first, adding that she had not known for certain that I was married until the time of the last visit.   She had been afraid to ask her mother or me for fear it would look as if she were "too interested."   But on that occasion she had said "I would not want to kiss an old married man" as a way to make me commit myself without her having to ask a direct question. When, from the way I replied, she saw that I was married, she felt considerably perturbed over the fact that she had allowed herself to get into such a state of mind concerning me. She felt it wrong to have such thoughts about a man who was married though as long as she had not known for certain that I was married she had not particularly reproached herself. The belief that such things were wrong gave rise to a resistance which caused what had been a normal expression of the libido to be transformed into heart symptoms and anxiety.

The discovery of the existence of this transference to me now explains why the patient had displayed a desire to belittle and make fun of me. This impulse was a reaction against her sentimental interest, and was intended to conceal it.

These and other transference phenomena which manifested themselves in immediately succeeding visits were just the material I needed to corroborate my analysis of the dog dream and my explanation of her symptoms derived from that analysis. As I explained to her, the sentimental feelings she had had toward me were not new and did not refer to me actually, but represented a transference and re-edition of feelings, perhaps more intense originally, that she had had toward some one else without being willing to realize them. In other words, what was now taking place *consciously* with regard to me, had previously taken place unconsciously in regard to some other person who for the time being I represented. This person I was quite disposed to think was Mr. Densmore. She could no longer deny that she was capable of sentimental feelings, because she had had them toward me; while, since she had had them toward me, it was probable they had also occurred elsewhere, even admitting that she might not have been aware of them. Her apparent detestation of Mr. Densmore, was, I thought, analogous to her impulse to belittle me. Her heart symptoms and the fear associated with them, that she would die—a fear which, if she had had her own way, would have prevented her from coming to my office, served, obviously enough, as a protection against developing sentimentality and expressed her wish not to see me in order to get over any interest in me. They were in perfect analogy with her fear of riding on cars and of going out alone, which had prevented her from reaching the office, where she would see Mr. D—— daily. In short, her reactions of interest, compensatory disparagement, and defensive fear symptoms intended to protect again an increase of interest by preventing her from seeing me, gave in miniature a view of the reactions that had taken place with greater intensity and extent in respect to Mr. Densmore.

But here again, as in reference to the dog dream, Miss S——, though admitting the plausibility of my explanations, was by no means convinced by them. She protested that she had always disliked Mr. D—— and could not believe that either consciously or unconsciously she had ever experienced toward him any sentiments of a more tender sort.

But, finally, after much hesitation she stated that one day, perhaps a year before the beginning of her illness, she was with him in a crowded subway train and, when to steady her he put his hand on her arm, she experienced a sudden flash of intense sexual feeling. This sort of feeling, she acknowledged, had frightened her, for she thought such emotions depraved and sinful. She would not admit, however, that it was her objection to such feelings that prevented her from having them more frequently, stubbornly maintaining that it was not that she was repressing such a tendency but that the tendency did not exist. She did admit that after the incident of the subway her resistances against Mr. D—— had decidedly increased, but she refused to see that they were intended as a defense against an increase of sex interest in him.

During the period this discussion was going on Miss S—— opened the conversation at one of her visits with the laughing remark "I have made a new transference; you are not in it any more." She went on to explain that there was a young doctor who had paid her some attention of late and on the Saturday night preceding this visit she had attended a dance where he was present. He danced with her a number of times, held her quite close, and gently squeezed her hand while they were dancing. Toward the close of the evening he took her to a side room which happened to be empty and in a very gentle and tender way put his arms around her and kissed her. She had been quite well aware of what was coming when he took her to this room, and submitted to the caress

with very little protest. On the whole she quite
enjoyed the experience. She had expected to feel
a little more thrill in response to the caress than
actually took place, and, though a little disappointed in this respect, she viewed the experience
as a very pleasurable one. She found herself
afterward thinking about it and about the doctor
with considerable sentimental interest.

This affair with the doctor continued. Miss
S—— displayed an increasing interest in him, had
many daydreams about him, and allowed him to
kiss her occasionally. His kisses were of a tender
sort and gave no evidence of passion. Miss
S——'s feelings seemed to correspond to his. She
liked him and his attentions, but neither actually
nor in her daydreams did she experience any feelings that were definitely sexual in the popular
sense. This, she said, was just the way she wanted
things to be. She asserted that if she had had any
physical sex sensations, she would have felt so
guilty that she would have had to stop seeing him.
Even as it was she felt a little guilty about allowing herself to be kissed.

About this time the analysis was interrupted for
a considerable period because of my absence from
the city. Miss S—— had improved a good deal.
She could not go out alone yet, but could ride on the
cars if there was some one with her, which as a
rule, she had not been able to do before. She was
almost free from the anxiety attacks, general nervousness, and depression from which she had previously suffered even when she did not go out.
For about a month after I left she kept what she

had gained, and then she got worse again. I learned after the analysis was resumed that this relapse had taken place when her friend the doctor left New York under circumstances that led her to believe that he was not likely to return. Until the analysis was resumed, she remained in about the same condition. At no time, however, were her symptoms as bad as when she first came to me.

Her friendship with the doctor quite obviously had been a factor in her temporary improvement. He was a sort of compromise between Mr. Densmore and me. He resembled me in being a doctor and Mr. Densmore in that he was not much older than the patient. Her feelings toward him were not sufficiently "physical" for her to object to them and for this reason he represented an emotional outlet which, while she had it, made easier the suppression of any love feelings toward Mr. Densmore or me. In a sense, it was a case of *similia similibus curantur.* By encouraging herself to take an interest in the young doctor she attempted to cure herself of the attraction Mr. D—— exerted upon her, one motive for so doing being her reluctance to admit the definitely sexual feelings that Mr. D—— seemed able to inspire in her in spite of her resistances. But when the safety valve represented by her friendship with the doctor was closed by his leaving New York, her libido, thus dammed up, reverted to its earlier channels, namely to Mr. D—— and myself. By getting worse she restored her defense against Mr. D—— and at the same time had a reason for continuing under my care.

All this was explained to her when the analysis was resumed; and, though she said she could not believe it to be entirely true, she gave the impression that she was more nearly convinced than she would admit. The analysis then continued for some little time without much real progress, although she had immediately improved a little as soon as the treatment was resumed—obviously a transference phenomenon. Then Miss S—— had the following dream, which shows a reason for the standstill and at the same time discloses a piece of new information about the factors which had operated to produce her neurosis. This is her dream.

"I was riding on a train or subway car. A fat man who sat near me dropped something and ordered me to pick it up for him. I resented being asked to wait on him and, seeing a key on the floor, I picked that up, with the thought that instead of doing what he wanted I was doing just the opposite. Then, I ran and, getting off the train, hid in a house to get away from him. After a time the scene changed, and it seemed that I had started out to enlist in the German Army. Finally, I found myself in an office, where sat a man who seemed to be a priest, but was also King James II. The man said, 'Tell me about the key,' and I began to do so. He listened with great interest, but he kept having to answer the telephone, and other interruptions occurred, so that the dream ended with my story unfinished."

This dream is too long to be interpreted here in all its details. I shall tell only the most important of the patient's associations to each element of the dream, and explain them without taking up all the reasons upon which the explanation is based.

The first thought in the dream, "I was riding on a train," led the patient to remark: "Well, that is just what I cannot do now." We may, therefore, regard the fantasy "I was riding on the train" as the equivalent of the thought "Before I was taken sick"—thus, a sort of subordinate time-clause, which introduces the main part of the dream.

The fat man in the dream proved to be the patient's employer, who, in fact, is very stout. His dropping something and asking her to pick it up and her resentment at this request have the following explanation.

Soon after she began to work for him, she had reasons to be not altogether satisfied with the step she had taken. For, though outside of office hours her employer maintained his usual attitude of thoughtfulness and consideration, yet in the office he treated her like any ordinary stenographer,—ordered her around, scolded her for mistakes, swore in her presence, and heaped an enormous quantity of work upon her. This made her both unhappy and resentful, and, had it not been for the fear of hurting his feelings and the danger of the considerable material loss that might result if she incurred his displeasure, she would gladly have given up her position. In fact if anything had presented itself which would have furnished a good excuse for her leaving his employ, she would have been happy to take advantage of it. The inconsiderate attitude of her employer during business hours and her consequent resentment are expressed in the dream by her resentment at being asked by the fat man to pick up something he had dropped. Gallantry prescribes that gentlemen should pick up things for ladies; in the dream just the opposite takes place, and a lady is asked to pick up something for a man. In this way is represented the attitude of her employer in the office, which was just the opposite of gallant.

But in the dream she picked up a key which she saw lying on the floor, with the thought that she was doing just the opposite of what he wanted. Now, what does the key mean? Asked to associate, the patient remarked, "A key is something you use when you want to get into things—Yesterday my mother tore her dress on a key in the bureau. She was very much exasperated, but I told her she must not blame the key, because it was herself, through her carelessness, that was at fault. I meant that she had made of the key a sort of excuse."

The key which the patient picked up in the dream was, then, according to her associations, *something that could be made a sort of excuse, something upon which the blame could be placed when one's self was really at fault,* and perhaps also something which, like a key, could be used not only when one wants to get *into* things but, in a different sense, *when one wants to get out of them.* Now, as we know, the patient wanted to get out of working for her rich benefactor. She would have been glad of an excuse to withdraw from his employ. But we have already seen that her neurosis brought about this withdrawal, or in other words was the excuse she wanted. In short, the thing that she picked up in the dream, and that her associations indicated was an excuse, was as a matter of fact her neurosis. She could use it to get out of things. She could blame it when what was actually at fault was her wish to shirk responsibilities.[1]

The first part of the dream is, therefore, historical, and its meaning or latent content may be summed up as follows. "Before I became ill, my employer treated me during business hours with so little gallantry and consideration that I wished to leave his employ; so instead of trying to please him, I did just the opposite by developing a neurosis, which enabled me to escape from the office and hide myself at home."

The rest of the dream refers to the question of treatment, for in the dream after she had hidden in the house for some time the scene changed and she started out to join the German Army. Her associations, which I need not repeat, indicated that to join the German Army meant to be brave, and in her case thus represented an attempt to overcome her fear, or, in other words, an effort to be cured of her neurosis.

At any rate, after setting out to join the German Army, or, as we know it, after taking up medical

[1] The "Secondary function" of neurotic illness. See Freud's "Sammlung Kleiner Schriften Zur Neurosenlehre," Bd. II.

treatment, she found herself, as has been said, in the office of a man who was King James II, but at the same time seemed to be a priest.   What does this mean?

Her associations concerning King James II finally led, without her realizing the drift of them, to her speaking of a certain man of about my age whom she had often mentioned to me because it seemed to her we were so remarkably alike.   Now, this man's name was James.   But, since I was so much like him, she could regard me as a second James, or in other words, as James the Second. I, then, was the king in her dream.   In view of this there is no real incongruity in the fact that James II in her dream seemed to be a priest and sat in an office equipped with a telephone.   She looked upon me as a priest because she had to confess to me.

The King's request, "Tell me about the key," was my request for her to tell me about her neurosis.   The interruptions which occurred in the dream so that it ended with her story unfinished represent the wish fulfillment.   She feared that if she got well she would have to go back to work for her former employer.   Hence she wished interruptions or anything else to occur which would put off the completion of the analysis.   In short, the dream shows that a wish to get out of working was not only a factor in producing her neurosis but would also delay her recovery.   She wished to retain some of her symptoms, for in this way she could avoid having to go back to work.   She acknowledged also that she enjoyed coming to me

and that this had furnished a motive for wishing
to defer her recovery. I must add that one feature possessed by the fat man in the dream—a
feature which for reasons of discretion I may not
describe—suggested that the dream also referred
in some way to Mr. Densmore. We shall learn
later that this was true, and that her dislike of
work meant more than at first appeared.

After this dream and its analysis had been discussed—and this time Miss S—— accepted my explanations almost *in toto*—things began to progress much more rapidly. Though she admitted
that she was not at all enthusiastic about returning to work, she remarked that she did not intend
to let this interfere with her recovery, for, as she
said, if she could not become resigned to working,
she could doubtless find some way to avoid it even
if she were well.

At this period the patient rarely saw Mr. Densmore, though he formed a frequent theme in our
conversations. She still protested that she disliked him, and as of old she ridiculed and made fun
of him. If any of her friends spoke of him she always took pains to refer to him in terms of de-
rision and contempt. Nevertheless, it seemed to
me that she was beginning to realize that, as I had
explained to her, these reactions were merely a
compensation for a real and strong attraction
which he exerted upon her, and which, in my opinion, was definitely sexual in the ordinary accep-
tation of the word.

That it was sexual in this sense seemed to be the
chief reason why she would not let herself like

him.   In spite of all I could do she had not yet appeared to be able to overcome the feeling that sex was essentially sinful.   Though now admitting that she was not entirely sexless and that sex impulses must be normal, she asserted that she had never experienced such a base longing as that for physical sex relations with a man and she hoped she never would.   But these statements were soon to be contradicted.   About this time Miss S——'s mother, who all along had felt that perhaps some uterine trouble was responsible for Miss S——'s illness, expressed a desire to have the girl examined by a gynæcologist.   Miss S—— told me about this; and though she felt that such an examination was unnecessary she thought perhaps she might better have it merely to satisfy her mother.   I gave her the name of a friend of mine to whom she could go for the examination (which, however, was never made); and then she asked if it was all right to go, meaning, might not her hymen be ruptured. I of course told her that the doctor would take care to avoid anything of the kind, and she seemed satisfied.   A night or two after this she dreamed that on my recommendation she had gone to a man, apparently a doctor, for some sort of treatment. She found herself in a room reading a large book which apparently the doctor, who seemed to be a negro, had given her.   From the title page she saw that the book was by a Professor F. R. E. D. —— (the name of a man who will be mentioned later).   The treatment seemed to consist in the reading of this book.   She saw in the book something about ''plenty of cracked ice and exercise.''

While reading she kept glancing at the clock, the idea being that at a certain time the doctor's office hour would be over and then she would go.

In view of what has been said the meaning of some parts of this dream are almost self-evident, though on the whole the dream is obscure. The person to whom in the dream she went for treatment apparently has some connection with the gynæcologist we had spoken of and who she was afraid might rupture her hymen. But the man seemed to be a negro. A negro, to most American girls is, in their dreams at least, a symbol or personification of masculine sexual aggression. Thus, the patient dreams that through my recommendation she finds herself in a situation where apparently she is exposed to a certain danger of sexual aggression and rupture of her hymen. Just what this situation is will appear later.

The large book which she read in the dream brought to her mind a "Family Medicine Book" which her mother possessed. She now admitted that she had occasionally referred to this work in the hope of satisfying her sexual curiosity, and of obtaining some information about the relation of the sex impulse to nervousness. The words "Plenty of cracked ice and exercise" were a condensation of certain passages in this book which referred to the treatment of masturbation. The name which she saw on the title page of the book in the dream was a condensation of the name of Professor Freud, of a psychoanalyst to whom I told her she could go if during my absence from the city she needed advice, and of another man

whom she regarded as an authority on sex. At
any rate, the reading of the book, which seemed to
be a sort of treatment, apparently represented the
doing of something that would satisfy her sexual
curiosity. What this something was, together
with additional associations with regard to the
book, was brought out in discussing the idea which
appeared in the dream that at a certain time the
doctor's office hour would be up and she could go.
When asked for associations on this point she soon
reverted to the theme of books, and at length told
me of having read an erotic novel entitled "His
Hour." The substance of the part that impressed her was as follows. A woman who had
been married is alone in the house of a man who is
in love with her. He suggests intercourse but she
refuses and is prepared to defend herself with a
revolver. He knows she will not kill him and sits
down as if to tire her out. At length, she faints.
When she recovers consciousness she finds her
clothing torn and disarranged and so concludes
that the man had had intercourse with her while
she was unconscious. Not until the end of the
book does she realize that this is not so and that
during her faint her lover "did but kiss her little
feet."

In reading this book the patient had experienced considerable sexual pleasure. The idea of
the helplessness of the woman during the fainting
attack strongly appealed to her, and she fantasied
herself in a similar situation, in which more happened than the kissing of feet. Now this, as
shortly appeared, had been a determinant of her

neurosis. The time when the man chased her on the street, on the day preceding her first fainting attack, she was still under the influence of the erotic excitement occasioned by the reading of this book. Her inability to run was due to her assault fantasies, which now, though in a not very acceptable way, seemed about to become realities. That is to say, her wish to be caught (not by this particular man, of course) operated as a counter wish to impede her.[1]

It is clear that the fainting attack which occurred on the day after her fright was in imitation of the woman in the story. It occurred when she knew Mr. D—— was near at hand, and it served to bring him to her side and cause him sympathetic concern about her. Now in the dream she is, at my suggestion, in a situation which apparently exposed her to sexual aggression and the loss of her hymen, but which is some sort of treatment, and has to do with the gratification of sexual curiosity. Her looking at the clock, etc., suggests that it is "His Hour." Expressed in this way, the dream is not difficult to interpret. The idea of treatment is associated with the idea of gratifying sexual curiosity. And the best way to gratify such curiosity is by actual experience. From what I had said with regard to repressed wishes being pathogenic, the patient concluded that one way to get well was to fulfill these wishes. Hence she dreams that she is having a "His Hour" experience—that as a means of getting well she ful-

[1] This is an excellent example of the utter disregard which wishes of the unconscious have for reality.

fills her sexual wishes. The idea that I was responsible for her undergoing this sort of treatment corresponds to her wish to shift responsibility for what she thought was wrong. It is evident too, that she was making of the psycho-analysis a substitute for the wish for sexual experience with, presumably, Mr. D——, and that she had thought of me, in his place, as the hero in an assault phantasy.

It will be remembered that the patient's chief symptom was a fear that if she went out alone or in the subway she would get weak, faint, and die. But we can now interpret this by saying that she had been afraid that if she continued well and able to work at the office she would get weak in the sense of giving way to Mr. D——'s charms, and that "her hour" would come, in the sense of ultimate sexual relations. Thus, as I had suspected at the beginning of the analysis the fear of death was actually a fear of love, or rather of her repressed longing for it.

The discussion provoked by the analysis of this dream marked the first pronounced relaxation of her resistances. I could point out to her a sequence that showed most convincingly the existence of a relationship between her symptoms and repressed sexuality. First, was the sudden flash of sexual feeling toward Mr. Densmore in the subway. Then came the reading of the white slave reports which led her to asking questions and resulted in a condition in which in spite of herself the theme of sexual relations gained for her a fearful fascination. Next was the reading

of the erotic book which, together with what the
girl had told her, provoked fantasies of fainting
and assault and caused a condition of considerable sexual tension. Then the incident of her
being chased by the man in the street. Her inability to run was determined by her assault fantasies which now, though in a not very acceptable
way, seemed about to become a reality. On the
following day (the day of her first attack) she
was expecting to make a visit to the scene of her
homosexual experience and this expedition would
have led, had it not been for her resistances, to
her indulging in pleasant recollections or fantasies
of a homosexual coloring. But in reacting against
this tendency, her libido reverted more strongly
to Mr. D—— and she fainted, the motive on
the one hand being a wish to escape from sexuality, which seemed to be on all sides of her, and
on the other for erotic experience corresponding
to that of the woman in the book, but with Mr.
Densmore in the rôle of the hero.

To this interpretation of the situation Miss
S—— gave partial confirmation. She admitted
that probably I was right in supposing that her interest in Mr. D—— was greater than she had been
willing to acknowledge. Soon after she declared
that she had been in love with him all along but
that she had tried to avoid admitting to herself
that such was the case. She stated too that she
was sure that if she were willing to "let herself
go" her love would rapidly increase. But though
she now admitted these things she was not content with them. Though admitting that Mr.

Densmore appealed more strongly to the passionate side of her nature than any one else that she
had ever known, she felt that that sort of an appeal was not right, and that she should care for a
man in a "spiritual way" only.   Even marriage,
to her mind, failed to legitimatize physical sexuality, and she continually argued that the fact that
Mr. D—— inspired "lustful" feelings in her was
the very reason she ought to keep away from him.
I pointed out, of course, that the impulses she was
trying to suppress were something perfectly normal and possessed by everybody, and that the sort
of love she thought she ought to have was really
an infantile sexuality.   Her conviction that sexuality was essentially wrong and debasing was
traced in various ways to earlier experiences particularly with regard to her parents—for instance,
it was pointed out that when her parents had concealed their sexuality from her she had assumed
that it did not exist and had based her ideal of
what she ought to be on this false assumption, ad-
hering to it in the face of the information she
gained at fourteen that all parents had intercourse
and that such was the way children came to exist.
Instead of viewing this information as evidence
that her sexual idea needed modification and that
there was nothing inherently disgraceful about
having sexual desire and gratifying it, she had repressed the information that might have served to
correct her false notions and persisted in clinging
to them in spite of it.   In these and other ways
effort was made to overcome her pathological
resistance against her sexuality but without meet-

ing with any pronounced success. She continued
to assert that everything sexual was repugnant
to her, and that though she did have sexual feelings she could not accept the view that they were
normal and inevitable. It seemed to me at times
however, that she was more nearly convinced than
she was ready to admit.

At length there occurred the following dream
which marked a definite change in her attitude.
She saw flying in the sky an enormous bird, which
mounted higher and higher, and upon which she
looked with feelings of awe and wonder but not
of fear. She tried to point out this wonderful
sight to her mother, who stood by, but the latter,
as if blind or stupefied, failed to look where the
bird was and kept repeating "I can't see it, I
can't see it." After a time, however, her mother
was induced to look in the right direction and said
"Oh, yes, I do see it after all." In the dream she
felt much surprise that she had so much difficulty
in making her mother see the bird, for it seemed
so plainly in sight and impossible to overlook.

As we began the analysis of the dream the patient said, "I don't know what the bird could represent. I've never seen anything like it. It seemed
to me so wonderful and amazing." Here she
paused, and when I asked her what she had in
mind she replied "I've thought Nature wonderful and amazing too." She meant by this, as she
at length explained, reproduction and all it signified. The bird therefore could be regarded as a
symbol of reproduction.[1] On the day preceding

[1] The bird is a familiar penis symbol—cf. Jones' paper, *Die*

the dream we had spoken of the biological meaning of the sex instinct and I had taken occasion to
use some matter that came up to support the proposition that sexuality could not be essentially
"bad." She demurred and later I said "Perhaps
you do not want to see these things." Still later
I had used the phrase "There are none so blind
as those who won't see." This was the source of
the dream material. In the dream she gazes on the
forces of nature, or of sex, in wonder and awe.
Her mother to whom she tries to point out the remarkable sight, seems blind or stupid. In the
dream the mother represents that phase of her
personality which is identified with her mother;
the same phase from which arose the sex resistances I had been combating. At last in the dream
she did get her mother "to look in the right direction," or in other words, she finally became willing to see the sexual life as something fine and
wonderful instead of as "dirty" and debasing.

The stimulus which had resulted in this dream
was, I learned, as follows: It seems that across
the court in the apartment house where she lived
there was a young married couple whom she had
often watched from her bed room. They had
seemed to her to be singularly sweet and tender
with one another, and she had regarded them as
strikingly "good" young people. On the day of
her dream she had learned that this young woman
had given birth to a baby, and in the face of this

Empfangnis der Jungfrau Maria durch das Ohr. Jahrbuch der
Psychoanalyse 1914. Also, children are told that babies are
brought by a bird, the stork.

conclusive evidence that they must have had intercourse, she said to herself that surely if such sweet and innocent appearing young people practiced coitus there could hardly be anything really wrong about it.[1] The dream shows that there had been in existence two phases of her personality; the one caused in her by her mother's apparent attitude toward sex matters (a foreconscious trend), and another which secretly sided with me (essentially of the Unconscious).

The interpretation of this dream the patient readily accepted and her resistances appeared greatly decreased. She had been slowly improving up to this time but now her improvement became much more rapid, and she felt as if soon she would be entirely well. But then one morning, she came late for her appointment and reported that she had felt so badly that she had been almost afraid to make the trip to my office thinking she would probably die on the way. She felt much disappointed, for the night before she had been thinking that on this day for the first time, she would try to make the trip to my office alone. During the night she had dreamed that she was in a wedding dress and about to be married. Then suddenly she changed her mind and felt that she did not wish to marry and that she would die if she did. She told this to her mother, who stood by in the dream, but her mother urged her to go ahead. The girl would not do so, however, and was about to run away when she awoke.

[1] Another element in the life of these young people also affected her, as we shall hear later.

The general meaning of the dream is plain enough. She had regarded herself as just on the point of getting well. In the dream she is just on the point of getting married. Apparently she had identified the two things. Her illness had expressed her resistances against marriage, and to get well meant to overcome these resistances, and, in this sense, to be ready to marry. The dream thus shows that she has changed her mind; that she still had some resistances toward the idea of marriage, or, what was equivalent, toward Mr. Densmore.

After this her resistances against sex seemed to return somewhat for she again began to repeat her earlier assertions that such things were dirty. She decided that she did not want to see Mr. Densmore and let herself become more fond of him, because of her repugnance to the dirty things that marriage would involve.

She said also that there was another and equally important reason why she did not want to marry him and of this she began to talk a good deal. It seems that Mr. Densmore had a woman relative who had divorced her husband. Miss Sunderland asserted that she was unwilling to marry into a family where such a thing had taken place. She felt, she said, that the whole family was somehow tainted, and that the tendency to infidelity and cruelty [1] which she supposed had been displayed

[1] She had no definite information as to what were the grounds upon which the divorce was obtained. The divorce occurred in another state, and that infidelity and cruelty were the grounds for it, Miss Sunderland merely assumed.

by the divorced husband would sooner or later crop out in Mr. Densmore. This fear that he might be cruel had arisen on a certain occasion when she heard him order a waiter around rather roughly.

I could not convince myself that a girl as intelligent as Miss S—— could be deterred from marrying a man she loved merely because there was a divorce in his family, nor could I believe that she was really sincere in supposing that the assumed brutal and immoral tendencies of the divorced man could have been transmitted to Mr. Densmore and the rest of his family—Mr. Densmore was not a blood relative of the man, but only a connection by marriage. Nor did I think that a little roughness in her husband—such, for instance as Mr. D—— displayed toward the waiter—would be altogether distasteful to her. She seemed to have a rather strong masochistic tendency and a certain degree of masterfulness in a man would, in my opinion, have appealed to her. The fact was unquestionable, however, that these resistances, against Mr. D——, absurd as they seemed, were not to be removed by pointing out their very apparent absurdity. That the resistances were real, there seemed to be no doubt, though I could hardly believe that they arose from the source to which the patient attributed them. At no time would she admit their unreasonableness and absurdity.

There came to my mind finally an observation I had made in certain other cases which seemed to afford a possible explanation of this resistance,

namely, that when a person is vacillating between
two divergent courses and can not bring himself
to give up the attractive features of either one in
favor of the advantages of the other, he has a
tendency to see, or to imagine that he sees, in one
course *disadvantages* that really belong to the
other, where, however, he is loath to see them.
Thus, for example, if a man were trying to find
excuses for staying in the city in the summer, he
might say to himself, ''Oh those country houses
are so terribly hot and ill ventilated, etc.,'' while
as a matter of fact, the heat and the lack of air
circulation is one of the most disagreeable features of remaining in the city, and one of the
strongest reasons for going to the country.

On this basis I began to suspect that the patient
wished to follow some course contrary to that of
marrying Mr. Densmore but against this course
the stigma of divorce and of the possibility of
cruelty arose, not as an imaginary but as a real
objection, and that it was the *attractive* features
of this course which were the *real* sources of that
resistance against marriage with Mr. Densmore
which we have been discussing.

This conclusion was finally confirmed by the
analysis of the following dream. ''I was somewhere in a fine house. A woman was showing me
beautiful dresses which I was to try on. It
seemed I was about to marry a rich man, who
was giving me all these things and who could
give me anything I wanted. Then, I realized that
the man I was marrying was a foreigner, perhaps
a Chinaman, and I ran away, feeling that I could

much more easily do without the things he could give me than get them at such a price.''

The idea of a Chinaman brought to the patient's mind a newspaper story she had recently read about a wealthy Chinese who had a beautiful white girl as his mistress. Then came something she had never mentioned before.

She confessed that before she became ill she had met at a dinner a very wealthy foreigner who immediately became impressed with her and paid her most conspicuous attentions. She was quite disposed to think he would ask her to marry him if she gave him the least encouragment. She did not love the man but the idea of a rich marriage strongly appealed to her.[1] On the other hand, Mr. D——, as she now admitted, had less money than almost any of the other young men she knew. Though his prospects were good, she knew her life, if she married him, would at first be anything but luxurious, and she would have to consider herself lucky if she had a servant to help her with the work. Such a prospect was not altogether to her fancy.

After this disclosure there came a still more interesting item. The foreigner had already been married and his wife had divorced him, on the ground of infidelity. In the newspaper accounts of the divorce which Miss S—— had read there were some more or less definite charges of cruelty. These were the facts that had caused the patient

[1] Her desire for a rich marriage was partly the result of her experience with her rich employer. The foreigner was a substitute for him.

to exaggerate the significance of a divorce having occurred in Mr. D——'s family and to persuade herself that he might be cruel. Her wish for wealth was the motive. If she could make herself believe that the objections to the foreigner also applied to Mr. D——, then there would be that much less reason for not taking the one who had the most money. Dirt is often a symbol for money and this may have had something to do with her resistance to marrying Mr. D——, which she rationalized by saying that sexuality is dirty. It was really the *attraction* of dirt—filthy lucre—from another quarter which was the source of this resistance.[1]

In the light of all this the meaning of her dream is evident. To marry the rich foreigner would be to make of herself a sort of prostitute—hence her identification with the white slave mistress of the rich Chinaman. The dream shows that Miss S—— had decided to give up the idea of obtaining wealth in this way.

After the dream, Miss S—— went on to explain that Mr. D—— had begun to pay her attentions, and she to like him, before she met the foreigner.[2] But when she did meet him, and began to believe that all his wealth would be at her disposal if she wanted it, she commenced to repress her interest

---

[1] The dream about the bird which seemed to be connected with thoughts about the young couple next door and which marked a relaxation of her resistances must be connected with an idea gained by watching the young people that one could be happy without wealth.

[2] The foreigner was 40 years of age—one of her alleged objections to Mr. Densmore was that he was too young—"a mere boy," though he was eight years older than she.

in Densmore, and to try to like the foreigner, without however meeting with entire success in either direction. Then she made up her mind that she would not attempt to decide the matter either way, but that instead, she would go to parties and dances as much as she could, in the hope that she might meet some new man who on the one hand would be as rich as the foreigner and on the other as lovable as Densmore. But at this point came the outbreak of the neurosis. It was a sort of resultant of all these conflicting forces. On the one hand it interfered with the social activities she had planned and thus served to keep her faithful to Mr. Densmore. On the other, it kept her from seeing so much of him that she would become deeply enough in love to renounce the money, and in like manner it kept her from seeing much of the foreigner.

Her morbid fear that if she went out alone she would "fall" (in a faint, etc.) which, as we know, came on shortly after her reading about white slavery in the papers, is really connected in a more intimate way with the idea of white slavery. If she married the foreigner merely for his money she would in a certain sense fall. Her act would be a form of prostitution and she a white slave. On the other hand, if she married Mr. Densmore she might regard herself as being a white slave in quite another sense—that is she might have to work harder than was to her liking. We now see that these matters were dealt with in the dream of King James II. Her running away from the fat man who ordered her around referred

on the one hand to her wish not to have to work
(as the wife of Mr. Densmore) and on the other
to her impulse to escape from the wealthy man
(the foreigner who was concealed behind her employer) because she did not like him as a husband.

After the analysis of this dream the patient
improved with great rapidity. She seemed now to
understand what her illness meant, and felt confi-
dent that she would soon be well. Of her own accord she came to my office alone, and she experienced no fear or other unpleasant symptoms on
the way. At last, she told me of a plan she had
devised to get Mr. Densmore to renew his attentions—she had not been seeing him for some
time, for he apparently had given her up in de-
spair—and at the same time announced that she
did not feel it necessary that she should come to
me any more. I saw her a month later and she
reported that Mr. Densmore had promptly responded to her scheme and that she was having
a most delightful time with him. She felt that
she loved him and that everything would be well.
I saw her a few other times at long intervals and
each time she reported herself to be in the best
health and spirits. She married Mr. Densmore a
year or more after the completion of the analysis,
and when I last heard from her, she was well and
happy.

For the sake of completeness, I might add that
my experience with later and more deeply analyzed cases indicates that morbid fears of attacks
of unconsciousness—fainting, epilepsy, etc.—have
reference to a period of bed-wetting in the child-

hood of the patient and possess as one of their oldest and deepest roots a certain urethral-erotic tendency and the corresponding unconscious fantasies. Though this was not definitely worked out in the case of Miss Sunderland, considerable of the material brought out in her analysis (not all of which I have reported) strongly suggests that such was one of the determinants of her symptoms, e. g. her dream of urinating on the ground, the history of bed-wetting, her notion that the sex relations are dirty, etc.

The only state of unconsciousness and irresponsibility which children know about is that of sleep, and it must be a rather impressive experience for them to find that a condition is possible in which they do, without knowing about it and without being held very much to blame, a thing which if done voluntarily and in the conscious state would win them severe punishment. It is not surprising then that in later years when there break out conflicts with wishes which, if acted upon voluntarily would expose the individual to social censure or punishment or to the misery of self reproach, there should arise a wish (or fear) of sleep-like states in which the repressed desires could be conceived of as being *involuntarily* fulfilled.

Furthermore, the teasing and ridicule over not having control of their sphincters, and the occasionally none too tolerant attitude of the parents, have, in certain cases, the effect of laying the foundation for a feeling of inferiority and sensitiveness which may persist throughout the individual's life and forever act as an inhibition upon the normal expression of the sexual activities.

CHAPTER X

IF the reader has closely followed the preceding chapters, he may complain, on having finished them, that certain of the items set forth in the discussion of theory were not brought out concretely by the two case reports which have been given. These cases did not, for instance, demonstrate the infantile factors to be as important as perhaps he had been led to expect, nor did they show beyond all peradventure the neurosis to be the negative of the perversion. The matter of transference, though it came up, apparently did not play the dominant rôle which the reader might have been prepared to find it occupying.

Such complaints would not be unjust, for, as I am well aware, the reports I have given do possess these defects, as well as other similar ones. On the other hand the fact that I have chosen them for reporting is not without justification. As I originally planned this book, I had intended that the last chapter should consist of a report of a case so completely analyzed as fully to illustrate all the points raised in discussing the theoretical aspects of the neuroses. I thought by this means to make up for the defects of the two earlier cases, which I had felt would serve an introductory function better than others more elaborately analyzed. But I know now, from having failed at it, that I had set myself an impossible task. That is to say, my later and better analyzed cases, which gave full illustration of the theories here set forth, represented such an enormous mass of intricate and almost endless detail that, without destroying their scientific value, I could not compress any one of them into a narrative short enough to be included within this volume. I therefore decided to complete this book with a chapter on the theory of the psychoanalytic treatment and to endeavor to make up for the fact that my two cases here reported fail to fulfill all that might be desired of them as illustrative material by writing a supplementary volume which would be devoted to a single detailed case report. For, as a matter of fact, the full report of any case which is completely analyzed deserves a volume by itself and cannot be accurately presented by anything short of it.

In the twenty-five years that have elapsed since Breuer and Freud published their first paper on hysteria, the theory and technique of psychoanalytic treatment have passed through a number of evolutionary changes. The method had its beginning in 1880 when, in studying the case of an hysterical girl, Brezier found that the symptoms of her malady vanished when she could be made to remember in full detail the situations and associative connections under which they first appeared. When ten years later Breuer and Freud together took up the investigation, which in the

meantime had been neglected, there was developed
the so-called cathartic method of treatment.
They came to the conclusion that certain pathological experiences, to which the patients had in-
adequately reacted, played the rôle of psychic traumata, causing the neurotic symptoms analogously
to the physical traumata which Charcot had regarded as causative for hysterical paralysis.   The
technique of the treatment then was to restore to
the patient, by means of hypnosis, a perfect memory of these pathogenic experiences and of the setting in which the symptoms first appeared, affording in this way free discharge to the previously
strangulated affects.   (Abreaction.)

After a time Freud abandoned hypnosis as a
means for filling out the gaps in the patient's
memory, and adopted instead the method of free
association.   The patient was asked to concen-
trate his mind on some given symptom or on some
point where his memory of connections or of
events was obviously incomplete, and then to relate all the thoughts that came to him.   The physician sought to divine from the associations thus
produced the missing material that the patient
was unable to remember.   The resistances which
had kept this material unconscious and prevented
recall were then to be circumvented by the physician's imparting to the patient the reconstruc-
tion derived from the study of the associations.
Abreaction, upon which so much emphasis had
been laid earlier, now retired from the foreground
and its place seemed to be taken by the expenditure of energy required of the patient in resisting

the censorship over his incoming associations. The doctrine of complexes came into vogue, and the physician bent his energies to figuring out what complexes were behind each given symptom and describing them to the patient as soon as the discovery was made.

Then came a further change which brought the technique into the form which is in use to-day. The physician no longer concentrated upon the symptoms themselves or strove to discover and as soon as possible to impart to the patient a correct interpretation of them. Instead of making an attack upon some definite manifestation of the disorder, the physician now assumed a more passive and expectant attitude, and, directing the patient to talk about whatever came to his mind, waited for him to unfold his personality to view without being concerned as to what manner and what order the different constituents took in making their appearance. Instead of using the interpretation of free associations, dreams, etc., as a means of getting hold of the submerged psychic material and dragging it to the surface while the resistances were still in force, these procedures were principally employed in attacking the resistances themselves, which were interpreted and explained to the patient so that through understanding they might be overcome. For it was found that when, through successive interpretations, the resistances were worn away, the patient was then able, spontaneously and without effort, to recall and relate the forgotten situations, phantasies, wishes, connections and so on which were required for a complete picture of the ensemble of factors, conscious and unconscious, which had to do with the development and continuance of the disease.

As soon as the resistances became the first consideration in the technique, the transference, which is the source of the most stubborn and baffling of all resistance, became one of the most important problems.

The essential goals of these various techniques have remained the same from the start; on the one hand the overcoming of the repression resistances, on the other the filling out of the gaps of memory, the bringing into consciousness of the pathogenic material from the unconscious.

In thinking this over we come upon one of the most interesting and yet most baffling questions that analysis has yet presented. Why is it that when the resistances are overcome and the memory gaps filled out, the patient is then well? How does this cure him?

That a person can be cured in this way is indeed a remarkable fact. It is by no means self-evident why the overcoming of repressions or the filling out of gaps of memory should render a sick person well. In fact "common sense" would perhaps tell us that at least the latter feature (the filling out of gaps of memory, the bringing up of all sorts of unpleasant recollections out of the past) should tend rather to make him worse. Indeed the psychoanalytic cure seems to be without parallel in human experience. How are we to explain it?

As a matter of fact, a completely adequate explanation has yet to be formulated. Most psychoanalytic writers have made no very serious attempts to account for the results of analysis. Freud himself has said comparatively little about the question. The explanations of the cure which have been given amount to little more than saying: "It is the understanding of himself which the patient gains through the analysis which cures him" or "when the previously unconscious pathogenic trends are rendered conscious, the patient is then in a position so to dispose of them that they no longer work pathogenically." These explanations are perhaps correct enough as far as they go, but they by no means tell the whole story. *Why*, for instance, should the understanding of himself, which the patient gains in the analysis, have the effect of curing him?

To tell the truth, it seems to me that in the present state of our knowledge the analytic cure cannot be fully explained. The only explanations that can at present be advanced involve items which themselves require explaining, or give rise to questions which as yet no one is fully prepared to answer. On the other hand the cure which results from analysis is no absolute mystery. We can go a certain and perhaps a considerable distance toward explaining it—further, possibly, than any one has made any effort to go, for, as it seems to me, the question of why analysis does cure is one which, on the whole, has been rather neglected by psychoanalytic writers.

The explanation I should like to offer is some-

what more elaborate than those usually given,
though I cannot claim that it adds anything really
new to them. In attempting to set it forth I wish,
first of all, to emphasize, and to ask the reader to
bear in mind throughout, that, in point of view of
effect, the overcoming of resistance and the filling
out of gaps of memory are identical, or at least
inseparable. The filling out of memory gaps requires the overcoming of resistances; the overcoming of resistance requires gaps of memory to
be filled out. The two processes go hand in hand;
each is a part of the other. This fact of the con-
fluence or basic continuity between what, at first
glance, seem to be two essentially different processes gives, it seems to me, the indication of the
direction which any adequate attempts to explain
the psychoanalytic cure must at first take.

Let us look at the problem first from its dynamic side, namely, Why is it that a cure is brought
about through the overcoming of resistances? A
partial answer to this question may be given by
way of an analogy. It need hardly be said that
the state of a man having strong and continually
unfulfilled wishes and no prospect of fulfilling
them may, without the introduction of any additional factor, be one of considerable unhappiness.
The constant tension of desires unsatisfied is in
itself a source of pain. For instance, a man serving a term of life imprisonment is ordinarily a
very unhappy person, yet, save for the actual
physical discomforts of prison life (which certainly in most instances are not nearly so great as
those which a soldier in the trenches bears very

cheerfully) he has not much to worry him except his unfulfilled wishes. His unhappiness results for the most part we would say from his "lack of freedom." Almost everything he would like to do he cannot do. Nearly every wish he has must forever remain unsatisfied. And as is well known there results in a certain number of cases not only a state of great unrest and unhappiness, but of actual mental illness, the prison psychoses and other disturbances. In fact some of these conditions, much like the neurosis, represent an effort to ameliorate the unbearable state of tension from the non-fulfillment of all wishes by supplying a phantastic fulfillment—the delusion of a pardon and other psychotic wish-fulfillment formations.

Now the unhappiness, the suffering, the sense of being ill, which the neurotic suffers is in many respects analogous in origin to the unhappiness of a man in prison. A part of it corresponds to the pain of desires ungratified; the constant tensions of longings unassuaged. A part of it, too, corresponds to a sense of guilt, which of course may be a factor in the unhappiness of the prisoner in confinement. And though I have had no opportunity to study prison inmates, I am very much disposed to think that a sense of guilt is a much larger component in the misery which the scrupulously moral neurotic suffers, than in the unhappiness of the incarcerated criminal. For the one has a conscience which in many cases is over acute while the conscience of the other is as a rule subnormal. The one does not have to violate any important moral law in order to feel guilty, while the

other may violate almost any law without reproaching himself at all, providing he escapes
punishment.

But while in the case of the prisoner the restraints responsible for the pain of many wishes
chronically unfulfilled are physical and external
ones, those restraints which have the similar effect in the neurotic are endogenous and psychic
ones. The prisoner may struggle against bolts,
bars and chains, but the struggle of the neurotic
is against himself. His prison is his own mind,
he was condemned by his own laws and sentenced
on his own judgment; he himself is his own
keeper. He has therefore not only the miseries
that are much the same in origin as those suffered
by a person in prison (the pain of unsatisfied
wishes and the torment of a sense of guilt) [1] but
others more difficult to factor which arise from
the circumstance that the restraining forces are
psychic and a part of himself. Morbid fear, in
part at least, belongs to that category.

Now the codes according to which the neurotic
was sentenced and the psychic bars by which he is
confined are none other than the resistances which
the analysis overcomes. The analysis renders
him free to fulfill his wishes—not that, except to a
limited extent, he then fulfills them in their original form, for the analysis does not confer license;
the patient still has to adapt himself to reality, to

[1] The sense of guilt which may be a large contributor to the
neurotic's misery is by no means invariably perceived by him as
guilt. More often it is so subject to displacement or distortion as
to be regarded by him as some other sort of unpleasant feeling.

the demands of civilized existence. Rather the analysis makes practical the establishing of a minimum of non-fulfilled wishes and a maximum of wish fulfillment by making it possible for the patient to satisfy by way of sublimation many wishes of such a nature that previously they could only be expressed in symptoms. In this sense the overcoming of resistances releases him; he is now free to gratify in suitable manner a great number of wishes that previously were relatively unfulfilled. To some extent the analytic cure is then analogous to the relief which a prisoner experiences if he is declared innocent and let out of prison. There is done away with the constant urge of unsatisfied wish tensions, the torments of guilty conscience (if that had been an element in the case) and in addition that less easily defined factor which depends on the fact that the individual's struggle for freedom was against himself. But such an explanation as this tells only a part of the story and gives a very inadequate picture of what really takes place in the analytic cure. We must go into the matter further.

Let us now ask what are the resistances which the analysis overcomes. How are they constituted? What is their origin?

After a fashion we have answered these questions in earlier chapters. The resistances belong in the main to the higher psychic systems, especially to the foreconscious. In general they are trends which have an inhibiting, a repressing effect upon the primary tendencies of the individual, the instinctive and infantile, or, in other words, upon the unconscious. Furthermore they correspond to that in the personality which is acquired rather than to that which is innate [1]—they are the result of experience, of environmental influence, of training, even though to some extent their energy may be in part derived from primary tendencies that have been added to or modified by influences to which the individual was subject in the course of development. The resistances include many, if not all, of those functionings which we would set down to conscience. But the point to be remembered is that they are acquired, the result of experience.

It may well be of service to look at these resistances from a different angle from the one to which we have become accustomed. All organized responses that can be called forth in both man and animal, declare the behaviorists, fall under one or the other of two headings, instincts (including here the simplest forms of reflexes) and habits.[2] Both instinct and habit are analyzable into simple congenital reflexes. Instinct is defined by the behaviorists as "a complex system of reflexes which function in serial order when the organism is confronted by certain stimuli." In exactly the same terms do they define habit. "After habits are perfected they function in all particulars as do instincts." The only essential difference be-

[1] This must be accepted only as a general statement to which there are many exceptions. Some of the transference resistances with which one has to deal in the analysis may belong more to the instinctive or infantile part of the personality than to that part which comes from training.

[2] J. B. Watson: *Behavior*, Chap. VI.

tween habit and instinct is, then, that of origin.[1] In instinct the "pattern" (the number and localization of the different reflex arcs involved) and the "order" (the temporal relations of the unfolding of the elements of the pattern) are inherited, while in the case of habit both pattern and order are acquired during the lifetime of the individual. All organized behavior, whether it be "explicit" (action) or "implicit" (thought or feeling) is then from the behaviorist's point of view, the expression either of habit, of instinct or of the two combined.

Some of the important Freudian concepts are quite readily translatable into behavioristic terms. The unconscious (i. e. that which is primary in the personality, the instinctive and infantile) embraces the same functionings which the behaviorist calls "instinct." Likewise that which is acquired, and which controls and supplements instincts and is called " habit " by the behaviorist, is about the same as that which psychoanalysis conceives of as belonging to the higher psychic systems, especially to the foreconscious. Even though the correspondence between the "habit" of the behaviorists and the foreconscious of Freud

[1] L. c. That which the behaviorists and which Freud would call instinctive is about the same. Freud, however, uses the term instinct as the heading for large groups of tendencies, while the term impulse or wish applies to the subdivisions of the group. The behaviorists would call instinctive these or even finer subdivisions. I trust it is clear that the term habit as here employed has a much broader meaning than is given to it when in common speech we speak of a cigarette habit or the habit of twiddling one's thumbs.

is not absolutely perfect, yet for practical purposes they may be thought of as identical.

This being the case, it is not difficult to see that what we are accustomed to call a " resistance " might, in most cases at least, be called a habit.　At least this is true of all resistances, all repressions, that are acquired by the individual, and not innate. Even some of those resistances which have an hereditary basis can be regarded as instinct modified or reënforced by habit.[1]　All the repression or inhibitions which the individual develops because of training, everything in conscience which is acquired, can just as well be regarded as an expression of habit as of the foreconscious or of the libido.

Let us ask ourselves what is the significance of habit, with the intention of thereby enriching our understanding of what is meant by resistance. We may answer this question by considering an example of habit.　Young retriever dogs, when first taken hunting, will in many instances chew the birds they are to retrieve to such an extent as to spoil them.　A way to train a dog not to do this is to make him retrieve repeatedly a dead bird or a ball which has been thrust full of pins.

[1] The term "complex" does not quite coincide either with instinct or with habit.　Most complexes have an instinctive basis to which are added the effects of experience or training.　Minor complexes are perhaps pure habits but the major ones have both instinctive and habitual constituents.　Also, habit participates in the forming of fixations of instinct, and the infantile fixations though really representing the effect of experience upon instinct are considered from the psychoanalytic standpoint as belonging to the unconscious.

After the dog has pricked his mouth a few times by shutting down upon such an object, he learns to carry it so gently that in spite of the pins he will not hurt himself. He can then be trusted to carry with equal gentleness the game which the hunter shoots. A habit has been established by the use of pins which remains in force and inhibits the dog's original tendency to mouthe the birds while retrieving them. Because of this habit he now carries the game *as if it contained pins.*

Now this latter fact about the habit is an important one. The behaviorist seeks to formulate an individual's reactions in terms of external objects or conditions, of which the behavior is said to be a "function." Thus he asks concerning the animal or person to be studied, "What is he doing?" and the reply is supposed to be made in terms of immediate external circumstance. But in the case of a dog whose original tendency was to mouthe game, but who now, after the sort of training just described, carries it gently, the question "What is he doing?" cannot be completely answered by the statement "He is retrieving a bird." For such an answer quite obviously does not tell the whole story. He is retrieving a bird in a (for him) special manner, namely, *as if it contained pins.* His behavior is a function of something more than the bird he at the moment holds in his mouth. It is partly determined by past experience, without which he would be still mouthing the game. In other words, we cannot adequately formulate his behavior, when this

510 MORBID FEARS AND COMPULSIONS

habit is involved, if we employ terms only of the
present. To make an adequate picture of the
significance of the habit requires us to draw in it
phantoms of past pins.

Now much the same thing applies to habits generally.[1] Their significance cannot be expressed
without historical references. The question
"What is he doing?" cannot, when it is a case of
habit, be answered satisfactorily without bringing in terms of the past experiences which were
instrumental in integrating the reflexes which
constitute the habit. In short, in those responses
of an individual which belong to habit, he is behaving very much *as if he were still surrounded
by those same external circumstances to which the
actions which eventually became habitual were
originally an adaptation.*

The Bible says: "Train up a child in the way
he should go and when he is old he will not depart
from it." This is the equivalent of saying:
"Devise a system of rewards and punishments,
of praise and blame, which will lead your child to
react for a period in the ways that seem to you
best, and these ways of reacting will eventually
become habits which he will retain throughout his
life. In other words he will, even after you are
dead and buried, continue to act, to feel and to
think in response to certain stimuli, AS IF *you
were still watching over him;* AS IF *your orig-*

[1] Naturally I am thinking in this connection only of sensori-
motor habits—not of the sort which depend on some artificially
produced changes in the chemistry of the body such as occur with
the morphine or tobacco habit.

inal system of rewards and punishments were still in force.[1] To be sure he will soon cease to interpret his own behavior in any such light. When the habits that you instilled function in his adult life, he will very likely rationalize his actions, thoughts or feelings by saying for instance that now he has become a man, he sees that his parents were "right" in their training of him or that he believes or behaves in this or that way because one "ought to" or because his "conscience prompts it." But the whole business is but the manifestation of habit, or instinct plus habit.[2]

[1] Many parents have been grievously disappointed to find that, after they have devoted themselves assiduously to training up a child "in the way he should go," he departed from it with the greatest dispatch as soon as he left the parental fireside or ceased greatly to fear parental punishment. But this by no means alters the fact that the biblical statement expresses a perfectly correct general principle, and one which holds good to an even greater extent than superficial observation would consider possible. The general principle is that the effects of training tend to be permanent, whether they be in the direction of the way the child should go, or of the way he should not go. Many of the parental disappointments of the sort described depend upon the fact that the efforts that were made to train the child in the way he should go were really training him in very different directions, for example, to react with feelings of hate, rebellion and suspicion to all stimuli that would come under the head of "authority."

[2] I know very well how difficult it is for one to recognize in himself the functioning of deeply ingrained habits or instincto-habits for what they really are. The more fully a given response is the product of habit, or of habit grafted on an instinct, the more likely, generally speaking, is the individual to rationalize it into something else and thus to believe sincerely that he is acting in this or that way because it is "right" to do so, or for some similar reason. The people of this country, for instance,

But we are rapidly becoming in danger of losing sight of the questions that we set out to answer: What is a resistance? and why is it that the psychoanalytic cure results from the overcoming of resistances? In reality we have not wandered so far from these questions as perhaps might seem. And at the same time we have been getting into a position from which we can consider, with some prospect of answering it, the other question: Why is it that the patient becomes cured by the filling out of the gaps in his memory?

Whenever in the foregoing discussion I have used the word "habit," I might perhaps just as

feel that it is "wrong" for a girl to come unchaste to her husband, little realizing that what they think or feel in this matter is infinitely more dependent upon the influence of environment or, in other words, upon habit, than upon whatever rightness or wrongness may really inhere in the question. They would say that a girl self evidently "ought to be" chaste, and that their opinions and feelings in the matter depend upon the actual merits of the case and not upon habit and training. By way of contrast, then, I might mention that there are regions where just the opposite opinions prevail and just the opposite habits are developed. In Japan, for instance, at least in certain quarters, it is considered a moral disgrace for a woman to come to her husband uninitiated and untrained in matters of sex, and for this reason the young woman is prepared for marriage by spending a certain time in public brothels, where, in intercourse with strangers, she gains the experience in sexual affairs, without which, in the Japanese opinion, no girl is fitted to be a good wife. And just as an American girl not only *thinks* but *feels* it to be a disgrace if her chastity is violated (that is, she would experience the reflex efferent discharge producing the subjective feeling of guilt, a purely automatic and reflex functioning) so, presumably, the Japanese girl would, through an opposite sort of training, show the same reflex response under directly opposite conditions, that is, if she came to her marriage without having had extensive sexual experience.

well have said "resistance," or even "complex," in most instances. For whether one says habit or resistance, that which is thought of is the same. The two words correspond to different ways of thinking of it. The habit, which reduces to arcs and reflexes, coincides with the purely objective point of view; the resistance, which is analyzable into ideas, memories, impulses or wishes, takes into account subjective factors.

What I have desired to bring out is that the full significance of a habit, and consequently of a repression resistance (with the exception of those repression resistances which are purely instinctive, and these perhaps are never overcome, even in the most thoroughgoing analysis), can be expressed *only by employing terms of past experience.* The action, thought or feeling which, in a given individual, results when there is touched off one of those acquired integrations which we may call interchangeably habit or resistance, occurs in general *as if* he were surrounded by and reacting to the same conditions or objects which originally called forth this response. It is a question of the same principle as that with which we are already familiar from the discussion of the conditioned reflex (in the section on transference) namely, that a small *part* of the stimuli corresponding to an original sensory pattern may serve to excite the *whole* original motor pattern and efferent discharge—may, in short, cause the individual to react *as if* the whole ensemble of external factors from which proceeded the stimuli for the original sensory excitations were still present and still giving off stimuli. *The question, What is he doing? when acquired organized responses are involved (habit or resistance) cannot be fully answered without reciting the history of the experiences which produced the integrations now functionating.*

Now in the case of the dog in whom there has been built up, by the use of pins, a habit or resistance which inhibits his original tendency to mouthe game, we can describe his behavior in objective terminology by introducing the words *as if*. We take account of his habit and its history by saying that he now retrieves game *as if* he were trying to avoid getting his mouth hurt. A step beyond this, which would bring us nearer to the psychoanalytic way of looking at things, would be to say he was behaving *as if he thought* the game contained pins, *as if he desired* to avoid getting his mouth hurt.[1] In answering the question, What is he doing? we have now introduced the concepts of thinking, of wishing and of ideas. Now the psychoanalytic way of answering such questions goes still further than that just indicated. In matters of human behavior which involve the functionating of a habit, or a resistance, the answer runs not *"as if* he thought" nor *as if* he wished" so and so, but rather " he *does* think it, he *does* desire it," but in the main " *unconsciously.*" And this is not purely conceptional nor merely a convenient way of describing. As

---

[1] This way of expressing the facts is quite permissible even though we may know that the dog is incapable of "thinking," in any ordinary human sense, anything of the kind.

our previous chapters have indicated, the assumed unconscious thinking or wishing can with all reasonable certitude be demonstrated to have existed, even though the evidence is not wholly direct. The history of the past experiences which first called forth the responses which eventually became integrated as habit or resistance is preserved as memory traces in the mind of the individual. Some of these records are foreconscious and subject to voluntary recall; others are unconscious and can be reproduced only in the course of an analysis. But the point is, that there is contained in the individual's own mind that same historical material which, as we have said, is required to express the full significance of any item of acquired organized behavior—action, thought, or feeling.

It is now to be seen that we have stumbled upon an answer to the questions from which we set out. The filling out of gaps of memory is nothing else than a process of bringing to the surface the historical records of the experiences instrumental in integrating the systems of habits or resistances which are now functionating. It supplies the patient with the data which are required for him to see the whole meaning of his present behavior, implicit and explicit. *It shows him what he is doing, in the fullest possible sense.* We have said that when acquired integrations are functionating the behavior of the individual is the same as if there were still present the original conditions which first called forth these responses. He is reacting as if surrounded by phantoms of the past, though this he himself does not recognize. The filling out of the gaps of memory which takes place in the analysis allows him to see this, and to appreciate the significance of that part of his present acting, feeling or thinking for which habit is responsible. This, apparently, is what cures him. The reducing of acquired integrations to the terms of the original experiences frees the individual from their automaticity and enables him to adapt to the facts of the present instead, as previously, to phantoms of the past. When he knows in full detail what he really is doing, *then* he can do otherwise if his inner needs and external circumstances demand it. Habit, write Dewey and Tufts,[1] is a stage "of unconscious activity along the lines set previous action. Consciousness thus 'occupies a curious middle ground between hereditary reflex and automatic activities upon the one hand and acquired habitual activities on the other.'[2] Where the original equipment of instincts fails to meet some new situation, when there are stimulations for which the system has no ready-made response, consciousness appears. It selects from the various responses those which suit the purpose, and when these responses have become themselves automatic, habitual, consciousness 'betakes itself elsewhere to points where habitual accommodatory movements are as yet wanting and needed.' To apply this to the moral development we need only to add that this

[1] Dewey and Tufts: Ethics, page 9.
[2] Angell: Psychology, page 59.

process repeats itself over and over." The analysis is exactly the reverse of this. By it, consciousness, which had "betaken itself elsewhere" is brought back to the points at which "responses which have become themselves automatic, habitual" had origin; the individual is allowed to deliberate, to value, to choose anew. New, better, more intelligent ways of reacting to present situations are thus opened up to him to replace those in his repertoire of ready-made automatic responses, which, because they were integrated when his intellect had not yet reached its maturity, and when his capacities for analyzing and choosing were especially limited, do not fully utilize his adaptive possibilities or allow him to put forth his actual best.

The overcoming of resistances, as was indicated in the beginning, is inseparable from and almost identical with the filling out of the gaps of memory. The resistances, which maintain the repression against which the instinctive forces struggle, exist as it were in layers. The first resistances that present themselves in the analysis are overcome by explaining them; by filling out what is missing from the patient's consciousness to give him a full view of their significance; in short, by showing the patient what he really is doing when they act. In the breaking up of resistances the personal association of the patient with the physician plays an important part. The rôle of the analyst, as Ferenczi says, is that of "a catalytic ferment that temporarily attracts to itself the affects split off by the dissection.''[1] With one resistance, or one layer of resistances, out of the way there becomes accessible new historical material which is serviceable for filling out the gaps of memory that will lead the patient to an understanding of the next. Eventually, if this process is continued far enough, the purely instinctive and infantile levels are reached. Then with his unnecessary internal inhibitions dissolved the patient can make the adaptations that shall give him a maximum of wish-fulfillment, and do away with the damming up of the libido, without at the same time overstepping the requirements for a moral and socially commendable life. Morality and wishfulfillment are both easy and compatible when one's problems are simplified by the elimination of unreality and reduced solely to the question of adaptation to external facts.

In order that we be perfectly clear about all this it may be well to make some concrete applications. The orthodox Jew reacts negatively to ham. If he were compelled to eat it by force, he would doubtless be able to swallow ham but not however without some slight feeling of shrinking or of guilt. Such a reaction is not instinctive, but the result of training, of earlier experience. In other words it is the expression of a habit. But in perhaps most cases the individual himself would not spontaneously recognize this. If he were asked

[1] Ferenczi, "Contributions to Psychoanalysis," p. 34. He continues, "In a technically correct psycho-analysis the bond thus formed is only a loose one, the interest of the patient being led back as soon as possible to its original, covered-over sources and brought into permanent connection with them."

why he so reacted to ham, he would say it is because ham is *Träfe* and it is a sin to eat it. But this would be attempting to formulate his behavior in terms only of the present, which is quite inadequate to express the full significance of the habit which is functionating. He would not know what he was doing in any full sense of the phrase.

But I have been told by certain Jews who were orthodox as children but later abandoned their old religion in favor of some other, or no religion at all, that their first attempts to eat ham were attended by considerable feelings of aversion, and a vague sense of guilt, and this despite the fact that they were fully convinced that ham is a perfectly wholesome food, and that there was no reason at all why they should not eat it. In this case the habit was left functionating in a state of greater or less isolation by the individual's personality having passed on to newer developmental phases. But these men, however, knew something more of what the reaction meant (of what they were doing) than was true in the first cases. They would have said themselves: "I feel this way because of my bringing up. It is a matter of habit or training which I have not yet overcome." But this knowledge would not go very far toward breaking up the integration. The history of the integration would still be incomplete.

Now these particular Jews that I have in mind did eventually overcome their habit of reacting negatively to ham by the simple process of continuing to eat it. They never knew precisely what were the original experiences which caused the habit to be integrated. But I can very well imagine that there are other cases where in spite of the individual's being convinced intellectually that ham is something altogether desirable to eat, and in spite of his wishing to eat it, the old habit was not overcome, but continued to function indefinitely. Now an enormous number of habits we once have possessed have spontaneously ceased to function when, as we grow older, they ceased to serve any adaptive purpose. Were this not the case we would never be able to adapt ourselves to any later environment that was not almost identical with that in which we grew up. But other habits in many persons persist long after they have outlived their usefulness, and when instead of being of advantage to the individual they are of great disadvantage both in themselves and by way of interfering with his making the new adaptations that might readily come, once these old integrations were out of the way. Such is the case with the neurotic. He has been unable to shake off the old habits of childhood in favor of the new ones that would adapt him to adult life. In this case the analysis may intervene, and by breaking up the old integrations for him, allow him to express his instinctive energies in the manner best adapted to the requirements of his particular place in life.

If in the case of a Jew who continues the habit of reacting negatively to ham after he had abandoned his religion and really desired to eat ham, it should become highly essential that the habit be overcome artificially, he would have to be made to recall the actual experiences of his childhood which had brought the habit into existence, to be shown, in other words, what he was doing. When these memories were recalled, the unconscious elements belonging to the habit rendered conscious, he would then perhaps see that his reaction was only to a most limited extent a function of what ham is actually, but perhaps much more so a function, let us say, of his father—i. e. that what originally caused him to avoid those things called Träfe was that he was scolded and punished by his father when he did not.[1] When then he could see clearly that his negative reaction to ham was really conditioned by an unconscious, but still operative, fear of punishment from his father, it would without doubt cease.[2]

In the case of this habit, as that of any item of acquired organized behavior, the reaction of the individual represents a precipitate from certain past situations and experiences which continue to live as present ones in his unconscious memories. While these memories remain unconscious, his response to such present situations as contain stimuli for the constellation is for the most part a blind, unreasoned and automatic one. In other words, responses which come from habit do not take advantage of the possibilities for other and

[1] Of course the history of the integration of the habit could not be as simple as this, but what I have said is sufficient for our immediate purposes.

[2] This fear belongs to the foreconscious rather than to the unconscious proper.

perhaps more suitable and intelligent responses offered by the increases in knowledge, experience and intellectual development which have taken place in the individual subsequent to the time the habit was formed. Habit is static, unprogressive, retardative. But by bringing the unconscious memories to consciousness, by showing the individual in full exactly what he is doing, there is quite understandably restored to him adaptative flexibility and the opportunity to exchange the automatic habitual response for action from reflection and deliberation, which shall eliminate unreality and take advantage of whatever he has gained from maturity and increased knowledge and experience in the period succeeding the formation of the habit. We miss the full significance of this discussion of habit unless we keep continually in mind that there are habits of thought and feeling just as well as habits of conduct.

I will now attempt to illustrate some of our earlier points by reference to the analysis of a particular case, drawing meanwhile some parallels between it and the problems suggested by the matter of the Jews' reaction to ham.

A man came to me suffering from a mild neurosis. He had, as he expressed it, lost confidence in himself. A feeling of uncertainty attended everything he did; for instance he could no longer feel satisfied that his judgment of business matters was correct. He was continually apprehensive of making mistakes that would have some sort of serious consequences. He could not do his work either with the ease or with the enthusiasm

he had had formerly. In addition to this he felt
somewhat depressed the greater part of the time.
Everything seemed to have lost interest for him.
He could not enjoy himself at the theater, in reading or in any of the other recreations he had previously cared about. His trouble, though not a
serious one, was very unpleasant and hampering
and he had been unable to shake it off.

He very soon said that he himself had felt that
his difficulties were somehow connected with the
sexual problem. His symptoms had come on
gradually toward the end of the first year after
his marriage. He frankly admitted that his home
life was not in just the state he thought it should
be. Not that there was any open friction between
him and his wife, or that he had any just reason
for complaining of anything in her attitude
toward him. She was a very beautiful, intelligent, refined and good tempered woman, who, he
felt, should make an ideal wife and completely
satisfy him. Nevertheless he was not content.
He admired and respected her enormously, and
had for her a very deep affection. On the other
hand she did not, as he expressed it, appeal to
him in a "physical way." In spite of her personal beauty he felt little passion towards her and
their sexual relations gave him none of the full
sense of gratification and enjoyment that he had
known in his premarital experiences with other
women. Why this should be he could not understand. He had sometimes told himself that if
his wife were more passionate he would enjoy
himself better, yet at the same time he had to

acknowledge that on the one hand she was far from frigid, and on the other that in his premarital affairs he had experienced full enjoyment with women who showed even less signs of passion than she. But at any rate, and, as it seemed to him, in consequence of his lack of full sexual satisfaction with her, he had become more and more subject to a sense of unreasonable irritation against his wife and a certain distaste for her society. It had seemed to him that he was becoming less and less in love with her, and that at the same time this was somehow his own fault. Meanwhile he had found his mind continually dwelling on erotic phantasies about other women, either those he had known before his marriage or others he had met since. Sometimes they were about perfect strangers, as, for instance, some attractive looking woman he might see on the street. At times he found himself wishing that he had not married or were again free to pursue some of these women who seemed to have a stronger sexual appeal to him than his wife. Such thoughts distressed him profoundly. He felt that he ought to be perfectly satisfied with his wife and that longings and phantasies concerning other women should not enter his mind at all. He had made every effort to be content with his marriage and to resist these outside appeals, but even though he knew he had done his best, he continually felt guilty for not having succeeded. He had suspected, quite correctly, that his distrust of himself in business affairs, his lack of interest and his depression were merely diffusions of feelings of self-distrust and dissatisfaction that really arose in connection with his home.

The story which this man related is indeed a very common one, with the analytic significance of which I was familiar from previously studied cases. The patient mentioned during one of his early visits that he had not known anything about intercourse until, when he was some ten years old, another boy had described it to him, saying that was the way all babies were made. Like many other children in similar circumstances, he had refused to believe this explanation of reproduction, saying: "That may be true of *some* people, but I know my mother would never have done such a dirty thing."

When he had related to me this incident, I took it as a text upon which, with certain other material not mentioned here, to set forth the following explanation of his difficulties with his wife. His apparent lack of passion toward her and his inability to experience full satisfaction in their sexual relations was not, I said, the result of a real absence of sensual appeal, but was produced by an inhibition, a repression. The repressing or inhibiting agent was a habit, complex or resistance (whichever one might choose to call it) which had been integrated by certain incidents and educational influences to which he had been subject in the course of his bringing up. Though the details were lacking, it was possible to describe in general terms how this integration had been formed. No doubt, as a small child, he had gotten into trouble when he showed some infantile sexual interest in his mother. There were probably a large number of as yet unremembered incidents which led him to feel that all erotic interests were "dirty" and "bad" and therefore offensive to and to be concealed from his mother and all "good" women, who, naturally, were conceived of as having no feelings of so base a sort. In short through training there had been built up a resistance, or inhibition, a habit, in short) which caused him to react toward his mother in a way quite different from what would have been the case had he been left perfectly free to follow his primitive holophilic impulses.

Now it was this habit or complex which was responsible for his lack of complete satisfaction in his sex relations with his wife. For, not unnaturally, it was brought into action not only by the mother herself but by other "good" women who had certain traits in common with her which produced an unconscious identification. Thus such qualities as virtue, refinement and culture which caused him to hold a woman in high esteem did not reënforce the effect of her physical charms to excite *all* his holophilic impulses, but served rather to bring more or less fully into action the old repressive integration and thus to *inhibit* in some degree the more sensual components of love. And just as in the case of the Jews I have mentioned, the habit of reacting negatively to ham continued even after they were convinced intellectually that it is a perfectly wholesome food, so in this patient the inhibitive reaction upon his sensual erotic impulses continued to be exerted even after he had ceased intellectually to think that a display of passion would be offensive to the good woman (his wife) and could not meet with a corresponding excitement in her.

This explanation, when I had outlined it to the patient he said impressed him greatly and he felt convinced that it was entirely correct. In substantiation of it he remarked that now he came to think of the matter he realized that the women with whom in his premarital affairs he had experienced a high degree of passion and full sexual enjoyment were invariably ones whom he had reason to think "bad" even before he made advances to them. Furthermore, when he felt attracted by some woman he might pass on the street, it was always by one, as he now realized, who used a good deal of paint and powder, dressed flashily, showed her legs, or had some suggestion of "sportiness" about her which indicated to his mind that she was not overburdened with virtue nor likely to be offended by any sort of sexual display, provided it were made under favorable circumstances.

Now in the case of the Jew reacting negatively to ham after he had given up his religion, the individual was aware in a general way of why he so reacted. He would have said, if any one had asked him: "The reason I feel this way is because of my bringing up. It's a matter of habit or training." But in the case of this patient, the reason for the inhibition, or indeed the fact of its existence, was not understood until I had explained it to him. But after he had heard the explanation, his state was analogous to that of the Jew. He too could say and believe, "It's a matter of bringing up, of habit and training," but without being able to remember any but a small number of the incidents by which he was trained.

The Jews who abandoned their religion lost their negative reaction to ham through their continuing to eat it. The old habit spontaneously ceased to functionate. But this was not paralleled in the case of the inhibition suffered by this patient. The explantion given above had the effect of making his sexual relations with his wife slightly less unsatisfactory, but the change was by no means profound. The old integration continued in operation despite all the changes which had taken place in the patient's conscious thinking since the period in which it was formed and in the course of the analysis. He went right on reacting towards his wife in the same manner (if not to the same degree) that he had been *trained* to react toward his mother.

Now the analytic explanation I had given him had, in a certain sense, rendered conscious something that had previously been unconscious. He knew that there was an inhibition exerted upon the sex-impulses directed toward his wife, and, in a general way, what this inhibition sprang from —that is to say, from the training he had received in childhood, from various incidents of the past. But this explanation had merely placed him in about the same position as that of the Jew who continues a negative reaction to ham even when, having abandoned his old religion, he desires to eat ham and knows of no reason why he should not. The analysis had simply formulated the patient's problem, had diagnosticated his situation. The problem still remained to be solved, the trouble which was diagnosed had yet to be cured.

How then was this old habit or integration which still continued to functionate eventually broken up? Obviously the integration was produced by, and the continued habit was an effect of, certain earlier experiences which we would include under the head of "training." The number of individual experiences which had been instrumental in forming the integration quite obviously must have been large. And the same might be said of those experiences of religious training and family life which produced in the Jew a feeling of aversion to ham. But in each case only a small number of the integrating experiences could be spontaneously recalled in detail by the individual and observation goes to show that those which can be recalled are by no means invariably the most important or the ones which had the profoundest effects. In short the memories and records of the experiences which had served to build up these habits still remained in great measure unconscious. Now the way that the analysis eventually breaks up these integrations or complexes and frees the individual from the habits of reacting that have outlived their usefulness is, as we have said, *by reducing them to the original individual experiences through which they were built up.* They have, in one way or another, to be recalled. The individual is, as it were, taken back in memory to the original situations, allowed to review them in the light of new knowledge and to start from them afresh in such a way as to form new integrations better adapted to the demands of adult existence than were the old.

One could, then, divide the analytic work, on theoretical grounds, into two parts: the diagnostic, which discovers what complexes, resistances or habits are responsible for the patient's troubles and which formulates his problems for him, and the disintegrative or analytic proper, which breaks up the undesirable habits or complexes by making the patient re-live the original experiences by which they were built up. As a matter of fact, in practice there is no such distinction possible. Both diagnostic and disintegrative analysis occur together and are indistinguishable. Nevertheless the division I have suggested has a certain value. Some mild cases and some of the elements involved in severe cases require little more than a diagnostic analysis. Once the problem is clearly formulated for the patient he may be able to meet it unaided further, just as the Jew would overcome his resistance to ham by simply continuing to eat it. Perhaps a larger part of the analytic cure than we are wont to realize is brought about in this way. In fact if every troublesome complex and integration required as detailed analysis as do some of the most important ones, the already lengthy process of an analytic treatment would be really endless. In the case of Miss

S—— for instance, an adjustment was brought about and a cure resulted from an analysis that was more largely diagnostic than disintegrative. None of her complexes were reduced to the terms of the original integrating experiences with anything like the fullness of detail with which I am familiar from cases of a more severe type, and which is required in them to bring about a cure.

How then is the distintegrative living-over-again of the earlier complex-producing experiences accomplished? Apparently in two essentially different ways, the one by the patient's directly recalling these past experiences, the other by his re-living them in the form of transference.[1]

Let us first consider remembering. The analysis is begun when, after the history is taken at the first sitting, the patient is directed to talk of whatever presents itself to his mind (to think aloud, in short) relating whatever occurs to him, whether or not it seems to him important or trivial, pleasant or disagreeable. Many patients when started in this way, will produce a good deal of valuable material. Once they have begun to think over their past history and the story of

[1] In the original hypnotic analysis first used by Breuer and Freud this taking of the patient back to earlier experiences seemed much simpler than it does now. It was suggested to the patient that he was in this or that situation and he was then required to describe it and his feelings in detail. The most unfortunate feature of this otherwise very desirable method of procedure is that the physician does not always know what situations he should make the patient go back to, and that to some, against which the patient has strong resistances because they are in some way painful, he cannot be made to go back in spite of all suggesting.

the development of their symptoms, they will not
only remember and relate much that they had
known to be important at the time of its occurrence, but also many things the importance of
which had previously escaped them and is now
recognized for the first time. A good deal of this
material, which we could consider as belonging to
the unconscious, the patient assures us he knew
all along. "Only until now I didn't happen to
think of it." The "forgetting" of such material,
the repressing of it, had consisted merely in its
being isolated.[1] This sort of forgetting is particularly common in the compulsion neurosis. In
hysteria and anxiety hysteria an absolute forgetting is met with more frequently. There are also
"remembered" certain internal psychic processes
which as a matter of fact had never been conscious; phantasies, wishes, conclusions, perception of connections and relations all of which had
come into being without ever exciting awareness.

The memory material thus collected gradually
enables the patient to view his behavior and his
neurosis (which is a form of behavior) in a new
light and from the point of view of its history.
He can see more and more what he really is doing,
more and more that he is reacting *as if* persons
and conditions of the past were still present as
objects of environment. He even passes a little
way from the stage *as if I thought* to that of *I
realize that I have been thinking, unconsciously.*

Yet on spontaneous memory alone one can never

[1] Cf. Freud's *Weitere Rätschläge*, Int. Zeit. f. Arzt. Psychoa.
II, 1914.

rely for a complete picture of a neurosis. A good many gaps can be filled out in this way, in some cases. In others, as early as the first or second visit, the flow of associations stops and the patient declares nothing more occurs to him. But in every case memory sooner or later stops adding to the patient's understanding, the associations cease to flow freely, he no longer repeats with any fidelity what comes to his mind. Instead of becoming increasingly conscious, by way of the reproduction of associations, of what, in the larger sense, he has been doing, *he now goes ahead and does it*. I mean by this that he begins to *re-enact*, in the transference to the physician, what he has been unable to remember. Old patterns, which had previously found expression mainly in the symptoms, now come more fully to the surface, but with the physician in the rôle formerly occupied by some other person. Naturally the transference re-enactment does not take place entirely without distortion nor without seemingly logical connection with the actual facts of the immediate situation. In other words it appears to the patient as a product of the present, not as a relic of the past. As the two previously recorded cases did not illustrate this very fully, I will go on to relate what took place with the male patient last spoken of.

For a short time after I had given him my explanation of his lack of passion for his wife, he added more and more confirmatory material to it and seemed more and more satisfied of its correctness. But though he could plainly see that, as he himself expressed it, he was in a measure afraid to love his wife in any other way than he had been allowed to love his mother, yet he complained that he could remember very little of his early childhood, and of the period where it appeared that the events responsible for the integration of the inhibitory mechanism took place. He could not recall, for instance, that he had ever had an interest other than a "pure" affection for his mother, to say nothing of remembering any occasion when he had been scolded or punished for "improper" interests in her. The events which constituted his repressive training were, in short, completely lacking from his memory.

At length he began to doubt very much whether I had explained his inhibition correctly, saying that if there had occurred in his childhood training any punishments or other repressive events sufficient to have a lasting effect upon him, they surely would have made such a deep impression that he would easily be able to remember them. But as he was quite unable to recall any such occurrences he ceased finally to believe that any inhibition upon his sex impulses really did exist, declaring that he was now convinced that he was right in the first place when he thought that he and his wife were "sexually mismated" (i. e. that there was no attraction to inhibit and that she simply did not appeal to him in a physical way). Meanwhile his attitude of great interest in the analysis and of profound confidence in me changed into one of a sulky antagonism. Instead of being as at first perhaps over credulous he was now always on the defensive and ready to pick flaws in anything I might say, even though this was generally done in a somewhat hesitant manner, as if he were a little afraid of me.

After a considerable time the set of facts which explained this change was forthcoming. They belonged under two headings. In the first place there was a matter he was not telling me. Across the court in the apartment house where he lived were the rooms of a young woman. It was in the summer and he had discovered that she very often neglected to pull down the shades when she was undressing for bed. He had fallen into a habit of watching her. Apparently she was an actress, for she usually came in quite late in the evening, after he and his wife had gone to bed. He would tell his wife that he could not sleep, and, getting up, would go to the living room of his apartment, from which this girl's bedroom was plainly visible if her shades were up, and, sitting there in the dark, would watch her while she was disrobing. This would get him into a state of great sexual excitement and sometimes he would return to his bedroom and have intercourse with his wife, meanwhile imagining she were this girl, which added considerably to the pleasure he was accustomed to gain from his sexual relations.

He had not felt particularly troubled about what he was doing until one evening when he was watching the young woman there came upon him the thought: "What a contemptible picture you make—you, a married man—sitting here in the dark, peeping at this girl, like a nasty minded lit-

536 MORBID FEARS AND COMPULSIONS

tle boy! Suppose you told this to the doctor! He would give you hell! He might refuse to treat you if you did not stop it at once!"

But these feelings of mortification and self-reproach soon became mixed with a sense of resentment against me. "Why should I tell him about it?" the patient had thought, "What business is it of his? Am I not a man and can I not do as I please, without running to him and confessing?" And then at other times he would think: "Why should I be afraid to tell him? Suppose he does criticize me, he is not God. Why should I care? He is no better than I. Very likely he'd do the same thing if he got the chance!"

While this conflict was going on, a second arose. As he was sitting one day in my waiting room, he heard me laughing with the patient who preceded him and who was just leaving. As she passed the waiting room door, he saw that she was a good-looking young woman. "Aha!" he thought, "the doctor is very friendly with his lady patients! I'll bet there's something doing!" From that time on he was continually on the alert to find out something about me. If I was called on the telephone when he was in my office, he would listen to see whether he could figure out from the conversation whether the other person was a woman and whether there was anything "intimate" between us.

If I ever left the room when he was in my office, he would be assailed by a great curiosity to look at the letters and papers lying on my desk, and this temptation on one or two occasions he was unable to resist. On the street one evening he saw at some distance in front of him a man he took to be me, walking with a woman. He wondered whether this was my wife with me or whether I was out for a "party" with one of my patients. Overcome with curiosity to see whom I was with and where I was going, he hastily followed, keeping in the shadows of the buildings in order to escape observation himself, only to discover after he had gone some distance that the couple he had been watching were really perfect strangers.

He became consumed with curiosity about my private life. What sort of person was my wife? How did I get along with her? What were our sexual relations? Did I have affairs with other women? He had an impulse to picture to himself in phantasy intimate scenes of my home, feeling at the same time a certain envy, as if in some mysterious way everything sexual in my existence must be somehow superior to and different from anything he could experience, and that I had unknown pleasures which would be forever denied to him.   Sometimes he felt hurt that I did not take him into my confidence and tell him all about these intimate things. I must, he thought, know a good deal about sex that he did not, and why had I to be so reserved? Why couldn't I tell him frankly of my own feelings and experiences and let him improve his relations with his wife by copying me instead of through the disagreeable and lengthy process of analysis?

All this took place with the greatest conflict. He felt himself utterly mean, dishonorable and

contemptible to be so continually suspicious of me
and to have such an irresistible curiosity about my
private affairs. That he had looked at my letters
or been willing to spy upon me on the street
seemed to him the lowest limit of sneaking con-
temptibility. But what is more to the point is
that he was mortally afraid of my anger if I
found out what he had done. "How can you," he
thought, "confess to the doctor how nosey you
have been? He would never forgive you! · He
never talks of his own affairs, and that should
have warned you how he would resent any one's
prying into them! What would he think if he
knew you had tried to picture his sexual relations with his wife; that you had tried to imagine
how she would look undressed; that your foul
mind had attempted to invade every nook and
corner of his privacy; that you had suspected
him of immorality with his women patients!
Suppose he were to discover some of these things
from one of your dreams. He would be furi-
ous!"

He not only feared my anger as such but also
what I would do if I were angry. "This man,"
he thought, "has no inhibitions or fears. In his
anger he would be absolutely merciless. There
is no telling what he might do to you. He could
cause a lot of harm if he told what he knows
about you, and he might not hesitate to do it.
Doubtless he has powerful friends among business men, and in his desire for revenge, he would
enlist their help and ruin you, or he might do you
some physical injury." These and other fears of

my vengeance (some of them quite fantastic), assailed and tormented the patient unspeakably. In spite of the great absurdity of most of them they were entirely real to him.

The material which I have here recited, with more of a similar tenor, was brought out slowly and fragmentarily, with every sign of the greatest resistance on the part of the patient. It seemed hardly to have occurred to him that there was any possibility of my not resenting his "prying" or of my failing to take action against him once I discovered it. And when he had, after great difficulty, told me one item, the fact that I took it quite indifferently seemed to give him no assurance that, when he had come to the next one, I would not resent that. At such times as he was about to tell me some one of these things, he would squirm about in his chair with every sign of the greatest uneasiness and apprehension. Invariably he would raise his hand to his face and turn his head from me at the moment of making the "confession." This, when I first called his attention to it, he said was because of mortification. He could not bear to look at me when he was relating things about himself which showed him to be such a "dishonorable sneak." Yet at length it dawned upon him that the real purpose of the gesture was *to ward off an unconsciously expected blow.*

It was only when this realization came to him that he began to see what was really meant by his feelings of guilt before me and his fears of my anger—namely that all these manifestations were transference phenomena and reproductions of the long-forgotten past. What he had experienced with me was really a living over again of unremembered incidents of his childhood, subject to enough distortion and rationalization to accord them with the present. The important episodes of his early corrective training which he had been unable to remember, he had reënacted with me. The inquisitiveness, the spying and the suspicions he had expected I would resent and avenge, corresponded to the infantile sexual curiosity that had been active in his childhood. His sense of guilt and his fear of me were a reproduction of what he had originally felt, on much more logical grounds, in connection with his father.

At last when he understood what all this really meant, there came the direct recollections of actual experiences, which had previously eluded us. When he was about five years of age, or perhaps even younger, he had been playing in a neighbor's garden with a little girl of seven. She had volunteered to show him "what papa and mama did," and after unbuttoning her clothing, and assisting him to do the same, they displayed to one another their buttocks and genitals, and urinated in each other's presence. She told him that all married people did this in their bedrooms every night. In the midst of the proceedings the little girl's mother spied them from the window, and, sending her daughter into the house, took the little boy home and told his mother what had been going on. Both children were severely punished and not allowed to play together again. In the transference, the spying on the young actress, about which the patient feared to tell me and over which he felt so very guilty, apparently corresponded to this episode. He unconsciously expected that I would take much the same attitude with regard to this adult experience that his parents had taken toward the earlier one.

Some little time later, shortly after his experience with the little girl and before the patient was six, he had hidden under the bed in his mother's room, hoping to see her use the chamber vessel. What the little girl had told him and what he had seen of her genitals had greatly excited his curiosity and at the same time puzzled and disturbed him. Why had she no projecting organ like his own? Was his mother that way too? And did married people really do at night what the little girl said they did? If so, why was it he had been so severely punished? He felt he must find out, and therefore embarked on the adventure in his mother's bedroom. But she discovered him in his hiding place, and seemed to divine at once what was his purpose in being there. She questioned him closely but he desperately maintained that he was merely "playing," and begged her not to tell his father as she had threatened to do. She seemed not to be fully convinced of his innocence but finally said she would not tell if he would promise to be a good boy.

After this, what attempts he made to gratify his sexual curiosity were carried on in the most crafty manner, and, though he did not at once abandon his investigations but for a time continued on the alert to find out anything possible as to what went on between his parents, this was all done with such an appearance of artless innocence that they were completely deceived. Never did he really satisfy himself as to what did take place between them and at length the somewhat deferred latency period set in, and the whole history of this period of investigation was almost completely lost to his conscious memory, so that when he was later told about intercourse, he was sure his mother would not do such a "dirty thing." It is easy to see, however, that his transference curiosity about my sexual life, his desire to have me describe to him my own feelings and experiences, his thoughts about my wife (whom he had never even seen), his uncertainty as to my morality, etc., coincided with the early inquisitiveness and uncertainty about his parents, while his antagonism toward me and his ideas about how, in my anger, I would take revenge on him, were descendants of the early and well-founded fear of punishment from his father.

With the filling out of memory gaps that came from the transference itself and from the additional memory reproductions which occurred after the transference had ceased to act as a resistance, the patient became at last not only fully convinced that his lack of contentment with his wife was due to the functioning of a compound habit which exerted an inhibition upon the more sensual components of the love life, but he could now see the constituents of this habit, its unconscious factors, and the *why* of its continued operation. It became clear to him that an important constituent of this habit or inhibition was an unconscious [1] fear, on the one hand, of punishment from the father, and, on the other, of exciting the disapproval of the mother (his wife)—that he was reacting as if the original conditions, which through exciting such fears had served to suppress his sex impulses in childhood, were still present and still to be feared. With this vision of what he really was doing came the freedom to make new and more satisfactory adaptations.

As must now be clear, the curiosity or looking impulse was strongly developed in this patient. But it had been very much inhibited in his relations with his wife. For instance, if he came into the room when his wife was partially dressed, he would quite automatically look away from her or act as if he had not noticed that she was not fully clothed. What exposure of her person took place with the performance of their sexual relations he seemed almost to ignore. Though previously he had not recognized this, he at length saw that whatever gratification of his looking impulse he had allowed himself in his relations with his wife was accomplished in a furtive manner and in such a way as to conceal from her the fact that he had any desire to look. He behaved with her, in short, just as if she would react, should she catch him looking at her, as his mother would have reacted. Unconsciously he expected she would scold him

[1] Strictly speaking, foreconscious.

or give him over to punishment. But this inhibition had functioned so subtilely that he had not realized what was taking place.

Instead of being aware that really he had a strong desire to look at his wife's person, and could derive great pleasure from doing so were it not for an inhibition, he felt that she did not interest him physically, that her bodily charms were not of the special sort that could appeal to him. In short, he could freely gratify his looking impulse only in phantasies of sexual scenes with other women, or, as in his premarital experiences, when his inhibition was overcome by the woman's making manifest that she was not overburdened with modesty, and that, like the "bad" little girl in his childhood, she would take pleasure in being looked at, instead of resenting it. The fact that in his unconscious the looking desire included a wish to witness the excretory process of the female, in short, to repeat what, as a child, he had experienced with the neighbor's little girl, of course made the inhibition upon the looking impulse even more difficult for him to overcome than might otherwise have been the case.

What I have related of the analysis of the inhibiting habits that functionated in the patient's love life is of course only a part of the whole story, but the rest is not required for our purposes here. The inhibition on the looking impulse was completely paralleled in respect to others of the patient's sensuously erotic tendencies. As the analysis drew to a close he was able to see clearly

that, as he had at first surmised, the doubts, resistances and inhibitions that he met with in his
business life were merely a diffusion or displacement of affects that really had their immediate
origin in his life at home—for instance, his fear of
making a mistake that would have most serious
consequences was really a descendant of the old
fear of being punished by his father for the expression of (now repressed) sexual interests. It
need hardly be said that, once the interfering inhibitions were broken up, the patient was enabled
thoroughly to content himself with his wife, while
the phantasies about other women and his desire
to be free to pursue them disappeared entirely.

The integrations which functioned in his relations with me had been set in motion by many
other sorts of stimuli and in many other contacts
in his life. But outside of the analysis, however,
the system of habits, the complex, had worked for
the most part from beneath the surface, so to
speak. Even when its influence was profound,
only a small part of the entity appeared in consciousness, and even this was rationalized into
accord with the immediate situation. In the
analysis, however, as the constellation was stimulated and rose to the surface, it was caught and
held. Instead of being permitted, as ordinarily,
again to recede to unconscious levels, it was hauled
out further and further, and at last delivered in
its entirety from the depths of the non-perceiv-
able and surrendered to examination into its every
part. Then and only then was it deprived of

autonomousness and independence of action and
rendered assimilable with the results of adult experience and the requirements of adult life.

The breaking up of the pathological integrations which function either as repression resistances or as fixations of instinctive tendencies is
accomplished, as has now been illustrated, by making the patient live over again the experiences
which were instrumental in forming the intgera-
tions. These experiences he may re-live either in
memory, which he does not confuse with the present, or in the form of transference, which he feels
arises from the present. By this re-living of the
past he can see what he is really doing in the
present, namely, that he is reacting as if much
of the past were still in existance. We have said
that when he *knows* what he is really doing he is
then free to do otherwise if adaptation demands
it. But I must now state that this knowing has
to be of a very special sort. It must be a knowing that comes from *re-living,* either in memory,
or in transference. A mere intellectual knowledge of the significance of a habit, a resistance
or a symptom ordinarily does not break up the
integration, or prevent it from continuing to functionate. In this particular case, for example, I
was able to divine quite completely from dreams,
symptoms, and associations, what sorts of occurrences had taken place in the patient's childhood
to create the repression resistances that were functioning. I told him a good part of what I had
discovered, and for a time at least he agreed that
in all probability I was correct. But this did

not have either the effect of bringing to his consciousness the actual recollections of the incidents in question, nor of producing any amelioration of the symptoms. When the physician gives to a patient a perfectly correct explanation of the unconscious ideas or wishes which are responsible for a symptom or resistance, he merely introduces into the patient's consciousness *new* ideas *having the same content* as the unconscious ones. This is not the same as bringing the unconscious ideas into consciousness, and the explanation has no great effect upon the symptom unless it serves (as it may do) to bring up this missing material from the unconscious.

This shows that the explanation that has been here given of the effect of psychoanalysis does not explain very extensively. Certainly it is not any ordinary kind of "knowing" or "understanding" that cures the patient. It is a living-over-again of that which had subsided from consciousness that has the therapeutic effect, but just what this really consists in, or why it should have just this effect, is, to my mind at least, decidedly obscure. Obviously, an important fact is that the patient is released from depending on ready-made and outworn responses to meet present situations, and gains thereby an enormous freedom to make new adaptive reactions—he becomes flexible, while before he was crystallized—but exactly what takes place inside of him we can express only in terms of ideas. What changes are made in the integration of reflex paths, and exactly how they come to be made, we can hardly even guess.

It is clear, however, that psychoanalysis is a re-education, in the very fullest sense. As Burrow has remarked, education, as it is ordinarily carried on, really belies its name. The word implies a leading out; the process is largely a pressing in. Familial, and to a less extent, school training have not been predominantly devoted to discovering what were the special tendencies with which instinct had endowed each individual, and to leading out these energies along the lines that would give them fullest and most advantageous expression. The training most children receive, in the home especially, has generally been somewhat in imitation of the mythological Procrustes who had a bed in which he would invite travelers to sleep. If the guest were too short for the bed, the host would stretch him until he was long enough to fill it; if he were too long for the bed, enough of his person would be chopped off to make him fit it perfectly. Education has shown similar tendencies. There has been a disposition to fit the child to the training, rather than to fit the training to the child. This has been especially true in regard to the developing sex impulses. Scoldings, punishments, and other repressive measures are applied with the greatest energy toward making the sexuality of the growing individual conform to fixed and predetermined standards of what should be, and which, incidentally, are in many instances founded more largely upon prejudice, superstition and ignorance, than upon any accurate knowledge of sexual psychology and physiology, or upon sympathetic common sense.[1] Where familial influence and training have established habits which inhibit normal sexual tendencies from expressing themselves, or which maintain fixations of others that, for the adult, are really abnormal, psychoanalysis performs a truly educative function. The pathogenic habits, inhibitions, or resistances are overcome and the individual's instinctive energies led out to express themselves in the fullest measure possible, either in the form of normal love activities or by way of sublimation.

It is evident in the case of the patient we have just considered that the habits established by the moral training received in childhood, the purpose of which was to withhold him from immoral action when he grew up, formed the very factor which interfered with his making a moral adaptation and bid fair to drive him into immorality (in-

[1] It is very commonly true that parents, in bringing up their children, do not utilize much of the knowledge and good sense they really possess, but instead fall into an unconscious identification with, and consequent imitation of, their own parents. Thus they not only reproduce with their own children practically all the mistakes of their own bringing up, but fail to take advantage of what opportunities for advance are offered to the newer generation.

The fidelity of such unconscious imitations is not only in many cases most striking but at times reaches the point of the ludicrous. I am acquainted with a man who, not entirely without reason, considers his father an utter fool, whose opinion on any subject under the sun could by no chance be correct or worth a moment's consideration. Nevertheless this man, in training his own son, unconsciously reproduces, with absolute fidelity, the training his despised father gave him.

The psychology of parenthood, as well as the psychology of childhood might be studied with profit by those who are working for educational advance.

fidelity to his wife) in the search for a field in which his sex impulses could secure free outlet. That which saved the patient from this danger and made it easy for him to be content with a perfectly moral marital life was really the overcoming of certain moral impulses. In other words, as this case exemplifies, the resistances which are dissolved in the analysis are in part moral resistances, habits which have been instilled by ethical training.

If psychoanalysis dissolves certain moral inhibitions the effect, one would think, must be to make it easier for the individual to be immoral. In a measure this is true. But on the other hand, as in the case we have considered, the effect is likewise that of making it easier for the individual to be *moral,* and to feel content in so being, while according to all experience the moral course is that which after the analysis he ordinarily pursues. Thus the result of overcoming certain moral inhibitions may really be the attainment of a higher degree of morality than was possible while they were in force. Now really the purpose of psychoanalysis is practically identical with that of moral instruction and moral codes (if viewed according to their basic significance), namely, the highest welfare of the individual as a member of the social group, the best possible adaptation of himself to his environment. If psychoanalysis led to a real immorality, it would defeat its own purpose. Its prime rôle really is to step in and do for the individual what the ordinary moral forces had tried to do for him but failed. The analysis does not seek to overcome morality but rather certain moral inhibitions or habits which have outlived their usefulness, and defeat their proper purpose by interfering with, rather than furthering, the welfare of the individual and his adaptation to life. It assists him to abandon these old moral inhibitions in favor of newer controlling and adaptive machinery more efficient than the old. It tries to perfect, to improve upon, that intricate system of "habits not only of acting, but of feeling and believing about actions, of valuing or approving and disapproving"[1] which the individual calls his conscience and which has as some of its basic constituents certain pathological resistances and inhibitions which result from ignorant, if well intended, parental efforts to shape the child's personality according to standards that take no account of the natural.

Sexuality, even perfectly normal sexuality, gives rise to most serious and difficult adaptive problems, and may easily be the spring of actions which will end in pain or misery or disaster for the individual. But for this very reason, and quite apart from the question of making the most of the instinct's great potentialities for happiness and for good, all efforts toward establishing habits that shall control and direct the erotic energies need to be undertaken in the most carefully considered and enlightened manner that is humanly possible. Man's effort to overcome the imperious domination of sexuality has been at-

[1] Dewey and Tufts, *Ethics*, p. 173.

tempted, as Hinkle remarks, "by lowering the instinct, and seeing in it something vile or unclean, something unspeakable and unholy. Instead of destroying the power of sexuality this struggle has only warped and distorted, injured and mutilated the expression; for not without destruction of the individual can these fundamental instincts be destroyed. Life itself has needs and imperiously demands expression through the forms created. All nature answers to this freely and simply except man. His failure to recognize himself as an instrument through which life is coursing and the demands of which must be obeyed, is the cause of his misery—"[1] Ignorant and too rigorous early repressive training, bad family influences, or unnatural ideals establish in the child such habits "of feeling and believing about actions" that when he becomes an adult he can not without pain and horror see himself as he actually is. Tendencies which are innate and inevitable become sources for the development of tormenting affects of guilt; energies that are normal and deserving of direct expression, and energies that, though not normal, could become so, are fruitlessly and wastefully confined and repressed. Instead of securing outlet in the form of activities that are compatible with the requirements of social existence, and which could be given them once they were faced and understood, many of these fundamentally normal and natural impulses remain as skeletons in the closets of the

[1] B. M. Hinkle, Introduction to Jung's *Psychology of the Unconscious*, p. xlii.

individual's psychic household, which whenever he gets a glimpse of them, excite him to spasms of morbid fear. The overcoming of resistances which occurs with analysis reëducates him to new points of view. It enables to see the whole of himself as it actually is; to face his defects, whatever they may be, without horror or self reproach, but simply as matters of biological fact; and to develop the energies at his disposal along the lines that will most fully adapt him to his place in life. This is accomplished not so much by teaching him new standards as by unteaching old, erroneous and distorted ones.

BIBLIOGRAPHY:

CHAPTER I

Ellis, H.—Autoerotism; Analysis of the Sexual Impulse; Love and Pain; Erotic Symbolism; Sexual Inversion, in the *Studies in the Psychology of Sex*, F. A. Davis Co.

Freud, S.—Three Contributions to the Sexual Theory, 2d Edition, translated by A. A. Brill, *The Journal of Nervous and Mental Disease Monograph Series*, No. 7.

Triebe und Triebshicksale, *Internationale Zeitschrift für ärztliche Psychoanalyse*, Vol. III., 1915.

Beiträge zur Psychologie des Liebeslebens II., *Jahrbuch für psychoanalytische und psychopathologische Forschungen*, Bd. IV., Hft. I., 1912.

Ueber Infantile Sexualtheorien, *Sammlung kleiner Schriften zur Neurosenlehre*, Bd. II., S. Karger, Berlin.

The Origin and Development of Psychoanalysis, *American Journal of Psychology*, Vol. XXI., No. 2, 1910.

Analyse der Phobie eines fünfjahrigen Knaben, *Jahrbuch für Psychoanalytische und Psychopathologische Forschungen*, Bd. I, Hft. 1, 1909.

Frink, H. W.—The Sexual Theories Formed in Early Childhood, and Their Rôle in the Psychoneuroses, *New York Medical Journal*, November 15, 1915.

Hug-Hellmuth, H. von.—Aus den Seelenleben des Kindes, F. Deuticke, Vienna.

Jones, E.—Die Empfängnis der Jungfrau Maria durch

das Ohr, *Jahrbuch der Psychoanalyse*, Bd. 6, 1914.

Jung, C. J.—Experiences Concerning the Psychic Life of the Child, *Analytical Psychology*, translated by Constance Long, Moffat, Yard & Co.

Moll, A.—The Sexual Life of the Child, Macmillan Co.

Reitler, R.—Eine infantile Sexualtheorie und ihre Beziehung zur Selbstmordsymbolik. *Zentralblatt für Psychoanalyse*, Bd. II, Hft. 2, 1912.

Watson, J. B.—Behavior, Henry Holt & Co.

CHAPTER II

Freud, S.—Das Unbewusste, *Internationale Zeitschrift für Arztliche Psychoanalyse*, Bd. III., Hft. 4–5, 1915.

De Verdrängung, Ibid., Hft. 3.

Zur Einführung des Narzissmus, *Jahrbuch der Psychoanalyse*, Bd. VI., 1915.

Einige Bemerkungen über den Begriff des Unbewussten in der Psychoanalyse, *Internationale Zeitschrift für Arztliche Psychoanalyse*, Bd. I., Hft. 2, 1913.

The Interpretation of Dreams, Chapter VII., The Macmillan Co.

The Psychopathology of Everyday Life, Macmillan Co.

Frink, H. W.—What is a Complex? *Journal of the American Medical Association*, Vol. LXII., p. 897.

Hart, B.—The Conception of the Subconscious, *Journal of Abnormal Psychology*, Vol. IV., No. 6, 1910.

"The Psychology of Insanity," Cambridge University Press.

Holt, E. B.—The Freudian Wish, Henry Holt & Co.

Jones, E.—The Significance of the Unconscious in Psychopathology, *Review of Neurology and Psychiatry*, Vol. XII., No. 11, 1914.
Pfister, O.—The Psychoanalytic Method, Part I, Moffat, Yard & Co.
Putnam, J. J.—Human Motives, Little, Brown & Co.

CHAPTER III

Abraham, K.—Dreams and Myths, *Nervous and Mental Disease Monograph Series, No. XV.*
Bleuler, E.—Das autistiche Denken, *Jahrbuch für psychoanalytische und psychopathologische Forschungen*, Bd. IV., Hft. I., 1912.
Brill, A. A.—Dreams, Chapter II. of *Psychoanalysis*, W. B. Saunders Co.
Ferenczi, S.—The Psychological Analysis of Dreams, and Stages in the Development of the Sense of Reality, Chapters III. and VII. of *Contributions to Psychoanalysis*, Richard G. Badger.
Freud, S.—Formulierung über die zwei Prinzipien des psychischen Geschehens, *Jahrbuch für .psychoanalytische und psychopathologische Forschungen*, Bd. III., Hft. 1, 1911.
The Interpretation of Dreams.
On Dreams, The Rebman Co.
Die Handhabung der Traumdeutung in der Psychoanalyse, *Zentralblatt für Psychoanalyse*, Bd. II, Hft. 3, 1912.
Jones, E.—Freud's Theory of Dreams, Chapter XV of *Papers on Psychoanalysis*, William Wood & Co.
Jung, C. G.—Concerning Two Kinds of Thinking, Chapter I., of *The Psychology of the Unconscious*, Moffat Yard & Co.

CHAPTER IV

Ferenczi S.—Introjection and Transference, Chap. II. of *Contributions to Psychoanalysis.*

Freud, S.—The Psychopathology of Everyday Life, Macmillan Co.

The Interpretation of Dreams, Chap. V.

Zur Dynamik der Ubertragung, *Zentralblatt für Psychoanalyse,* Vol. II., 1912.

Jones, E.—Papers on Psychoanalysis, Chapters I., III., XII., XIX., and XX.

Jung, C. G.—The Significance of the Father in the Destiny of the Individual, Chapter III., *Analytical Psychology,* Moffat, Yard & Co.

Pfister, O.—The Psychoanalytic Method.

Rank, O.—Das Inzest-Motiv in Dichtung und Sage, Deuticke, Vienna.

Watson, J. B.—Behavior.

CHAPTER V

Brill, A. A.—Psychoanalysis, W. B. Saunders Co.

Cannon, W. B.—Bodily Changes in Pain, Hunger, Fear and Rage, Appletons.

Crile, G. W.—Man, an Adaptive Mechanism, Macmillan Co.

Darwin, C.—The Expression of the Emotions in Man and Animals, D. Appleton & Co.

Ellis, H.—The Problem of Sexual Abstinence, Chapter VI. of Sex in Relation to Society, Vol. VI. of the *Studies in the Psychology of Sex,* F. A. Davis Co.

Ferenczi, S.—Introjection and Transference, in his *Contributions to Psychoanalysis,* Richard G. Badger.

Freud S.—Selected Papers on Hysteria and other Psychoneuroses, *Nervous and Mental Disease Monograph Series.*

Frink, H. W.—The Freudian Conception of the Psycho-neuroses, *Medical Record*, Nov. 29, 1913.

Hitschmann, E.—Freud's Theories of the Neuroses, Moffat, Yard & Co.

Jones, E.—The Pathology of Morbid Anxiety, in his *Papers on Psychoanalysis.*

The Relation between the Anxiety Neurosis and Anxiety Hysteria, *Journal of Abnormal Psychology*, Vol. VIII., No. 1, 1913.

Jung, C. G.—Analytical Psychology, Moffat, Yard & Co.

Seif, L.—Zur Psychopathologie der Angst, *Internationale Zeitschrift für ärztliche Psychoanalyse*, Bd. I, 1913.

CHAPTER VI

Brill, A. A.—Anal Eroticism and Character; and The Compulsion Neuroses, Chapters IX and IV of his *Psychoanalysis.*

Freud, S.—Bemerkungen über einen Fall Zwangsneu-rose, *Jahrb. f. psychoanal. u. psychopath. Forsch.*, Bd. I, Hft. 2, 1909.

Die Disposition zur Zwangsneurose, Int. Zeit. f. ä. Psychoanalyse, Bd. I, 1913.

Das Unbewusste, Int. Zeit. f. ä. P.A., Bd. III, 1915.

Triebe und Triebschicksale, ibid., Bd. III, 1915.

Drie Abhandlungen zur Sexualtheorie, 3d edition, 1915, p. 54, ff.

Selected Papers on Hysteria and other Psychoneuroses, Chapters V and VII.—*Nervous and Mental Disease Monograph Series.*

Jones, E.—Einige Fälle Zwangsneurose, *Jahrb. f. psychoanal. u. psychopath. Forsch.*, Bd. IV, 1912.

Hass und Anal-erotik in der Zwangsneurose, ibid., Bd. I, 1913.

CHAPTER VIII

Freud, S.—Analyse der Phobie eines fünfjährigen Knaben, *Jahrb. f. psychoanal. u. psychopath Forsch.*, Bd. I, Hft. 1, 1909.

Die Verdrangung, *Int. Zeit. f. ä. P.A.*—Bd. III, 1915.

Das Unbewussten, ibid.

Jones, E.—The Relation between the Anxiety Neurosis and Anxiety Hysteria, *Journal of Abnormal Psychology*, Vol. VIII, No. 1, 1913.

Stekel, W.—Nervöse Angstzustände und ihre Behandlungen, Urban & Schwartzenberg, Berlin.

CHAPTER X

Burrow, T.—The Meaning of Psychoanalysis, *Journal of Abnormal Psychology*, Vol. XII, No. 1, 1917.

Conceptions and Misconceptions in Psychoanalysis, *Journal of the American Medical Association*, Vol. LXVIII, Feb. 3, 1917.

Dewey and Tufts—Ethics, Henry Holt & Co.

Ellis, H.—Sexual Education, Chapter II, of Sex In Relation to Society, Sixth Volume of the *Studies in the Psychology of Sex.*

Freud, S.—Weitere Rätschläge zur Technik der Psychoanalyse, Nos. I, II, and III, *Int. Zeit. f. ä. Psychoanalyse*, Bd. I, II, and III, 1913–15.

Uber "wilde" Psychoanalyse, *Zentralblatt f. Psychoanalyse*, Bd. I, 1911.

Origin and Development of Psychoanalysis, *American Journal of Psychology*, Vol. XXI, No. 2, 1910.

History of the Psychoanalytic Movement, *Psychoanalytic Review*, Vol. III, No. 1, 1916.

Beiträge zur Psychologie des Liebenslebens, II.—

Uber die allgemeinste Erniedrigung des Liebeslebens—*Jahrbuch f. psychoanal. u. psychopath.
Forsch*, Bd. IV, Hft. I, 1912.

Holt, E. B.—The Freudian Wish.

Jones, E.—The Therapeutic Action of Psychoanalysis,
Chapter XIV of *Papers on Psychoanalysis*. See
also Chapters XIX and XX.

MacCurdy, J. T.—The Ethics of Psychoanalysis, *Johns
Hopkins Medical Bulletin*, 1915.

Reik, T.—Einige Bemerkungen zur Lehre vom Wider-
stande, Int. Zeit. f. ä. Psychoanalyse, Bd. III, 1915.

Watson, J. B.—Behavior.

INDEX

INDEX 567

Repression, 45
a protective mechanism, 49
brought about by foreconscious, 61
failure of, 75
failure of, a condition of neurosis, 221
primarily affects ideas, 144
Resistance, 47
overcoming of, identical with filling of memory gaps, 502, 517
origin of, 505
might be called habit, 508
Retention of feces, 9

Sadism, 13
in antivivisectionism and chivalry, 137 n.
in lynching, 140
unconscious, causes compulsive self-reproach, 290
repressed, 291
Sadistic-masochistic impulse, 12, 18
Sadistic perversion, 141
Sadistic impulse in compulsion neurosis, 300
Secondary defense measures, 295, 307
Secondary elaboration, 121
Secondary function of the neurosis, 307
Self-reproach, compulsive, 286
Sexual, the term, 3
Sexual emotion, 257
Sexual factor in neurosis, 223, 309
Sexual ideal in neurotics, 234
Sexual instinct, 2
development of, in education, 548
Sexual investigation, 22
Sexuality, human, three phases of, 8
effort to overcome, 551

SEXUAL SYNTHESIS, 1
Sexual theories, infantile, 21
Small penis complex, 185
Subconscious, 277
Sublimation, 19
Sublimation a kind of displacement, 146
Substitute activities, 282, 294
Substitute idea, 17
Superstition and compulsion neurosis, 301
Symbols in dream, 120
Symbols in dream not labeled, 102
Symptoms, neurotic, 124, 277
Synthesis, sexual, 1

THEORY AND MECHANISM OF THE PSYCHOANALYTIC CURE, 496
Thing-ideas, 145
Thinking, compulsive, 272
two kinds of, 89
Thought, omnipotence of, 302
Thumb-sucking, 9, 10
Transference, 192
positive and negative, 218
not created by analysis, 219
the most important problem, 500
as a re-living of complex-producing experiences, 531
phenomena, 540
Trauma, psychic, 498

UNCONSCIOUS, THE, 30
Unconscious is primitive, 66
Unconscious has no regard for reality, 66
Unconscious is infantile, 66
Unconscious is unoriented in time, 67
Unconscious is instinctive, 68
Unconscious contains no inhibition, no negation, no conflict, 70